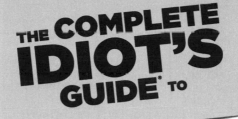

THE **COMPLETE IDIOT'S GUIDE** TO

Medical Terminology

by Veronica Hackethal, MD, MSc

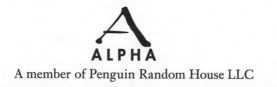

ALPHA

A member of Penguin Random House LLC

This book is dedicated to my mother, Dorothy Hackethal.

ALPHA BOOKS

Published by Penguin Random House LLC

Penguin Random House LLC, 375 Hudson Street, New York, New York 10014, USA • Penguin Random House LLC (Canada), 90 Eglinton Avenue East, Suite 700, Toronto, Ontario M4P 2Y3, Canada (a division of Pearson Penguin Canada Inc.) • Penguin Books Ltd., 80 Strand, London WC2R 0RL, England • Penguin Ireland, 25 St. Stephen's Green, Dublin 2, Ireland (a division of Penguin Books Ltd.) • Penguin Random House LLC (Australia), 250 Camberwell Road, Camberwell, Victoria 3124, Australia (a division of Pearson Australia Group Pty. Ltd.) • Penguin Books India Pvt. Ltd., 11 Community Centre, Panchsheel Park, New Delhi—110 017, India • Penguin Random House LLC (NZ), 67 Apollo Drive, Rosedale, North Shore, Auckland 1311, New Zealand (a division of Pearson New Zealand Ltd.) • Penguin Books (South Africa) (Pty.) Ltd., 24 Sturdee Avenue, Rosebank, Johannesburg 2196, South Africa • Penguin Books Ltd., Registered Offices: 80 Strand, London WC2R 0RL, England

International Standard Book Number: 978-1-61564-303-5
Library of Congress Catalog Card Number: 2013933131

17 16   8 7 6 5 4 3

003-192493-Aug2013

Interpretation of the printing code: The rightmost number of the first series of numbers is the year of the book's printing; the rightmost number of the second series of numbers is the number of the book's printing. For example, a printing code of 13-1 shows that the first printing occurred in 2013.

Printed in the United States of America

Note: This publication contains the opinions and ideas of its author. It is intended to provide helpful and informative material on the subject matter covered. It is sold with the understanding that the author and publisher are not engaged in rendering professional services in the book. If the reader requires personal assistance or advice, a competent professional should be consulted.

The author and publisher specifically disclaim any responsibility for any liability, loss, or risk, personal or otherwise, which is incurred as a consequence, directly or indirectly, of the use and application of any of the contents of this book.

Most Alpha books are available at special quantity discounts for bulk purchases for sales promotions, premiums, fund-raising, or educational use. Special books, or book excerpts, can also be created to fit specific needs. For details, write: Special Markets, Alpha Books, 345 Hudson Street, New York, NY 10014.

Publisher: *Mike Sanders*

Executive Managing Editor: *Billy Fields*

Executive Acquisitions Editor: *Lori Cates Hand*

Development Editor: *Heather Stith*

Senior Production Editor: *Janette Lynn*

Cover Designer: *William Thomas*

Book Designer: *William Thomas, Rebecca Batchelor*

Indexer: *Brad Herriman*

Layout: *Ayanna Lacey*

Proofreader: *Cate Schwenk*

Contents

Introduction

When I started medical school, most medical terms were a mystery to me. I looked at the mountain of terms thrown at me at a rapid-fire pace during the first semester, and I was scared. But I was also intrigued. Where did these words come from? How should I pronounce them? What was the hidden logic that could make memorizing them easier?

In medical school, I didn't have a book like this one. I had to come up with my own strategy for making sense of medical terminology. So I started making lists of related words, many of which share common origins in Greek and Latin. My father's stories about his own medical training made me realize the importance of these languages in forming the basis of medical terminology. When he immigrated to the United States, he had already completed his medical training. Like most foreign medical graduates, he had to retake his medical licensing exams in the United States. English was still a little shaky for him. He always said that the only reason he passed his exams was because he knew Latin.

When I first started writing this book, I thought that learning medical terminology was just like learning a foreign language. My past studies in French, Spanish, Italian, German, and Latin made me familiar with language acquisition. But I realized that learning medical terminology involves more than the rote memorization used in learning a foreign language.

Most medical terms have precise meanings that are intended to prevent errors and misunderstandings in the clinical arena. So acquiring a medical vocabulary entails developing a certain amount of understanding about the science and biological processes described by the terms, in addition to simply memorizing the terms themselves. This book reflects this way of learning. Each chapter contains lists of terms, their pronunciations, and their definitions that you can use for purposes of memorization. But there are also sections that provide a background to the subject. These sections describe the importance of these terms, the processes involved, and the biological functions each term describes. Knowing the why behind a term can aid in memorization and clear up confusion.

How This Book Is Organized

This book consists of five parts. **Part 1, Building Blocks for Learning Medical Terminology**, sets the foundation in the first three chapters for all the words and concepts to come. It focuses on such topics as the origins of medical terminology, word roots, pronunciation, and spelling. **Part 2, Human Anatomy: Terms for Body Parts and Systems**, takes you on a tour of the major organ systems in the body. **Part 3, Physiology: How the Body Works**, explains the words involved in bodily functions and processes. **Part 4, Pathophysiology: Disease and Injury**, provides you with words that describe what's wrong with the body when it breaks down due to illness or injury. **Part 5, Diagnostic Testing and Treatment**, covers the terms for medical tests and treatments.

Extras

The following helpful, informative sidebars are scattered throughout the book.

STUDY TIP

These reminders and pointers make learning medical terms easier.

WORDS OF WARNING

Medical terminology can be tricky. These notes alert you to possible points of confusion.

WORD ORIGINS

Information about the Greek, Latin, and other origins of various medical words makes them easier to remember.

DID YOU KNOW?

These facts ground the terms in medical history and help make learning them fun.

In addition, you'll find that terms defined throughout the book have been placed in bold to draw special attention to them.

Acknowledgments

This book could not have been possible without teamwork. Thanks to my editors Lori Hand and Heather Stith for their helpful guidance throughout the process, as well as to the production team for all their hard work. Thanks also to my agent Marilyn Allen for having faith in me. Nick Cheung, clinical laboratory supervisor at Columbia Presbyterian Hospital in New York City, provided his expertise for the chapter on clinical laboratory medicine. The pronunciations were adapted from the style used on Dictionary.com.

When I first began work on this book, a dear friend of mine passed away. Thanks to my friend Luca Caddeo for being there at the right moment to keep me company. Thanks also to my family, especially my sister Claudia Hackethal, who still has time for phone calls despite her busy life as a physician and mother. Above all, thanks to my mother, Dorothy Hackethal, whose unwavering support and love is a miracle.

Special Thanks to the Technical Reviewer

The Complete Idiot's Guide to Medical Terminology was reviewed by an expert who double-checked the accuracy of what you'll learn here, to help us ensure this book gives you everything you need to know about medical terminology. Special thanks are extended to Katharine O'Moore-Klopf, ELS, of kokedit.com. She is a board-certified editor in the life sciences (see BELS.org).

Trademarks

All terms mentioned in this book that are known to be or are suspected of being trademarks or service marks have been appropriately capitalized. Alpha Books and Penguin Random House LLC cannot attest to the accuracy of this information. Use of a term in this book should not be regarded as affecting the validity of any trademark or service mark.

Building Blocks for Learning Medical Terminology

Part 1 is divided into three chapters and provides a general overview to learning medical terminology. Chapter 1 covers the Greek and Latin origins of medical terms. Chapter 1 also provides a brief overview of Western medical history, starting in the ancient Middle East—especially Greece and Rome—where Western medicine originated. Grounding medical terms in their own history can be fun. It also explains why terms exist in their present form today. Though Western medicine has come a long way in treating human disease, ancient physicians like Hippocrates and Galen knew a surprising amount about human disease, and modern medicine provides significant continuity with past medical knowledge. Chapter 1 also describes medical terminology and knowledge that comes from cultures other than Greek and Latin, explains the importance of having a common medical language, and describes various types of health-care workers who all use the common medical language. The various medical specialties are also described and defined.

Chapter 2 provides an introduction to medical word parts: word roots, prefixes, and suffixes. It gives guidelines on forming plurals of medical terms as well. Tips on how to figure out unknown medical terms by breaking down word parts are also provided.

Chapter 3 covers how to pronounce and spell medical terms. Tricky words like homonyms, which are words that sound like each other but have different meanings, are also presented. Medical eponyms are also demystified. These terms can be can be hard to remember. Because they are named after their discoverer, there can seem to be no rhyme or reason to them. Knowing who's who in medical history can help you decipher these terms.

The Purpose of a Medical Vocabulary

In This Chapter

- Where and when medical terminology began
- Who uses medical terminology
- What different types of medical specialists are called

Though several longstanding medical traditions exist across the world, such as Ayurvedic medicine in India and traditional Chinese medicine, the Western medical tradition is the system of scientific and medical understanding that has spread most widely. The terminology of Western medicine varies based on country of origin, but many of the root words remain similar. That is because Western medical terms stem from common origins, mostly ancient Greece and Rome, where Western medicine began.

Learning medical terminology is like learning a foreign language. But medical terminology is more than a foreign language. Medical terms have precise meanings and refer to specific disease processes, conditions, or body parts. Medical terminology conveys more exactly than lay terms what is going on with a patient. For this reason, various kinds of health-care professionals communicate via a shared medical language. Knowing this language facilitates easier communication and should help promote improved patient care, the ultimate aim of any health-care professional. By mastering some of the basics of medical terminology, you can build a medical vocabulary that can be used and understood in many different settings and locales, as well as with many different health-care professionals.

Origins of Medical Terminology

Although some modern medical practices, such as surgery, obstetrics, and gynecology, existed in early forms in Babylon, Mesopotamia, and Egypt, Western medicine as we know it began to take form in ancient Greece around the fifth century B.C.E. (the so-called Golden Age of Greece). The Romans continued the tradition, preserving and expanding on the medical knowledge discovered by the Greeks. For this reason, many of the terms in modern Western medicine have Greek and Latin origins.

Hippocrates, who is considered the father of modern medicine, was the first to apply scientific principles of experience, observation, and experimentation to the practice of medicine, which had previously been closely tied to religion and the supernatural. Together with Aristotle, who is considered to be the father of the modern science, Hippocrates established principles that are part of the modern scientific method.

Hippocrates taught his followers and treated patients. He also established the Hippocratic oath, a series of ethical principles that all medical doctors and many other health-care providers recite when graduating and entering their professions. Hippocrates and his followers created a body of knowledge that covered many of the major fields of modern medicine, such as surgery, pediatrics, and internal medicine. Many medical terms originate from this body of ancient Greek medical knowledge.

Physicians in ancient Rome preserved the medical knowledge of Hippocrates and his followers and added to it. In particular, the Roman wars and gladiatorial combats may have offered ample opportunity for ancient Roman physicians and surgeons to study human anatomy.

It was Galen, a Greek living in the Roman Empire who was a physician and surgeon to the gladiators, who first theorized about the heart and the circulatory system. Galen wrote in Greek, and his writings on medicine became the standard for the medieval medical curriculum. In the 1500s, the Belgian physician Vesalius translated Galen's writings from Greek into Latin, which had become the language in which medicine was taught in medieval medical schools. Modern medical terminology preserves the legacy of these two languages, with some words originating from Greek and others originating from the Latin.

Dioscorides was another physician who lived in the Roman Empire at about the same time as Galen. Dioscorides is famous for his contributions to the herbal treatment of illnesses. His *De Materia Medica* (On Medical Substances) laid the groundwork for the classification and organization of various classes of medications, a system which is still used in modified forms today.

> **DID YOU KNOW?**
>
> Physicians from other cultures and areas of the world also contributed to the formation of modern Western medical terminology. In Spain in the twelfth century, Jewish physician Maimonides wrote several books about medicine in Hebrew and Arabic, which were later translated into Latin. Averroës was a Muslim physician from the same era who wrote an influential encyclopedia about medicine. Averroës wrote in Arabic, and his writings were later translated into Hebrew and Latin.
>
> The Persian physician Avicenna lived around 1000 C.E. He wrote the *Canon of Medicine,* which became an integral text in medieval medical education. It was originally written in Arabic and was subsequently translated into Latin and Hebrew.

As the Western medical tradition took root and began to spread around the world, the common language of medical terminology, with its Greek and Latin roots, spread with it. In this sense, medical terms truly do form a type of foreign language. Though variations exist, many medical terms in foreign languages maintain their Greek and Latin roots. More technical terms, such as those used for medical procedures or tests and made up of combinations of Greek and Latin word parts, can be very similar across languages.

This similarity doesn't mean that, having gained a mastery of medical terminology in English, you will be able to walk into any hospital anywhere in the world and be understood. There are enough variations in enough terms to make foreign language medical terminology classes, such as Spanish for Health-care Providers, popular among health-care professionals. At the same time, learning medical terminology in English lays an excellent groundwork for expanding your knowledge of medical terminology into other languages.

Different Speakers, Same Language

Health-care is a broad arena that encompasses many different fields and types of professions. Across medical disciplines, people need to be able to communicate with and understand each other. Medical terminology serves as a common ground for discussions between health-care professionals from different fields and backgrounds.

Medical Doctors

Medical doctors have a Doctorate degree in medicine (MD). In the United States, obtaining an MD degree requires completing four years of medical school after graduation from an undergraduate college. To practice medicine in the United States, medical doctors also are required to complete at least three years of additional residency training in a medical subfield after graduation from medical school. Medical doctors work in hospitals, clinics, medical research, and public health. Some medical doctors also contribute to biomedical research and teach future doctors at academic medical centers. Medical doctors are primarily responsible for clinical care: diagnosing and treating patients both in and out of the hospital. They also hold supervisory and advisory positions in government, business, and public health projects.

> **DID YOU KNOW?**
>
> Although online interactive technology has replaced some aspects of anatomy lab, the dissection of a human cadaver remains a standard part of the curriculum. Yet this practice has been controversial throughout history. It was outlawed during Roman times. During the Middle Ages, the bodies of executed criminals were used. For centuries in England, only a few physicians and medical schools were allowed to dissect human cadavers. When the number of English medical schools increased in the 1800s, however, demand for cadavers outstripped the legal supply, leading to a thriving black market in cadavers (and the term **body snatcher**) and several infamous murders. England responded by easing restrictions on cadaverous dissections, which increased the supply.

The field of medicine is made up of many subfields, each specializing in a particular body system. Medical specialists are highly trained medical professionals who have completed a fellowship, which requires 2 to 5 years of further training beyond medical school and general residency.

Internal medicine is a broad-ranging branch of medicine dedicated to the pharmacological treatment of human disease. **Internists** specialize in subfields organized by body system or organ. Internal medicine subspecialties include the following:

- **Gastroenterology:** the study and treatment of gastrointestinal conditions
- **Cardiology:** the study and treatment of the heart and related blood vessels
- **Endocrinology:** the study and treatment of the endocrine system
- **Pulmonology:** the study and treatment of the lungs

- **Nephrology:** the study and treatment of the kidneys
- **Infectious disease:** the study and treatment of diseases caused by bacteria, parasites, fungi, viruses, and other pathogens
- **Oncology:** the study and treatment of cancer
- **Rheumatology:** the study and treatment of diseases of the connective tissue
- **Hematology:** the study and treatment of blood disorders

> **WORDS OF WARNING**
>
> Do not confuse the terms intern and internist. An **intern** is someone who, having just graduated from medical school, is working through the first year of residency. An **internist** is usually someone who has already completed training in internal medicine and has acquired a large store of specialized knowledge and skills. Medicine is traditionally a very hierarchical field, and those who have climbed to the highest rungs of the ladder (internists) don't always take kindly to being confused with newbies (interns).

Surgeons specialize in the treatment of human disease through mechanical means, such as cutting body tissues to remove a tumor or constructing an arterial bypass in a diseased heart. The surgical field consists of general surgery and several surgical subfields, including the following:

- **Cardiothoracic surgery:** surgery on the heart and chest
- **Orthopedic surgery:** surgery of the musculoskeletal system
- **Gynecology:** surgery of the female reproductive system
- **Urology:** surgery of the urinary system and male reproductive system
- **Neurosurgery:** surgery of the brain, spinal cord, and peripheral nerves
- **Plastic surgery:** surgery aimed at reconstructing and restoring function to damaged body parts

Pediatrics is a branch of internal medicine dedicated to the treatment of children and adolescents. **Pediatricians** specialize in the special developmental issues of childhood, and treating diseases particular to children and their growing bodies. Many of the subspecialties of pediatrics are the same as those of adult internal medicine.

Neurologists specialize in the medical treatment of diseases of the nervous system. Psychiatry is the treatment of mental illness. Because many neurological conditions also contain a psychiatric component, there is often overlap between neurology and psychiatry. However, traditionally the two fields have been kept distinct. Neurologists often deal with disorders of the brain and peripheral nervous system that can affect movement but don't necessarily cause mental illness. **Psychiatrists** deal with disorders of the brain that always produce mental illness.

Nurses

Nurses who practice in the United States are required to have completed either a two-year Associate's degree or a four-year Bachelor's degree in nursing. Registered nurses are required to complete further training after graduating from a Bachelor's degree program in order to become certified. Nurses are responsible for direct patient care in the hospital and in outpatient clinics. They work in settings such as the intensive care unit, the operating room, the emergency room, and outpatient general medicine and specialty clinics. Nurses are instrumental in monitoring the health status of patients. They provide nursing skills such as wound care, pain management, intravenous line insertion, and administering medications. They communicate and coordinate care with medical doctors and other professionals responsible for patient care.

Dentists

Though requirements may differ for dentists in other nations, dentists who practice in the United States hold either a DDS (doctorate of dental surgery) or a DDM (doctorate of dental medicine) from a four-year graduate school in dental medicine. Dental school is similar to medical school, and dental students study subjects that are standard in the medical curriculum, such as anatomy and dissection, physiology, microbiology, and biochemistry. Physical health is intimately connected to dental health, and dentists must know about systemic physical diseases that can affect the teeth and gums. They use the same medical language as other medical professionals in diagnosing and treating patients.

Some dentists specialize in dental subspecialties that require further training after graduation from dental school, such as **orthodontics**, oral surgery, **periodontics**, and pediatric dentistry. **Orthodontists** deal mainly with correcting and straightening crooked teeth through the use of braces and retainers. **Periodontists** deal with conditions that affect tissues that support the teeth, such as the gums and supporting bones and ligaments. Diseases of the supporting tissues of the teeth, such as **gingivitis** (gum disease), can cause tooth loss.

Pharmacists

Pharmacists have completed a four-year graduate degree in pharmacology (PharmD or doctorate of pharmacology). During graduate school, pharmacists also study standard medical subjects, such as biochemistry, organic chemistry, anatomy, physiology, microbiology, **pharmacodynamics** (the effects that medicines have on the body), and **pharmacokinetics** (how the body processes medicines). Pharmacists also learn about diagnosis and laboratory tests. They work in hospital pharmacies, outpatient offices that dispense pharmaceuticals, and pharmaceutical companies. As specialists in pharmacology, pharmacists are instrumental in patient care. They sometimes alert physicians when they have prescribed medications at doses that are too high, or when they have prescribed a combination of medications that could interact and harm the patient. Pharmacists use medical terminology on a daily basis in communicating with other medical professionals.

Allied Health Professionals

The allied health field spans a wide variety of disciplines. The following list is not exhaustive, but the allied health field includes the following professions:

Audiologists	Paramedics
Biomedical engineers	Personal and athletic trainers
Clinical psychologists	Phlebotomists
Dental hygienists	Physical therapists
Dietitians/nutritionists	Rehabilitation specialists
Health information technicians	Speech and language pathologists
Massage therapists	
Music therapists	X-ray technicians
Occupational therapists	

People who work in the allied health field have various educational backgrounds. Some have PhDs or Master's degrees and specialized training beyond graduate school. Others have completed degrees from four-year colleges, while still others have completed certification programs or two-year Associate's degrees. Regardless of their educational background, people who work in the allied health field communicate in the language of medicine. They use medical terminology in their daily interactions with colleagues and others responsible for the care of patients. Being able to communicate in the same medical language allows for better coordination of care and ultimately improved patient care.

Patients

These days more and more people are taking advantage of the opportunities provided by the internet to learn about and manage their own health. An abundance of internet health websites has sprung up, which can help patients prepare for a visit to the doctor, figure out what questions to ask, and learn about their own bodies and illnesses. There is currently a trend away from medical paternalism and toward doctors and patients working together to make medical decisions that are in the patient's best interest. This trend places a certain amount of responsibility on patients to become educated about their own body and illness. In this sense, medical terminology is no longer a specialized language spoken by a privileged few. Facilitated by the internet, medical terminology truly is for everyone. Learning some basic terms can help clear up the confusion and anxiety that sometimes accompanies a new diagnosis or a routine visit to the doctor.

The Least You Need to Know

- Modern Western medical terminology has its roots in ancient Greek and Latin.
- Many different types of health-care professionals use medical terminology as a common language by which to understand each other.
- Learning medical terminology can be a part of becoming more knowledgeable about personal health and can be helpful for everyone, even people who don't work in healthcare.

Medical Word Parts

In This Chapter

- Dissecting medical terminology
- Learning medical prefixes
- Learning medical suffixes
- Forming plurals

Learning medical terminology is easier when you realize that each term is made up of various word parts. The word parts come from Greek and Latin and include prefixes, suffixes, and word roots. Learning the word parts expands your medical vocabulary and helps you decipher unknown medical terms.

Certain rules apply to forming medical terms. Learning these rules helps you analyze how word parts are combined and helps you understand the overall meaning of the term. Medical terminology also has rules for forming plurals. Once you learn these rules, you can apply them to many types of medical terms.

Much of the information in this chapter requires memorization. But once you lay the groundwork, you will be able to expand on your medical vocabulary in subsequent chapters.

The Structure of Medical Terms

Most medical terms are made up of a distinct combination of word parts. Almost without exception, each term has a word **root**, which stems from a Greek or Latin term and provides the basic meaning of the term. A word root often falls in the middle of the term, but not always. Some medical terms have more than one word root.

Word roots vary from term to term. Basically the only way to know them is to memorize the common word roots. Because many related terms use the same word root, learning basic word roots allows you to decipher many related terms that use the same word root.

Many medical terms have prefixes. *Pre-* means "before," and that's exactly where prefixes are found, at the beginning of the word. **Prefixes** often modify or add meaning to the word root. They can indicate location, quantity, or make the word root mean its opposite. Prefixes are never stand-alone words and must always be added to other word parts in order to form a complete medical term.

Medical terms also contain **suffixes**, which are word parts that are added to the end of the word. Suffixes add to or change the meaning of the word root. Medical terms contain standard suffixes that are added to various word roots. Like prefixes, suffixes can't stand on their own as individual words. Adding standard suffixes to various word roots creates new words, all with different meanings.

STUDY TIP

Analyzing a medical term is a little like doing a word search puzzle. A good strategy is to look for the word root first. Once you find the word root, you will know the basic meaning of the term. Then look for the prefix and suffix, which modify the term. For example, in the word **periorbital**, once you find the word root (*orbit-*), you know that the term will refer to the eye socket. Looking at the prefix (*peri-*), you realize that the term will have something to do with the area surrounding the eye socket. Finally, when you look at the suffix (*-al*), you realize that the term means "pertaining to the area surrounding the eye socket."

Word Part Combinations

Once you are able to find and decipher the word parts that make up a medical term, you are more than halfway to mastering medical terminology. Understanding how the word parts are combined is the other half of mastery. The various word parts—word roots, prefixes, and suffixes—are usually formed by using **combining vowels**. The vowels don't have any meaning in and of themselves. Neither do they add any additional meaning to the word. They just help make the word easier to pronounce.

One of the most common combining vowels is *o-*, though sometimes *i-* or *e-* is used. The combining vowel plus the word root is called the **combining form**. Finding the combining vowel provides a clue to how the medical term is divided into its different word parts. For example, in the term **transesophageal**, the prefix is *trans* (across), the root is *esophag-* (esophagus), the combining vowel is *e-*, and the suffix is *-al* (pertaining to). So the overall meaning of the term is "pertaining to [being] across the esophagus."

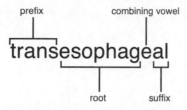

Medical word parts are combined to make a medical term.

When two word roots are combined, the combining vowel is usually retained. This still holds true when the root begins with a vowel, as in **gastroenterology**. However, this rule doesn't always hold true for suffixes. In general, if the suffix starts with a vowel, as in *-algia*, omit the combining vowel before adding the suffix. For example, the word **myalgia** is formed from the word root *myo-* (muscles) and the suffix *-algia* (pain).

Common Medical Prefixes

Medical prefixes can be easier to learn if they are categorized according to the type of meaning that they add to the word. The tables in this section list types of prefixes that are commonly added to medical word roots.

Location, for example, plays an important role in medical terminology. Prefixes that indicate location provide exact meanings about the position of pain, anatomical parts of the body, and other medical processes.

Location Prefixes

Prefix	Meaning	Example
ab-	away	abduction
acro-	top	acromegaly
ad-	toward	adduction
ambi-	found on both sides	ambidextrous
ante-	before, in front of	antenatal
circum-	around	circumorbital

continues

Location Prefixes   (continued)

Prefix	Meaning	Example
dextro-	on the right side	dextrocardia
endo-	within	endocrine
epi-	on, upon	epidermis
exo-	outside	exocrine
extra-	outside	extradural
infra-	below, beneath	infraorbital nerve
inter-	between	interstitial
intra-	within	intravenous
levo-	left	levothyroxine
medi-	middle	mediastinum
meso-	middle	mesothelium
meta-	after, behind	metacarpal
per-	through	percutaneous
peri-	around, surrounding	periumbilical
pre-	before	prediabetes
post-	after, behind	posthumeral
pro-	before, forward	prothrombin
re-	back	reflux
retro-	behind	retroperitoneum
sub-	below	subarticular
super-	above	superciliary
supra-	above, excessive	suprapubic
trans-	across, through	transurethral

In medicine, it is also important to succinctly describe the amount or extent of a disease or other medical process. Many medical prefixes indicate quantity or degree.

Prefixes That Indicate Quantity or Degree

Prefix	Meaning	Example
brady-	slow	bradycardia
diplo-	double	diplococcus
hemi-	one-half	hemiplegia
hyper-	above normal	hyperthyroidism
hypo-	below normal	hypothyroidism
iso-	equal	isotonic
macro-	large	macrocephaly
megal-, megalo-	large	megaloblast
micro-	small	microcephaly

Prefix	Meaning	Example
pan-	complete, pertaining to everything	pancytopenia
pauci-	few	pauciarticular
poly-	many	polymorphonuclear lymphocyte
olig-, oligo-	few	oliguria
super-	above, excessive	superior laryngeal nerve
supra-	above, excessive	supraspinatus
tachy-	fast, irregularly fast	tachycardia

Some prefixes change the meaning of a word root to its opposite, while others make the meaning of the word root more exact.

Other Common Prefixes

Prefix	Meaning	Example
a-, an-	without	anuria
anti-	against	antineoplastic
aut-	self	autologous
dys-	bad, difficult	dysphasia
isch-	restriction	ischemia
pseudo-	false	pseudoaneurysm

Common Medical Suffixes

As with prefixes, categorizing suffixes can make learning them easier. The tables in this section list types of suffixes that are commonly added to word roots.

Indicating relationships between diseases or medical processes and organs or organ systems plays an important role in medical terminology. Several common medical suffixes indicate relationship.

Suffixes That Indicate Relationship

Suffix	Meaning	Example
-ac, -acal	pertaining to	cardiac
-al, -eal	pertaining to	peritoneal
-ic	pertaining to	pediatric

WORDS OF WARNING

The suffix *-ical* is a combination of the suffixes *–ic* and *–al* that also means "pertaining to." For example, **immunologic** and **immunological** both mean "pertaining to the immune system." The trend in many medical textbooks and other medical written materials is to use the more modern, streamlined *-ic* suffix on its own. In clinical medicine, however, the more traditional, redundant *-ical* suffix is often still used. For this reason, this book uses the more common *–ical* suffix.

Suffixes that indicate medical conditions also are common in medical terminology. The same disease process can occur in different organs or organ systems. Combining the word root with the type of disease process precisely conveys what is going on with the patient.

Suffixes That Indicate Medical Conditions

Suffix	Meaning	Example
-algia	pain	fibromyalgia
-dynia	pain	pleurodynia
-emesis	vomiting	hematemesis
-emia	blood condition	anemia
-iasis, -asis	condition	hypochondriasis
-ism	condition, disease	aneurism
-itis	inflammation	ileitis
-osis	condition, disease	sarcoidosis
-pathy	disease, disorder	pyschopathy
-penia	deficiency	osteopenia
-philia	affinity for	hemophilia

Suffixes in medical terminology frequently indicate medical treatments or tests. Combining a word root with these types of suffixes pinpoints exactly what kind of test or treatment is being done.

Suffixes That Refer to Medical Treatments or Tests

Suffix	Meaning	Example
-centesis	surgical puncture	pleurocentesis
-cide, -cidal	killing	microbicide
-ectomy	removal of a body part	appendectomy
-gram	record or picture	arteriogram
-graph	devise used for measurement	electrocardiograph

Suffix	Meaning	Example
-plasty	reconstruction	rhinoplasty
-stomy	surgical creation of an opening	ostomy

Several other suffixes are used in medical terminology. Many of these provide additional meaning or further modify the word root.

Other Suffixes

Suffix	Meaning	Example
-ase	enzyme	lipase
-iatrist	specialist	psychiatrist
-logy	study of	hematology
-lysis, -lytic	destruction	hemolysis
-megaly	large	cardiomegaly
-oid	resembling, similar to	sigmoid colon

Word Roots

Word roots are the meat and potatoes of medical terminology. Every medical term contains at least one word root that provides the basic meaning of the term. Word roots are plentiful in medical terminology, and categorizing them also helps sort them out.

For example, almost every body part, body organ, or body region has a word root that describes it. Word roots that indicate medical conditions form another large category in medical terminology. Lastly, diagnosing disease and treating disease is what medicine is all about, so it's not surprising that many word roots refer to medical treatments and tests. The following tables list common word roots for each of these categories.

Word Roots That Indicate Anatomy or Regions of the Body

Word Root	Meaning	Example
adeno-	gland	adenitis
adren-, adreno-	adrenal glands	adrenopathy
amnio-	fetal sac	amniocentesis
angio-	blood vessel	angioplasty

continues

Word Roots That Indicate Anatomy or Regions of the Body (continued)

Word Root	Meaning	Example
arthro-	joint	arthroscopy
brachi-	arm	brachiocephalic vein
cardi-	heart	cardiomegaly
cephalo-	head	cephalosporin
derm-, dermato-	skin	dermatitis
dors-	back	dorsal
enter-	intestine	enteropathy
gyn-, gyneco-	woman	gynecology
lymph-	lymph	lymphedema
musculo-	muscle	musculoskeletal
myo-	muscle	myofascia
ophthalmo-	eye	ophthalmoscope
pleur-	ribs	pleurisy
pneum-	lungs	pneumothorax
splen-	spleen	splenomegaly
thorac-, thoracico-	chest	thoracentesis
ventr-, ventro-	belly	ventral

Word Roots for Medical Conditions

Word Root	Meaning	Example
alg-, algesi-	pain	analgesic
onc-, onco-	tumor	oncology
-paresis	partial paralysis	hemiparesis
-plegia	paralysis	quadriplegia

Word Roots for Medical Treatments and Tests

Word Root	Meaning	Example
pharmaco-	medication, drug	pharmacology
-scope	instrument	ophthalmoscope
-scopy	use of an instrument for visualization	arthroscopy

WORDS OF WARNING

In medical terminology, the basic rules for combining word parts and forming plurals usually work, but there are exceptions that prove the rules. Sometimes word roots and suffixes are merged together. For example, in the word **polycythemia**, the word root *hem* (blood) is merged with the suffix *emia* (referring to a blood condition). Notice that this word doesn't have any combining vowels, either. Being able to spot the exceptions is a sure sign that you have the rules down pat.

Some word roots stem from basic science fields like biology and chemistry. Terminology used in these fields also share common roots in Latin and Greek, so it's not unusual to have overlap between medical and basic scientific terms.

General Science Word Roots

Word Root	Meaning	Example
-cyte	cell	melanocyte
-genesis	origin, development	organogenesis
ovo-, ovi-, ov-	egg	ovum
sperm-, spermato-	sperm	spermatocyte

Other word roots look completely different from each other, but mean the same thing. That's because some of them come from Latin, while others come from Greek.

Greek and Latin Word Root Comparison

Meaning	Greek Root	Example	Latin Root	Example
abdomen	laparo-	laparotomy	abdomen-	abdominoplasty
bladder	cyst-	cystitis	vesic-	vesicouteral reflux
body	somat-, som—	somatosensory	corpor-	corporeal
bone	ost-, osteo-	osteoarthritis	ossi-	osseous
brain	encephal-	encephalopathy	cerebr-	cerebrospinal fluid
dead	necr-, necro-	necrosis	mort-	mortality
ear	ot-	otitis media	aur-	auricle
fat	lip-	lipogenesis	adip-	adipocyte
kidney	nephr-	nephrology	reno-	renal
vagina	colp(o)-	colposcope	vagin-	vaginitis

Plurals

Many medical terms are made into their plural forms in the standard English manner by adding an *s* or an *es* to the end of the word. But some medical terms don't follow the standard rules. The following table lists rules for forming nonstandard plurals.

Rules for Nonstandard Plurals

Word Ending	Rule	Singular Example	Plural Example
-a	keep the -a, add an -e	fistula	fistulae
-ex, -ix	replace –ex or -ix with -ices	fornix	fornices
-is	replace -is with –es	prognosis	prognoses
–on	replace -on with -a	ganglion	ganglia
-um	replace -um with -a	bacterium	bacteria
-us	replace -us with -i	staphylococcus	staphylococci

STUDY TIP

Some words that look like they should follow the nonstandard rules for forming plurals instead form plurals in the standard English manner. Watch out for these standard plurals. For example, the plural of the word **virus** is **viruses**, not virusi, which is hard to pronounce. Many medical terms are formed in a way that makes them easier to pronounce. If something is hard to pronounce, it might be wrong.

The Least You Need to Know

- Medical terms are made up of prefixes, suffixes, and word roots.
- Combining vowels link word roots together and make medical terms easier to pronounce.
- Categorizing prefixes, suffixes, and word roots can make memorizing them easier.
- Some medical terms form plurals in the standard English manner, but others follow special rules.

Pronunciation, Spelling, and Much More

In This Chapter

- Saying medical terms correctly
- Writing medical terms correctly
- Distinguishing between terms that sound the same or almost the same
- Identifying medical terms that are named after people
- Recognizing shortened medical terms

As you learned in Chapter 2, learning word parts and applying the rules for combining them can help you remember and figure out the meaning of medical terms. It also helps with spelling and pronouncing these terms. Pronouncing and spelling medical terms can seem tricky, but keeping your wits about you can help you learn how to do it.

Another tricky thing about learning medical terminology is that some medical terms sound and look like each other but have completely different meanings. Learning the difference between them is important in order to avoid confusion. Other medical terms don't come from Greek or Latin, so knowing word parts doesn't help you with their meaning. Instead, they are named after the person accredited with discovering them. You also learn about these types of medical terms as well as common medical abbreviations in this chapter.

Medical Pronunciation

Pronouncing common medical terms correctly can help you make a good impression at work. Throughout this book, new medical terms will be written with their pronunciations next to them. These pronunciations follow a certain format that was adapted from the style used on Dictionary.com. Uppercase letters indicate the syllable or syllables to stress when pronouncing the term. Letters in italics indicate which syllables receive the least stress, while letters in normal font receive an intermediate level of stress. The pronunciations are spelled out according to how they should sound when you say them out loud. For example, the word **pneumothorax** is pronounced noo-*muh*-THOHR-aks. The primary word stress is placed on the third syllable. Secondary word stresses are placed on the first and last syllables, and the second syllable receives the least stress.

Sometimes there is more than one correct way to pronounce a medical term. In such cases, both pronunciations are provided. For example, the word **duodenum** can be pronounced doo-*uh*-DEE-*nuhm*, with the main accent on the third syllable, or doo-OD-n-*uhm*, with the main accent occurring on the second syllable.

The Sometimes Silent Consonants

Some medical terms have strange-looking spellings, and it can be difficult to know how to pronounce them without some general rules. In words that start with *gn, mn, pn, ps,* or *pt*, the first consonant is usually silent, while the second is pronounced. Examples of these types of words include the following:

- **Gnathion** (NEY-thee-on or NATH-ee-on): part of the lower jawbone
- **Pneumonia** (*noo*-MOHN-*yuh*): infection or inflammation of the lungs
- **Psoas** (SOH-*uhs*): muscles on either side of the lumbar vertebrae that help flex and rotate the hip joint
- **Ptosis** (TOH-sis): drooping eyelid

On the other hand, if these same combinations of consonants fall in the middle of a word, both consonants are usually pronounced. Examples of these types of words include the following:

- **Orthoptics** (awr-THOP-tiks): exercises for the eye and eye muscles, used to improve vision
- **Prognosis** (prog-NOH-sis): prediction about the course of an illness and the likelihood for recovery
- **Dyspnea** (disp-NEE-*uh*, DISP-nee-*uh*): shortness of breath

Plural Pronunciation

Many medical terms follow the standard English rules for forming plurals by adding *s*, *ies*, or *es* to the end of a term. Plural medical terms that are formed by adding *s* to the end of the word are pronounced similarly to standard English. For example, the plural of **dermatome**, a region of the skin that corresponds to certain sensory nerves in the spinal cord, is **dermatomes**, which is pronounced DUR-*muh-tohms*.

Many medical plurals that are formed with an *ies* or *es* at the end of the term are pronounced with a long *eez* sound. For example, the plural of **ileostomy**, which is an artificial opening created between the small intestine and the abdominal wall, is **ileostomies** and is pronounced il-ee-OS-*tuh*-meez. The plural of **psychosis**, a state of having an altered sense of reality, is **psychoses**, which is pronounced seye-KOH–seez.

Some medical terms that end in *a* are formed by adding *e* to the end of the word. In this case, the plural is often pronounced with a long *ee* sound, as in **rugae** (ROO–gee), which are ridges or folds. Medical plurals that are formed with an *i* are usually pronounced with a long *eye* sound, as in **nevi** (NEE-eye), which are moles.

STUDY TIP

If a word ends in *a*, *is*, *ex*, *ix*, *on*, *um*, or *us*, that's often a clue that it forms a plural using the special rules found in Chapter 2. Watch out for exceptions, though, like the plural for hematoma. Even though it ends in *a*, the plural is hematomas not hematomae.

Spelling Medical Terms

Learning to correctly spell medical terms is crucial. Incorrectly spelling a medical term in a patient's record can convey incorrect information about the patient's condition and treatment plan. This mistake can cause misunderstandings among providers and can also be dangerous to the patient.

Most medical terms that refer to body organs use the common Latin and Greek word parts found in Chapter 2. Memorizing the common prefixes, suffixes, and word roots will help you spell many related medical terms. Understanding how combining vowels are used to create medical terms will also help you figure out how to spell unfamiliar terms. For example, the word root for stomach is *gastr-*. Knowing common prefixes and suffixes helps you spell a profusion of words all related to the stomach.

- **Epigastric:** upper middle region of the abdomen
- **Gastralgia:** stomach pain
- **Gastric:** pertaining to the stomach
- **Gastrin:** a digestive hormone secreted by the stomach
- **Gastritis:** inflammation of the stomach
- **Gastroscopy:** examination of the stomach and duodenum
- **Gastrostomy:** a surgical opening into the stomach
- **Hypogastric:** below the stomach
- **Perigastric:** surrounding the stomach

WORDS OF WARNING

Be careful about applying these rules across the board. Sometimes a word that looks like it contains a common word root uses that root in a different manner. For example, the word **gastrocnemius** looks like it might have something to do with the stomach. But don't be fooled. The gastrocnemius is one of the major muscles in the calf. It takes its name from the fact that it curves outward like a bulging stomach.

Some of the same disease processes affect different organs. Likewise, some of the same tests and treatments are used in different parts of the body. Knowing the spellings for common word roots that refer to body parts, medical conditions, treatments, and tests allows you to spell a long list of medical terms. For example, knowing the suffix *-itis* and some common word roots allows you to spell the following words.

- **Cholecystitis:** inflammation of the gallbladder
- **Colitis:** inflammation of the colon
- **Cystitis:** inflammation of the bladder
- **Encephalitis:** infection or inflammation of the brain
- **Hepatitis:** inflammation of the liver
- **Ileitis:** inflammation of the ileum
- **Mastitis:** inflammation of the breast
- **Neuritis:** inflammation of a nerve
- **Proctitis:** inflammation of the rectum
- **Prostatitis:** inflammation of the prostate

Medical Homonyms and Other Words That Are Easy to Mix Up

A **homonym** is a word that is pronounced exactly like another word, but has a different meaning. The two words are sometimes spelled the same, but they don't need to be. Sometimes variations in spelling don't change the pronunciation of a word, but they change the definition quite a lot. Medicine has numerous homonyms.

Common Medical Homonyms

Medical Term	Pronunciation	Meaning	Homonym	Pronunciation	Meaning
ilium	IL-ee-*uhm*	upper, flared portion of the hip bone	ileum	IL-ee-*uhm*	third portion of the small intestine
lice	LEYES	parasitic bug that sucks blood	lyse	LEYES	to break apart, often used in relation to cell destruction
peroneal	PER-UH-NEE-UHL	related to a specific area of the lower leg	perineal	PER-UH-NEE-UHL	related to the area of the body between the pubis and the anus
pleural	PLOO-R-UHL	pertaining to the membrane that lines the chest wall	plural	PLOO-R-UHL	pertaining to more than one
radical	RAD-I-KUHL	complete surgical removal, as in "radical mastectomy"	radicle	RAD-I-KUHL	small and rootlike, as in the the beginning of a nerve or blood vessel

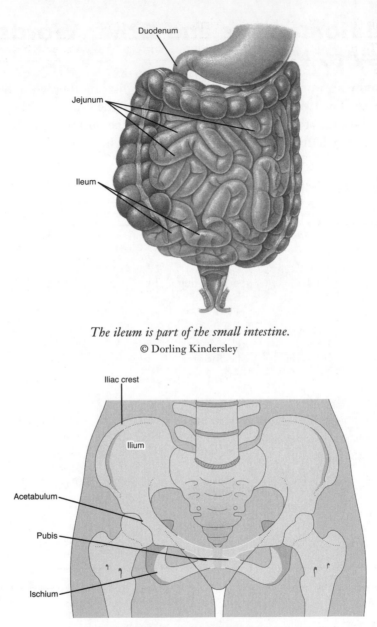

The ileum is part of the small intestine.
© Dorling Kindersley

The ilium is part of the hip bone.
© Dorling Kindersley

In addition to medical homonyms, which sound exactly the same, there are medical terms that sound nearly the same and are often mixed up. Learning them can sometimes be confusing, but it pays off to keep them straight. Using the wrong word, even though it sounds right, can cause real problems!

Medical Terms That Sound Almost the Same

Medical Term	Pronunciation	Definition	Similar Term	Pronunciation	Meaning
adherence	ad-HEER-*uhns*	sticking to something, like a medication regimen	adherents	ad-HEER-*uhnts*	biological things that attach to something else, as in adherent cell cultures
aphagia	*uh*-FEY-*juh*	pain in or difficulty swallowing	aphasia	*uh*-FEY-*zhuh*	inability to speak
diaphysis	deye-AF-*uh*-sis	the middle (long) part of a long bone	diathesis	deye-ATH-*uh*-sis	a tendency or predisposition for a certain condition
ecchymosis	ek-*uh*-MOH-sis	bruise	echinosis	ek-*uh*-NOH-sis	abnormal blood condition of red blood cells
facial	FEY-*shuhl*	pertaining to the face	fascial	FASH-*uhl*	pertaining to a band of connective tissue
flexor	FLEK-scr	a muscle that bends part of the body	flexure	FLEK-sher	a curve or a bend, especially in a tubular organ (such as the intestines)
peritoneal	per-i-tn-EE-*uhl*	related to the lining of the abdominal cavity	perineal	PER-UH-NEE-UHL	related to the area of the body between the pubis and the anus
viral	VEYE-*ruhl*	pertaining to viruses	virile	VIR-*uhl*	strong, energetic, masculine

Medical Eponyms

Not all medical terms come from Latin and Greek. These types of terms can make learning medical terminology tricky, until you realize why they came about. One way to remember them is that embedded in each term is a piece of medical history.

A medical **eponym** is a term that takes its name from a person or thing. Most often, medical eponyms take their names from the people who discovered them.

Some medical eponyms refer to parts of the body. For example, **Bartholin glands** are glands located near the posterior part of the vagina that produce lubrication. They were named after their discoverer, Danish anatomist Caspar Bartholin.

Other medical eponyms refer to medical treatments, surgical procedures, physical symptoms, or diagnostic tests. For example, the **Babinski sign** refers to a reflex found normally in newborns and abnormally in older people with brain damage that involves flexion of the foot. This term was named after the French neurologist Joseph Babinski.

Often medical eponyms refer to disease syndromes, which are a set of symptoms or abnormalities that are normally found together and are indicative of a particular underlying disorder. Medical eponyms are sometimes named after the person who first contracted the disease or brought attention to it. Such terms sometimes have two names—the eponymous name and a more precise, scientific one that is usually derived from Latin or Greek. For example, Lou Gehrig disease (progressive degeneration of the brain and spinal cord) was named after the famous baseball player Lou Gehrig, whose plight gained recognition for this disease. Lou Gehrig disease is also called **amyotrophic lateral sclerosis** (EH-mee-oh-TROH-fic LAT-er-*uhl* skli-ROH-sis) in the scientific literature.

Sometimes medical terms are named after places or organizations, as in Lyme disease (which was discovered near Lyme, Connecticut) or Legionnaires' disease (which was named after this disease broke out at a convention of the American Legion). Strictly speaking, though, medical terms that take their names from places or organizations are not considered to be medical eponyms.

Medical eponyms came about as a form of recognition. They reward accomplishment in science and medicine or recognize the person who suffered from the disease or disorder. Assigning a person's name to the disease, syndrome, body part, or other medical discovery preserves that person's name for posterity. Assigning medical eponyms to constellations of disease symptoms became popularized before science was advanced enough to investigate the underlying causes for the disease and before a more precise scientific term could be assigned. The practice is part of the annals of medical history, with hundreds of medical eponyms persisting today.

DID YOU KNOW?

Many controversies surround the use of medical eponyms. Some diseases have several different eponyms, and different countries may use different eponyms to describe the same disease, which makes for a lot of confusion. Sometimes eponyms reward credit to the wrong person or to people responsible for nefarious deeds. For example, Reiter syndrome (an autoimmune inflammation of the joints that occurs in response to bacterial infection) is named after Hans Conrad Julius Reiter, a Nazi physician who was convicted of war crimes for authorizing forced human experimentation at the Buchenwald concentration camp during World War II. The replacement term for this disorder is **reactive arthritis**.

Common Medical Eponyms

Eponym	Source of the Name	Definition	Alternate Name
Baker cyst	William Morrant Baker	a walled-off collection and buildup of fluid behind the knee	popliteal cyst, bulge-knee
Crohn disease	Burrill Bernard Crohn	a form of inflammatory bowel disease that affects all parts of the gastrointestinal tract, from mouth to anus	regional enteritis, ileitis, granulomatous ileocolitis
Graves disease	Robert James Graves	an autoimmune disease causing the thyroid to become overactive	diffuse thyrotoxic goiter
Hodgkin disease	Thomas Hodgkin	cancer of the lymph tissue	none
Huntington disease	George Huntington	an inherited genetic disorder caused by brain degeneration and characterized by abnormal movements and psychiatric symptoms	Huntington's chorea
Reye syndrome	R. Douglas Reye	an illness that causes brain and liver damage; primarily affects children and is associated with recent viral illness and aspirin use	none

Medical Abbreviations

By now it may be obvious that many medical terms can be lengthy and difficult to write in a hurry. In the interest of lightening the workload, many medical abbreviations have come into use. Here are a few common ones:

- **b.i.d.:** twice a day (Latin: *bis in die*)
- **CBC:** complete blood count
- **Dx:** diagnosis
- **Hx:** history
- **IM:** intramuscular
- **NPO:** nothing by mouth (Latin: *nil per os*)
- **PO:** by mouth (Latin: *per os*)
- **PRN:** as needed (Latin: *pro re nata*)
- **q.h.s.:** at bedtime (Latin: *quaque hora somni*)

The Least You Need to Know

- Knowing common medical prefixes, word roots, and suffixes will help you figure out how to pronounce and spell medical terms.
- Learning the difference between medical terms that sound similar can make a huge difference in patient care.
- Medical eponyms are usually named after the person who discovered the body part, procedure, or syndrome.

Human Anatomy: Terms for Body Parts and Systems

Part

2

Part 2 covers anatomy. Because many anatomical terms describe the position of one body part in relation to another, Chapter 4 provides a general introduction to positional and directional terms. Much of medical school is taught from the systems perspective, which means that subjects are broken up into body systems, such as the cardiovascular or gastrointestinal system. The rest of Chapter 4 explains the systems perspective, starting with microscopic cells up to body systems.

The remainder of Part 2 is also organized according to the systems perspective. Each chapter provides medical terms related to the body systems covered in that chapter. Because anatomical terms are easier to remember by understanding the role and function of body parts, each chapter explains body systems from the perspective of functional anatomy.

Chapter 5 covers the musculoskeletal system, which provides protection, enables locomotion, and provides movement for various vital processes in the body. Skin is also included in this chapter because it plays an important role in protecting the body from the external environment, although skin also performs many other important functions for the body.

Chapter 6 covers the cardiopulmonary, blood, and lymphatic systems, which are all intimately connected. Chapter 7 covers the digestive system: the intestines and associated organs. Chapter 8 covers the urinary, reproductive, and endocrine systems. The endocrine system provides hormones for the body and is included in Chapter 8 because the reproductive system is closely linked to the endocrine system, although hormones are vital to many other types of bodily processes (like growth and digestion). Chapter 9 covers the brain, nervous system, and sensory organs like the eyes and ears.

Body Positions, Systems, and Structures

In This Chapter

- Describing locations and positions of things in the body
- Grouping terms by organ system
- Learning basic biochemical terms
- Building a vocabulary for genetics

Medical professionals use positional and directional terms to organize and describe human anatomy. These terms communicate where in the body a disease process or body part is found in relation to the rest of the body.

The study of human anatomy follows an organizational framework, starting at the microscopic level with cells. These are organized into tissues, which work together to function as organs. In turn, organs work together to form organ systems. Many medical terms are based in human anatomy. This book follows the same approach and presents new terms based on organ systems.

Medical terminology contains many words from biochemistry and genetics. Because these fields play important roles in normal health and disease, it helps to know some biochemical and genetic terms.

Positional and Directional Terms

Positional and directional terms describe where in the body a disease process or other medical issue is occurring. Using these terms helps locate the organ or medical problem in relation to other parts of the body.

Abduction vs. Adduction

The terms **abduction** (ab-DUHK-*shuhn*) and **adduction** (ad-DUHK-*shuhn*) can be confusing. They look and sound similar, but mean the opposite of each other. Abduction refers to an action that brings part of the body away from the midline. Adduction refers to an action that brings part of the body closer to the midline.

One way to remember these two words is to think of the hip abductor/adductor machine at the gym. When you are using the hip abductor part of the machine, you are using your hip abductor muscles to spread your legs apart. When you are using the adductor part of the machine, you are using your hip adductor muscles to bring your legs together.

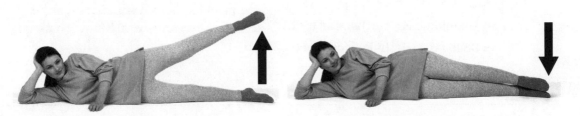

In hip abduction, the legs are pulled apart.
Steve Gorton © Dorling Kindersley

In hip adduction, the legs are pressed together.
Steve Gorton © Dorling Kindersley

Front and Back in Medical Terms

Some directional terms indicate relative location in relation to the front and back of the body. Most of us know where the back and the front of the body lie, but in medical terms back and front have to do with how the body forms during fetal development.

Dorsal (DAWR-suhl) refers to the part of the body that becomes the spinal cord. This part corresponds to the **posterior** (pah-STEER-ee-er, poh-STEER-ee-er), or back, in humans. So dorsal and posterior usually refer to the same area: the back part of the body.

DID YOU KNOW?

Pictures of the human body are often shown in the **anatomic position**. This position provides the standard reference for directional terms. In this position, the body is standing up with arms placed at the sides and palms facing forward.

Ventral (VEN-truhl) refers to the part of the body that develops into the abdomen. This part corresponds to the **anterior** (an-TEER-ee-er), or front, in humans. So ventral and anterior usually both refer to the front part of the body.

Ceph- means head in Greek, so **cephalad** (SEF-*uh*-lad) refers to the part of the body that becomes the head and means "toward the head." This often corresponds to the front, or anterior/ventral, part of the body.

Caud- means tail in Greek, so **caudad** (KAWD-ad) refers to the part of the body that becomes the tail (in creatures that have a tail) and means "toward the tail." This often corresponds to the back, or posterior/dorsal, part of the body.

General Directional Terms

Other directional medical terms are more general and indicate the location of one body part in relation to another. The following table lists some of the most common directional medical terms.

Common Directional Terms

Term	Pronunciation	Meaning
superior	*suh*-PEER-ee-er; *soo*-PEER-ee-er	above something else, upward
inferior	in-FEER-ee-er	below something else, downward
distal	DIS-tl	far from a reference point, or far from a point of origin
proximal	PROK-*suh*-*muhl*	near a point of reference, or near a point of origin
lateral	LAT-er-*uhl*	pertaining to the side
medial	MEE-dee-*uhl*	pertaining to the middle
median	MEE-dee-*uhn*	located in the midline
unilateral	yoo-*nuh*-LAT-er-*uhl*	located or occurring on only one side
bilateral	beye-LAT-er-*uhl*	located or occurring on both sides
superficial	soo-per-FISH-*uhl*	located near the surface
deep	DEEP	located far below the surface
anteroposterior	an-TAIR-o-pah-STEER-ee-er; an-TAIR-opoh-STEER-ee-er	in the direction from front to back, as in an x-ray taken from front to back
posteroanterior	pah-STEER-o-an-TAIR-ee-er; poh-STEER-o-an-TAIR-ee-er	in the direction from back to front, as in an x-ray taken from back to front

Anatomic Planes

Directional medical terms also use the concept of a plane, which is an imaginary surface that runs between two points and cuts straight through an object. Planes divide the body and organs into different sections. Organs look different in respect to other organs when viewed in different sections.

The key anatomic planes are the following:

- **Frontal** (FRUHN-tl)/**coronal** (*kuh*-ROHN-*l*, KOR-*uh*-nl) **plane:** This imaginary surface runs vertically and divides the body or organ into front and back.
- **Lateral** (LAT-er-*uhl*)/**sagittal** (SAJ-i-tl) **plane:** This imaginary surface runs vertically and divides the body or organ into right and left.
- **Midsagittal** (mid SAJ-i-tl) **plane:** This imaginary surface runs vertically through the midline and divides the body into right and left halves.
- **Transverse** (TRANZ-vurs; tranz-VURS)/**axial** (AK-see-*uhl*) **plane:** This imaginary surface runs horizontally and divides the body or organ into upper and lower parts, similar to a cross-section.

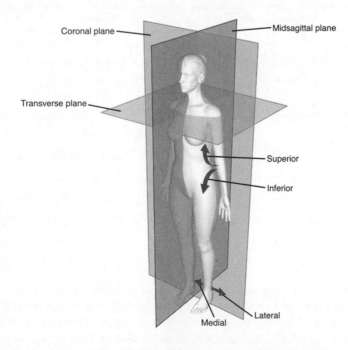

Terms for body locations often refer to anatomical planes.
Zygote Media Group © Dorling Kindersley

Body Cavities

Body cavities are spaces that contain organs. Dividing the body into body cavities is a good way of making sense of anatomy because interrelated organs often fall within the same body cavity (though not all do). The following table describes common body cavities. Note: the mediastinum is not a true cavity—it is more like a sac—but it is included in the following table because it forms a space inside the body.

Common Body Cavities

Body Cavity	Pronunciation	Location	Organs Contained
cranial	KREY-nee-*uhl*	head, space surrounded by the skull	brain, pituitary, related nerves and blood vessels
oral	AWR-*uhl*	head	teeth, gums, tongue
mediastinum	mee-dee-a-STEYE-*nuhm*	chest	heart, esophagus, trachea, bronchial tubes, related blood vessels and nerves
pleural	PLOOR-*uhl*	chest	none; potential space between the two membranes that line the lungs
thoracic	thaw-RAS-ik, thoh-RAS-ik	chest	lungs, heart, trachea, bronchial tubes, esophagus
abdominal	ab-DOM-*uh*-nl	below the chest cavity and above the pelvic cavity; abdomen	stomach, liver, gallbladder, small and large intestines, kidneys, spleen
peritoneal	per-i-tn-EE-*uhl*	abdomen	none; potential space between the membranes that cover abdominal organs and the abdominal wall
spinal	SPEYEN-l	back	spinal cord
pelvic	PEL-vik	below the abdomen, inside the pelvic bones	bladder, ureters, urethra, uterus, ovaries

STUDY TIP

The diaphragm is a muscle that lies just above the liver. The diaphragm is usually not under conscious control. Its contractions help expand the chest cavity to aid in breathing. A good way to remember the difference between the chest and abdominal cavities is that the chest cavity lies above the diaphragm, and the abdominal cavity lies below it. Basically, the diaphragm is the dividing point between the chest and abdominal cavities.

Some spaces inside the body aren't really cavities at all. Instead, they are considered "potential spaces," which means that they are empty but have the potential to be filled. One example is the pleural cavity, which is formed by two membranes that normally lie right next to each other. In lung disease, fluid sometimes collects in the pleural cavity. This condition is called a **pleural effusion** (PL*OOR-uhl* ih-FYOO-*zhuhn*). The peritoneal cavity is another potential space that is formed by two membranes. In liver and other diseases, fluid can collect in this space, a condition called **ascites** (*uh*-SEYE-teez). Medications are also injected into the peritoneal cavity.

Body Regions

For purposes of description, medical professionals also divide the body into different regions based on anatomy. These regions sometimes correspond to the various body cavities, but not always.

Body Regions

Region	Pronunciation	Description
cephalic	*suh*-FAL-ik	head, including the skull, face, eyes, ears, and related structures
thorax	THAWR-aks, THOHR-aks	chest, area of the body above the abdomen and below the head
cervical	SUR-vi-*kuhl*	division of the spinal column corresponding to the neck
thoracic	thaw-RAS-ik, thoh-RAS-ik	division of the spinal column corresponding to the chest
lumbar	LUHM-bahr	division of the spinal column corresponding to the waist
sacral	SEY-*kruhl*, *SAK-ruhl*	division of the spinal column corresponding to the lower back
coccygeal	kok-SIJ-ee-*uhl*	division of the spinal column corresponding to the tailbone
umbilical	uhm-BIL-i-*kuhl*, uhm-*bi*-LEYE-*kuhl*	central area of the abdomen surrounding the umbilicus (belly button)
epigastric	ep-i-GAS-trik	upper region in the abdomen, above the umbilicus (belly button)
hypochondriac	heye-*puh*-KON-dree-ak	upper abdominal regions to the right and left of the epigastric region
hypogastric	heye-*puh*-GAS-trik	lower abdominal region, below the umbilicus (belly button)

Region	Pronunciation	Description
suprapubic	SOO-*pruh*-PYOO-*bik*	lower abdominal region, below the umbilicus (belly button) and above the pubic region
pubic	PYOO-*bik*	lower abdominal region above the external genitals
inguinal	ING-*gwuh*-nl	lower sides of the abdomen on either side of the pubic region
iliac	IL-ee-ak	lower abdominal regions corresponding to the right and left iliac crests (hip bones)
abdominal	ab-DOM-*uh*-nl	region below the diaphragm and above the pelvis
pelvic	PEL-vik	region below the abdomen

The abdomen and pelvis are sometimes combined into one region for purposes of description. This combination is called the **abdominopelvic** (ab-DOM-*uh*-noh-PEL-vik) region. If you imagine this region to be divided by two imaginary perpendicular lines that cross at the belly button, you get four quadrants:

- **Left Lower Quadrant** (LLL): the area to the left and below the belly button
- **Left Upper Quadrant** (LUQ): the area to the left and above the belly button
- **Right Lower Quadrant** (RLQ): the area to the right and below the belly button
- **Right Upper Quadrant** (RUQ): the area to the right and above the belly button

Body Positions

Certain body positions have special medical terms. These positions are important because some medical tests and treatments can be done only on patients in these positions. Knowing the name of the position helps in learning how to do the test or treatment. These body positions include the following:

- **Decubitus** (dih-KYOO-bi-*tuhs*): lying down
- **Supine** (soo-PEYEN): lying face up on the back
- **Anatomic** (an-*uh*-TOM-ik): standing, with arms at the sides and palms facing forward
- **Prone** (PROHN): lying flat, face-down

- **Recumbent** (ri-KUHM-*buhnt*): lying down
- **Lateral recumbent** (LAT-er-*uhl* ri-KUHM-*buhnt*): lying on the side
- **Dorsal recumbent** (DAWR-*suhl* ri-KUHM-*buhnt*): lying on the back in bed with knees bent and feet flat on the bed
- **Semirecumbent** (SEM-ee ri-KUHM-*buhnt*, SEM-eye ri-KUHM-*buhnt*): lying on the back in bed with the head of the bed raised 45 degrees

Organ Systems

The body is organized into cells, tissues, organs, and systems. Some of the smallest individual body units are cells. Cells are specialized into different types, such as muscle, nerve, skin, bone, blood, and immune cells. Similar types of cells work together to form tissues. Each tissue has a particular function, such as muscle tissue, connective tissue, and epithelial (skin) tissue. Different kinds of tissues work together to form organs. In turn, organs work together to form organ systems, which carry out the task of keeping the organism alive.

Some organ systems work together, such as the muscle and skeletal systems. Others have functions that overlap. The skin is one example of this. The skin functions as a protective barrier in maintaining fluid and temperature balance, as well as a sensory organ. Because of this overlap, organ systems aren't always grouped in the same way.

The standard way of teaching medicine is by organ system. This method makes sense because many (though not all) human diseases occur in particular organ systems. The next few chapters follow this tradition and present medical terminology by organ system. These organ systems include the following:

- **Integumentary system:** skin (Chapter 5)
- **Musculoskeletal systems:** bones and muscles (Chapter 5)
- **Cardiovascular and lymph systems:** heart, blood vessels, lymphatics (Chapter 6)
- **Blood and immune systems:** red blood cells, white blood cells, lymph nodes (Chapter 6)
- **Pulmonary system:** lungs, bronchi, bronchioles (Chapter 6)
- **Gastrointestinal system:** stomach, small intestine, large intestine, liver, pancreas, gallbladder (Chapter 7)
- **Urinary system:** kidneys, bladder, ureters, urethra (Chapter 8)
- **Female reproductive system:** ovaries, uterus, vagina (Chapter 8)

- **Male reproductive system:** penis, testes, prostate (Chapter 8)
- **Endocrine system:** hormones and glands (Chapter 8)
- **Nervous system:** brain, spinal cord, and nerves (Chapter 9)
- **Sensory system:** eyes, ears, nose, tongue, skin (Chapter 9)

Common Biochemical Terms

Biochemistry is the study of chemistry as it applies to living organisms. Because biochemistry is integral to the proper functioning of cells, tissues, organs, and organ systems, it's worthwhile to learn a few biochemical terms.

Biochemical Terminology

Term	Pronunciation	Meaning
amino acid	*uh*-MEE-noh AS-id	a molecule from which proteins are made
carbohydrate	kahr-boh-HEYE-dreyt, kahr-b*uh*-HEYE-dreyt	a class of compounds that includes sugars, starches, and steroids
collagen	KOL-*uh*-*juhn*	a long, durable protein; the primary component of hair
DNA	DEE-en-ey	a compound (deoxyribonucleic acid) that carries the genetic information of an organism
enzyme	EN-zeyem	protein that speeds chemical reactions
glucose	GLOO-kohs	sugar, a compound made up of several carbohydrate molecules
hemoglobin	HEE-*muh*-gloh-bin	a group of proteins found in red blood cells that helps bind oxygen
lipid	LIP-id	a water-insoluble compound that is a fat, wax, sterol, or a fat-soluble vitamin
neurotoxin	NOOR-oh-tok-sin, NYOOR-tok-sin	compound that interferes with nerve cell function
protein	PROH-teen	type of compound made from amino acids; includes enzymes, hair, and cartilage

Common Genetic Terms

A gene is the basic hereditary unit of an organism. Genes are necessary for life because they carry the information necessary to make a new organism. Without genes, humans would not be able to reproduce. Because many human diseases occur when genes become defective, it makes sense to learn some genetic terminology.

Genetic Terminology

Term	Pronunciation	Meaning
allele	*uh*-LEEL	different versions of a gene; often refers to a gene that has mutated
chromosome	KROH-*muh*-sohm	a structure that carries genetic information
dominant	DOM-*uh*-*nuhnt*	used to describe a gene that determines outward appearance
gene	JEEN	a hereditary unit, found in a particular location on a chromosome
genome	JEE-nohm	all the genes carried by an organism
genotype	JEN-*uh*-teyep, JEE-n*uh*-teyep	the genetic makeup of an individual
phenotype	FEE-n*uh*-teyep	outward characteristics of an organism that are produced by the genotype
recessive	ri-SES-iv	a gene whose presence is masked by a dominant gene

The Least You Need to Know

- Medical professionals use many different types of terms to describe position, direction, and location of body parts and disease processes.
- Ranging from small to large, the human body is organized into cells, tissues, organs, and organ systems.
- Because biochemistry is a vital part of living organisms, medical terminology uses many biochemical terms.
- Genes carry the hereditary information of an individual. Medical terminology also uses many genetic terms.

Skin, Bones, and Muscles

In This Chapter

- Skin functions
- Skin layers and other structures
- Bones, joints, cartilage, and ligaments
- Voluntary and involuntary muscles

Skin, bones, and muscles are, to a certain extent, interconnected. Skin is the outermost layer of the body and has many functions. One major function is to provide sensory information about the outside world, so skin is sometimes grouped with the sensory organs such as the eyes, ears, and nose. But skin also plays a major role in protecting the human body against harmful things in the environment. Bones and muscles also serve a protective function, so skin is grouped with these other two organ systems in this chapter.

Because many health issues involve the skin, bones, and muscles, it makes sense to learn some basic terms for normal anatomy involving these organ systems before learning their related diseases in Part 4 later in this book.

The Skin

The skin, also known as the **integumentary system** (in-teg-*yuh*-MEN-*tuh*-ree SIS-*tuhm*), is the largest organ system in the body. Skin is a great multitasker and serves many functions in the body. To fulfill all these functions, it has many different structures.

Functions of the Skin

Skin serves as a protective barrier against the outside world. You can think of skin as your body's seal against harmful things in the environment. Microorganisms such as bacteria and viruses have difficulty crossing the skin to the inner parts of the body. The fat in skin acts as a type of padding that protects the body's muscles and organs.

Skin also functions in **homeostasis** (hoh-mee-*uh*-STEY-sis), which means maintaining conditions that are optimal for the proper functioning of the body and its organs. Skin protects the body from dehydration by minimizing the amount of body water lost to the environment.

> **DID YOU KNOW?**
>
> A third-degree burn involves all layers of the skin and is very serious. In third-degree burns, the skin appears white or black. The skin often feels numb due to destruction of nerve cells. People who have third-degree burns over the majority of their bodies have difficulty maintaining their body temperatures. They also have problems with dehydration because the protective function of skin has been lost. They also are at risk for infections because the skin can no longer serve as a barrier against outside organisms.

Skin also helps regulate body temperature. When the outside temperature is hot, the skin dissipates the heat by perspiration. (Waste products also are released from the body through perspiration.) Perspiration is created and regulated through sweat glands, also known as **sudoriferous** (soo-*duh*-RIF-er-*uh*s) **glands**, in the skin. Each sweat gland leads to a **pore** (POHR), which is the opening through which sweat flows to the outside world. When outside temperatures are chilly, blood vessels in the skin contract. Blood then can be redirected to vital organs, such as the liver, kidneys, heart, and brain, to keep the body alive during frigid temperatures.

Skin contains a compound called **melanin** (MEL-*uh*-nin) that is made by cells called **melanocytes** (*mel*-AH-noh-seyet). Melanin causes the skin to tan when exposed to sunlight and protects the skin from sunburn. In response to sunlight, skin also produces vitamin D, which is vital for proper bone formation and immune function. Skin serves as a storage area for vitamin D as well as water, fat, and sugar.

Skin also works as a sensory organ. The hairs in the skin help detect sensory information. Nerves in the skin convey information about temperature, touch, pressure, and pain to the brain. The skin is organized into **dermatomes** (DUR-m*uh*-tohms), which are regions of the skin that correspond to certain sensory nerves in the spinal cord.

Medical professionals, especially neurologists, use their knowledge of skin dermatomes to diagnose certain medical conditions on physical examination. Surgeons use
their knowledge of dermatomes to decide where to make an incision. Cutting across
a dermatome can result in poor wound healing and an ugly scar. Cutting along the
direction of a dermatome often results in the least scarring.

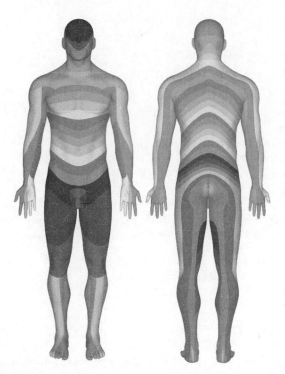

Each shaded area in these anterior and posterior views highlights
a different dermatome.
© Dorling Kindersley

Layers of the Skin

The skin consists of these three layers:

- **Epidermis** (ep-i-DUR-mis): This waterproof, uppermost layer primarily
  serves as protection.
- **Dermis** (DUR-mis): This middle layer contains nerves; blood vessels; sweat
  glands; oil glands; and hair **follicles** (FOL-i-*kuhls*), which are hair roots.

• **Hypodermis** (heye-p*uh*-DUR-mis): This bottom layer contains fat, nerves, blood vessels, and immune cells.

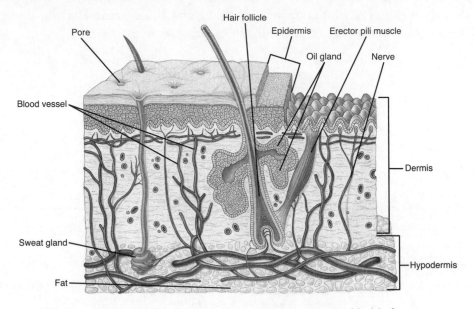

The layers of the skin contain many structures to serve several bodily functions.
Debbie Maizels © Dorling Kindersley

Structures in the Skin

Several structures play a role in helping the skin accomplish its various functions. Some of these are listed in the following table.

Skin Structures

Structure	Pronunciation	Meaning, Function
adipocyte	AD-*uh*-poh-seyet	fat cells
arrector pili/erector pili	ah-REK-ter peye-leye, ih-REK-ter peye-leye	muscle attached to a hair follicle that can contract and make the hair "stand on end"
hair	HAYR	fiber formed by hair follicles that has sensory and heat-conserving functions
keratinocyte	KER-*uh*-tin-oh-seyet	cell that makes keratin

Structure	Pronunciation	Meaning, Function
nail	NEYL	hard plate made of keratin that grows on toes and fingers and protects them
sebaceous gland	si-BEY-*shuhs* gland	gland that makes oil to lubricate the skin so it doesn't dry out

Descriptive and Other Terms Related to the Skin

Medical terminology contains many other terms that pertain to skin. Some of the most common ones are in the following table.

Common Skin-Related Terms

Term	Pronunciation	Meaning
cicatrix	SIK-*uh*-triks	scar
comedo	KOM-i-doh, kom-EE-doh	whitehead or blackhead
cyanosis	seye-*uh*-NOH-sis	blue skin due to cold or lack of oxygen
cyst	sist	a liquid-filled sac that is walled off from surrounding structures
diaphoresis	deye-*uh-fuh*-REE-sis	heavy sweating
erythematous	er-*uh*-THEM-*uh-tuhs*	red
furuncle	FUH-ruhng-*kuhl*, FYOOR-uhng-*kuhl*	boil
indurated	IN-*doo*-reyt-ed	hardened tissue
jaundice	JAWN-dis	abnormal yellowing of the skin, usually due to disease
keratin	KER-*uh*-tin	protein in hair and nails that makes them hard
nevus	NEE-*vuhs*	mole
pallor	PAL-er	pale
pruritic	*proo*-RIT-ik	itchy
purulent	PYOOR-*uh-luhnt*, PYOOR-*yuh-luhnt*	filled with pus
sebum	SEE-*buhm*	oil
turgor	TUR-ger	characterized by fullness

The Skeletal System

The human skeletal system is made up of bones, joints, cartilage, and ligaments. One of the major functions of the skeleton is to provide protection to various body organs. For example, the skull protects the brain. The ribs protect the heart and lungs. And the spinal column protects the nerves in the spinal cord.

The skeleton provides a framework and support for various other body structures. For example, the pelvic bones support the organs in the pelvis. Many muscles attach to bones, which give them something to contract against in order to generate movement.

The skeleton also has other functions. Bone marrow, which is found in the middle of many bones, produces red blood cells. Certain immune cells are formed inside bone marrow as well. Bone marrow stores iron, and bone itself serves as a storage site for calcium.

Bone also interacts with the endocrine system. **Calcitonin** (kals-*uh*-TOH-*nuhn*) and **parathyroid** (pair-*uh*-THEYE-roid) hormone are the major hormones that act on bone and play a role in bone formation and remodeling. Bones even release their own hormone called **osteocalcin** (os-tee-*uh*-KAL-sin), which plays a role in blood sugar regulation and bone formation.

Bones

There are 206 bones in the adult human body. (Newborns have more bones than adults because their bones grow together and fuse as they age, decreasing the number of total bones in their bodies.) The human skeleton is divided into the axial skeleton and the appendicular skeleton.

DID YOU KNOW?

Certain bones are shaped differently in men and women. This is how forensic scientists and anthropologists can figure out whether a skeleton belonged to a male or a female. The major difference lies in the pelvis. Female pelvises are flatter than those of males, and the hip bones flare outward more widely. The **pelvic inlet** (the central, circular opening where pelvic organs are found and through which a baby passes during childbirth) is round in females and heart-shaped in males.

The **axial** (AK-see-*uhl*) skeleton is made up of bones found along the central vertical axis of the body. Another way to think of the axial skeleton is as the "core" of the body, to which the pelvis, arms, and legs attach. The axial skeleton supports the head, chest, and spinal column, which makes human upright posture possible.

Main Bones of the Axial Skeleton

Term	Pronunciation	Common Name or Location
cranium	KREY-nee-*uhm*	skull
auditory ossicles	AW-di-tohr-ee OS-i-*kuhlz*	middle ear
hyoid bone	HEYE-oid BOHN	the bone that anchors the tongue
sternum	STUR-*nuhm*	breast plate, breast bone
costal	KOS-tl, KAWS-tl	pertaining to the ribs
vertebral column	VUR-*tuh-bruhl*, vur-TEE-*bruhl* KOL-*uhm*	spinal column

The **appendicular** (ap-*uhn*-DIK-*yuh*-ler) skeleton consists of the rest of the bones outside of the axial skeleton. A good way to remember the appendicular skeleton is that it is the part of the skeleton that contains the **appendages** (arms and legs). The appendicular skeleton makes walking possible. Because the pelvis plays a role in walking, it is part of the appendicular skeleton.

Major Bones of the Appendicular Skeleton

Term	Pronunciation	Common Name or Location
clavicle	KLAV-i-*kuhl*	collarbone
scapula	SKAP-*yuh-luh*	wing bone
humerus	HYOO-mer-*uhs*, YOO-mer-*uhs*	upper arm bone
ulna	UHL-n*uh*	forearm bone
radius	REY-dee-*uhs*	forearm bone
carpal	KAHR-*puhl*	wristbone
metacarpal	meh-*tuh*-KAHR-*puhl*	hand bones
phalanges	*fuh*-LAN-jeez	fingers
ilium	IL-ee-*uhm*	flared, upper portion of the hip bone
ischium	IS-kee-*uhm*	sit bones
pubis	PYOO-bis	bone that forms the front, lower part of the pelvis

continues

Major Bones of the Appendicular Skeleton   (continued)

Term	Pronunciation	Common Name or Location
femur	FEE-mur	thighbone
patella	*puh*-TEL-*uh*	kneecap
tibia	TIB-ee-*uh*	lower leg bone; shinbone
fibula	FIB-*yuh-luh*	lower leg bone
medial malleolus	MEE-dee-*uhl mal*-EE-*oh-luhs*	inner anklebone
lateral malleolus	LAT-er-*uhl mal*-EE-*oh-luhs*	outer anklebone
tarsal	TAHR-*suhl*	foot bone
metatarsals	meh-*tuh*-TAHR-*suhls*	toes

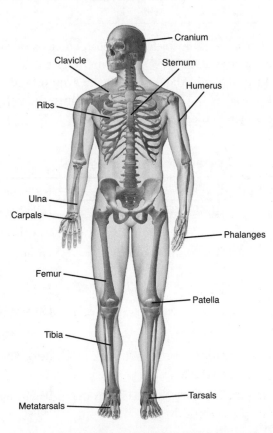

This anterior view shows major bones of the axial and appendicular skeletons.
Raj Dashi © Dorling Kindersley

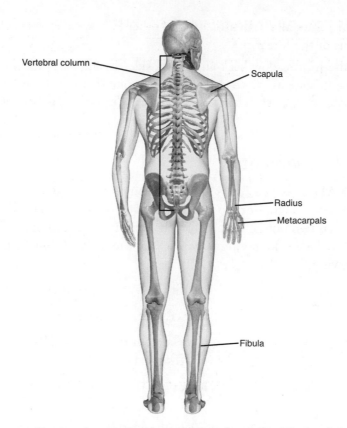

This posterior view shows major bones of the axial and appendicular skeletons.
Raj Dashi © Dorling Kindersley

Joints

A **joint** is the area where two bones **articulate** (ahr-TIK-*yuh*-leyt) or come in contact with each other. The human body contains different kinds of joints. The major categories include the following:

- **Ball-and-socket joints** have a wide range of motion including rotation, as in the shoulder and hip joints.
- **Condyloid** (KON-dl-oid) **joints** allow movement along two planes, but no rotation, as in the jaw and fingers.
- **Gliding joints** allow bone surfaces to glide past each other. Movement directions are limited, as in the bones in the wrist and ankles.
- **Hinge joints** allow motion along one plane only, as in the elbow.

- **Pivot joints** allow rotation around other bones, as in the neck bones and radius of the forearm.
- **Saddle joints** allow back-and-forth, side-to-side motions but no rotation. A major bone in the thumb is a saddle bone that enables humans to use their thumbs more adeptly than other animals (known as opposable thumbs).

Cartilage and Ligaments

Cartilage (KAHR-tl-ij) cushions joints and sometimes holds them together. Cartilage is made of a tough, flexible material. It acts like a shock absorber and reduces friction between two bones, which protects them from grinding each other down over time. Cartilage is found in many places in the body, including in the knee, ear, and the following:

rib cage	**costal** (KAWS-tl) **cartilage**
nose	**alar** (EY-ler) **cartilage**
spinal column	**intervertebral** (in-ter-VUR-*tuh-bruhl*, in-ter-VUR-*tee-bruhl*) **disks**
bronchial tubes	**hyaline** (HEYE-*uh*-lin) **cartilage**

Ligaments (LIG-*uh-muhnts*) are tough, fibrous tissues that connect bones to bones. Ligaments help form joints and also stabilize them. Most bones have ligaments associated with them, but not all ligaments are attached to bones. For example, the uterus is supported by ligaments.

Muscles

The muscular system consists of several types of muscle, each of which serves a particular function. In general, muscle helps support the body, enables conscious movement (as in walking), and performs nonconscious bodily functions (as in breathing). Muscle is highly **vascularized** (VAS-*kyuh-luh*-reyezd), meaning that it contains many blood vessels. As such, muscles also play a role in blood circulation. Muscular movement is also a major source of heat generation in the body.

Voluntary Muscles

Voluntary muscle is under the conscious control of the brain. That means that in order for you to contract a voluntary muscle, you must first think about doing it. Sometimes voluntary muscles contract as part of a reflex to avoid danger, but in general they take a break whenever they can.

Voluntary muscle is arranged in regular, parallel patterns that appear as **striations** (streye-EY-*shuhnz*), or stripes, under the microscope. These stripes are what give voluntary muscle the ability to produce powerful, quick contractions. For this reason, voluntary muscle is also called **striated** (STREYE-ey-tid) muscle.

Because the muscles that attach to and move the skeleton are mostly voluntary muscle, this kind of muscle is also called **skeletal** (SKEL-i-tl) muscle. There are about 639 voluntary/skeletal muscles in the body. These are divided into **superficial** (soo-per-FISH-*uhl*) and **deep** muscles. Superficial skeletal muscles are found closest to the skin, and deep skeletal muscles are found farther from the skin and closer to the inside of the body.

Major Voluntary/Skeletal Muscles

Term	Pronunciation	Function
sternocleidomastoid	ster-*noh*-cley-*doh*-MAS-toyd	tilts and rotates head, flexes neck, and raises sternum during breathing
intercostals	in-ter-KOS-tl	move the chest wall in respiration
serratus	*suh*-RAT-*uhs*, *suh*-REYT-*uhs*	aids in elevating and lowering the ribs in respiration
diaphragm	DEYE-*uh*-fram	helps expand the rib cage, aids in respiration, and separates chest from abdominal cavity
abdominal obliques	ab-DOM-*uh*-nl oh-BLEEKS	compress abdomen and rotate torso
rectus abdominis	REK-*tuhs* ab-DOM-*uh*-nuhs	flexes trunk and lumbar vertebrae
transverses abdominis	trans-VURS-uhs ab-DOM-*uh*-nuhs	supports chest and abdominal organs

continues

Major Voluntary/Skeletal Muscles (continued)

Term	Pronunciation	Function
levator ani (a group of three muscles)	li-VEY-ter EY-*nay*	supports pelvic organs, helps control urine flow, and inhibits defecation
sphincter ani (group of muscles)	SFINGK-ter EY-*nay*	controls the anus
latissimus dorsi	*luh*-TIS-*i*-mus DOHR-seye	pulls the arm back and down
trapezius	*truh*-PEE-zee-*uhs*	moves the scapula
pectoralis major and minor	pek-*tuh*-RAL-is MEY-jer, pek-*tuh*-RAL-is MEYE-ner	moves the humerus (upper arm) and stabilizes the scapula
deltoid	DEL-toid	moves the shoulder
rotator cuff	ROH-tey-ter KUHF	group of muscles that rotates and abducts the shoulder
biceps brachii	BEYE-seps BREY-kee-eye	flexes elbow and rotates forearm
triceps brachii	TREYE-seps BREY-kee-eye	extends the forearm and adducts the shoulder
brachioradialis	BREY-kee-oh-REY-dee-al-*uhs*	flexes forearm
iliopsoas	IL-*ee*-oh-soh-*uhs*	flexes hip and rotates spine
gluteus maximus, gluteus medius, gluteus minimus	GLOO-tee-*uhs* MAK-*suh-muhs* GLOO-tee-*uhs* MEE-dee-*uhs* GLOO-tee-*uhs* MIN-*uh-muhs*	group of muscles that moves the hip
quadriceps femoris	KWOD-*ruh*-seps feh-MOHR-*uhs*	extends the knee
hamstrings	HAM-stringz	group of muscles that extends the hip joint and flexes the leg at the knee joint
gastrocnemius	gas-*truh*-NEE-mee-*uhs*	calf muscle that flexes the foot and the knee

STUDY TIP

Muscles that appear in groups of two often work to produce opposite motions from each other, such as flexion and extension. **Flexion** is the bringing of two body surfaces closer together, such as when you bend your elbow to bring your forearm closer to your upper arm. **Extension** is pulling two body surfaces farther apart, such as when you unbend your elbow by straightening your arm.

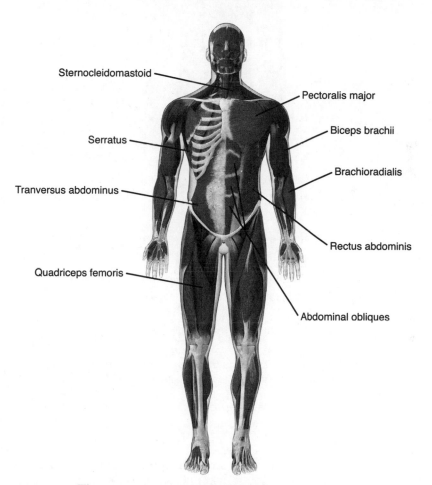

This anterior view shows the major voluntary muscles.
Raj Dashi © Dorling Kindersley

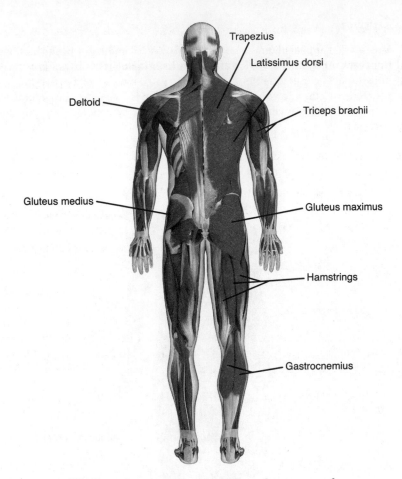

This posterior view shows the major voluntary muscles.
Raj Dashi © Dorling Kindersley

Involuntary Muscles

Involuntary muscle is also known as **smooth muscle**, or **nonstriated muscle**. That is because its fibers are not organized in regular parallel bands, so it does not contain striations. Involuntary muscle is capable of more prolonged contractions than voluntary muscle.

Involuntary muscle is not under conscious control. It operates on autopilot to maintain the necessary functions of life, such as digestion and breathing. Smooth muscle is found in many body organs, including the stomach, intestines, esophagus, bladder, and blood vessels. You will learn more about these organs in later chapters.

Cardiac Muscle

Cardiac (KAHR-dee-ak) muscle is a special type of muscle that is found only in the heart. Cardiac muscle is both involuntary and striated, meaning that its movements are not under conscious control but appear striated under the microscope. Heart muscle is an ultra-endurance athlete. It starts beating in early fetal life and continues for years without a break. Scientists estimate that an average heart beats 100,000 times per day, 35 million times in a year, and more than 2.5 billion times during an average lifetime.

Tendons

Tendons (TEN-*duhnz*) connect muscles to bone. They are made of tough tissue that can withstand the tensions that contracting muscles place on bone. Tendons also play a stabilizing role during muscle movements.

The Least You Need to Know

- Skin is the largest organ system in the body and serves many different functions.
- The skeletal system provides protection and serves as a framework for the body.
- Joints contain cartilage and are where bones come together (articulate).
- Muscle comes in three types: voluntary (skeletal, striated), involuntary (smooth, nonstriated), and cardiac (involuntary, striated).

Lungs, Heart, Blood, and Lymph

In This Chapter

- Upper airways, lungs, and diaphragm
- Heart and great vessels
- Blood functions
- Spleen, lymph nodes, and other lymphatic organs

The heart and lungs are vital for life. One of their primary functions is to make sure the body's tissues get enough oxygen. This process is achieved by means of the circulatory system, which delivers oxygen and nutrients to tissues and transports waste products away from them. Blood and lymph form the fluid part of the circulatory system, so they are also covered in this chapter. They provide the medium in which necessary materials are transported throughout the body.

Because the human body cannot exist for long if the circulatory system stops working, many medical terms are associated with organs and tissues involved in this system. This chapter defines the terminology for the anatomy of this system. Chapter 12 describes the physiology of circulation and breathing, and Chapter 16 introduces terminology for heart and lung disease. Chapter 17 covers blood disorders.

Pulmonary System

The **pulmonary** (PUHL-*muh*-ner-ee) system or **respiratory** (RES-per-*uh*-tawr-ee) system refers to the organs responsible for breathing and oxygenation of the blood. This system consists of the airways, lungs, and muscles used in respiration. The respiratory system is divided into the upper respiratory tract and the lower respiratory tract.

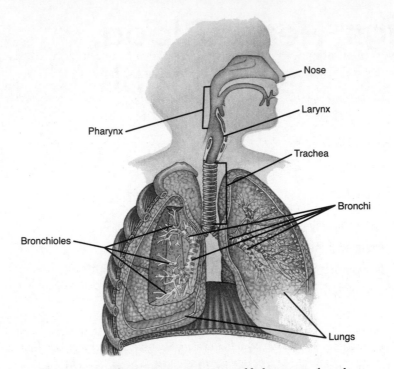

The organs in the respiratory system enable humans to breathe and oxygenate their blood.
Halli Verrinder © Dorling Kindersley

Upper Respiratory Tract

The upper respiratory tract consists of all the respiratory structures found above the chest cavity. These structures include the following:

- The **nose** is a structure used for breathing that is exposed to the external environment.
- The **nasal cavity** is the space above and behind the nose.
- The **paranasal sinuses** (par-*uh*-NEY-*zuhl* SEYE-*nuhs*-ez) are air-filled spaces that surround the nasal cavity.
- The **pharynx** (FAR-ingks) is part of the throat.
- The **larynx** (LAR-ingks) is the voice box, which is also part of the lower respiratory tract.

Lower Respiratory Tract

The lower respiratory tract consists of all the respiratory structures that exist inside the chest cavity. These structures include the following:

- The **trachea** (TREY-kee-*uh*) is the windpipe.
- **Bronchi** (BRONG-keye, BRONG-kee) are large air passageways.
- **Bronchioles** (BRONG-kee-ohlz) are small air passageways.
- **Alveoli** (al-VEE-*uh*-leye) are air sacs in the lungs that are specialized for gas exchange.
- **Lungs** are the main organs of respiration.

STUDY TIP

To remember respiratory structures, trace the pathway of air into the lungs. Air usually enters the body through the nose and then goes down the pharynx into the trachea. The trachea splits into two bronchi. Air flows through the bronchi into the smaller bronchioles. Bronchioles end in alveoli. Oxygen flows from the alveoli into the bloodstream. Waste products, like carbon dioxide, diffuse from the bloodstream to the alveoli, where they retrace the respiratory route and are exhaled through the nose.

Respiratory Word Roots

Root	Pronunciation	Meaning	Example
alveol-	al-VEE-*ohl*	air sac	alveolitis
bronch-	BRONGK	large air passageway, bronchus	bronchitis
bronchiol-	BRONGK-ee-ohl	small air passageway, bronchiole	bronchiolitis
laryng-	*luh*-RINJ	larynx	laryngitis
nas-	nas	nose	nasopharynx
pharyng-	*fuh*-RINJ	pharynx	pharyngitis
phren-	fren	diaphragm	phrenic nerve
pneumon-	NOO-*muhn*, NOO-*mohn*	lung	pneumonia
pulmon-	PUHL-*muhn*	lung	pulmonology
rhin-	reyen	nose	rhinitis
trach-	treyk	trachea	tracheitis

Muscles of Respiration

Several muscles help expand and contract the rib cage, which helps inflate and deflate the lungs:

- The **diaphragm** (DEYE-*uh*-fram) helps expand the rib cage, aids in respiration, and separates the chest from the abdominal cavity.
- The **intercostals** (in-ter-KOS-tlz) move the chest wall in respiration.
- The **sternocleidomastoid** (ster-*noh*-cley-*doh*-MAS-toyd) tilts and rotates the head, flexes the neck, and raises the sternum during breathing.
- The **scalene** (skey-LEEN) raises the first and second ribs and flexes the neck.

In normal health, muscles are not required to deflate the lungs during **exhalation** (breathing out). This is because the lungs are elastic and recoil when muscles are no longer acting on the ribcage to expand it. So most of the muscles involved in breathing are used only for **inhalation** (breathing in). Some diseases, like emphysema, damage the lungs, interfering with their elastic recoil and making exhalation difficult. In such cases, the abdominal and intercostal muscles come into play.

> **WORDS OF WARNING**
>
> Another word for inhalation is inspiration. Likewise, the equivalent word for exhalation is expiration. Be careful when using this last one, though, since expiration can also mean to die, or to take your last breath. The difference is usually clarified by the context in which it is used.

Cardiovascular System

The **cardiovascular** (kahr-dee-oh-VAS-*kyuh*-ler) **system** is also known as the **circulatory system** because it circulates the blood throughout the body. Basically, the circulatory system is the way nutrients and other necessary substances are transported throughout the body for use in processes that keep the body alive. The circulatory system also transports the by-products of these processes out of the body for disposal, which prevents build-up of waste products that could harm the body.

The circulatory system carries blood gases (like oxygen and carbon dioxide), hormones, proteins that clot the blood (or **clotting factors**), sugars, and immune cells.

It also helps to maintain body temperature and blood pH (PEE-EYCH), which is the amount of acid versus base the blood contains (its acidity versus alkalinity).

Blood follows a particular route when it circulates throughout the body. There are three main loops through which blood flows in the circulatory system. These are called **pulmonary** (PUHL-*muh*-ner-ee) **circulation**, **systemic** (si-STEM-ik) **circulation**, and **cardiac** (KAHR-dee-ak) **circulation**.

Pulmonary Circulation

Pulmonary circulation refers to the circulation of blood through the blood vessels in the lungs. The lungs are intimately connected to the heart through several large blood vessels. For this reason, this loop is also called the **cardiopulmonary** (kahr-dee-oh-PUHL-*muh*-ner-ee) **system**. Blood is **oxygenated** (OK-si-*juh*-neyt-ed), which means that it picks up oxygen, in the lungs. This blood then flows through the **pulmonary vein** (PUHL-*muh*-ner-ee VEYN) to the heart. Inside the heart, the blood flows through the left **atrium** (EY-tree-*uhm*), through the left **ventricle** (VEN-tri-*kuhl*), and then out the **aorta** (ey-AWR-t*uh*) to the rest of the body.

WORD ORIGINS

In ancient Rome, an atrium was the central part of the house. It was open to the sky and was used for collecting rain water. The atria of the heart are similar. They are open at the top, where blood flows in through the inferior and superior vena cavae and the pulmonary veins. The atria of the heart "collect" blood before the heart pumps to force it through the ventricles and out the aorta to be distributed to the rest of the body.

Deoxygenated blood from the body returns to the heart through the **superior vena cava** and **inferior vena cava**. The blood then flows through the right atrium into the right ventricle. From there blood flows through the pulmonary arteries back to the lungs, where it picks up more oxygen to start the process all over again.

DID YOU KNOW?

Oxygenated blood appears bright red; deoxygenated blood has a bluish color. For this reason, these are the standard colors used to indicate arteries (red) and veins (blue) in colored diagrams.

Systemic Circulation

Systemic circulation consists of the circulatory system outside the lungs and the heart. Blood leaves the left ventricle through the aorta and flows through progressively smaller channels until it reaches the capillaries, where gas, nutrient, and waste transport occurs. The forceful contraction of the meaty left ventricle provides almost all of the power necessary to push the blood through the body. Blood then returns via small veins that combine and become progressively larger until they reach the heart.

The major terms associated with the systemic circulation are as follows:

- An **artery** (AHR-*tuh*-ree) is a large blood vessel that carries oxygenated blood.
- An **arteriole** (ahr-TEER-ee-ohl) is a small blood vessel that carries oxygenated blood.
- A **capillary** (KAP-*uh*-ler-ee) is the smallest type of blood vessel; capillaries are grouped into beds and carry both oxygenated and deoxygenated blood.
- A **venule** (VEN-yool) is a small blood vessel that carries deoxygenated blood.
- A **vein** (VEYN) is a large blood vessel that carries deoxygenated blood.
- **Portal veins** (PAWR-tl VEYNZ) are a series of capillary beds that are connected by a vein. They are found in the liver and near the pituitary gland.

WORDS OF WARNING

The terms **vein** and **artery** are precise. Arteries carry oxygenated blood *toward* tissues. Veins carry deoxygenated blood *away* from tissues. One way to remember this distinction is through pronunciation: a vEYn flows awEY from an organ. Spelling helps with the other part: *ar*teries flow to*war*d an organ. There are two exceptions to this rule. The first is the pulmonary vein, which carries oxygenated blood. It is called a vein because blood in it flows *away* from the lungs. The other exception is the pulmonary artery, which carries deoxygenated blood. It is called an artery because blood in it flows *toward* the lungs.

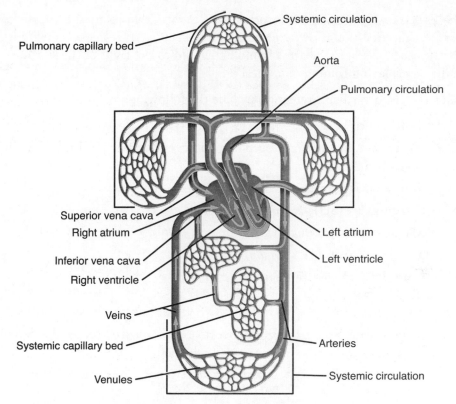

Here is the path blood takes through the systemic and pulmonary circulation systems.
© Dorling Kindersley

Cardiac Circulation

The heart has its own circulation, which is called cardiac circulation. Another term is **coronary** (KAWR-*uh*-ner-ee) circulation. *Coronary* means crown, and that's basically what most of these blood vessels do: they encircle and form a crown around the heart. Thinking of the term *coronation* or the *crowning* of a monarch helps this term make sense. Cardiac circulation caters only to the heart, delivering oxygen to the heart muscle and carrying away its waste products.

The heart is normally found under and to the left of the sternum. During fetal development, the chest and abdominal organs sometimes form on the opposite side of the body than where they are normally located. This condition is called **situs inversus**

(SEYE-*tuhs in-VURS-uhs*) or "inverted side." A term that refers specifically to the heart in this condition is **dextrocardia** (DEK-stroh KAHR-dee-*uh*), or right-sided heart. In such cases, the heart is found under and to the right of the sternum, which can be a perplexing finding on a chest x-ray.

Major vessels in cardiac circulation include the following:

- Left and right coronary arteries
- Posterior and anterior descending/**interventricular** (in-TUR ven-TRIK-*yuh*-ler) arteries
- Left and right marginal arteries
- **Circumflex** (SUR-*kuhm*-fleks) artery
- Great cardiac (coronary) vein
- Coronary **sinus** (SEYE-*nuhs*)
- Anterior and posterior cardiac veins
- Small cardiac veins

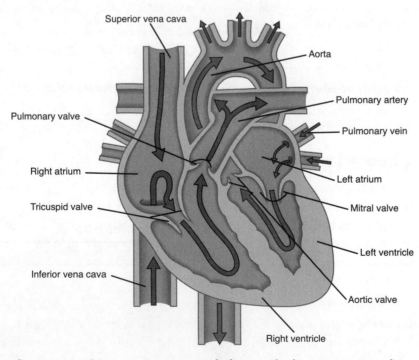

Coronary circulation carries oxygen to the heart and takes away waste products.
© Dorling Kindersley

DID YOU KNOW?

Coronary arteries sometimes become diseased and atherosclerotic. **Atherosclerosis** (ath-*uh*-roh-*skluh*-ROH-sis) is the buildup of hard, fatty material inside the arteries. When this happens, the arteries narrow and restrict blood from flowing easily. As a result, the heart muscle starts to suffer from lack of oxygen. When the arteries narrow too much or completely obstruct blood flow, a heart attack can happen. To prevent this, surgeons sometimes perform a **coronary artery bypass graft** (abbreviated as CABG, pronounced like *cabbage*). They take a blood vessel from another part of the body and use it to create another passageway through which blood can flow freely, bypassing the diseased artery so that oxygen can reach the heart muscle.

Other Major Blood Vessels

The following are major blood vessels in the body:

- The **carotid** (k*uh*-ROT-id) **artery** supplies the head and neck.
- The **jugular** (JUHG-*yuh*-ler) **vein** drains the head and neck.
- The **subclavian** (suhb-KLEY-vee-*uhn*) **artery** supplies the arms; the **subclavian vein** drains them.
- The largest artery in the body, the **abdominal aorta** (ey-OR-*tuh*) supplies most of the abdomen and lower half of the body.
- The **renal** (REEN-l) **artery** supplies the kidneys; the **renal vein** drains them.
- The **femoral** (FEM-er-*uhl*) **artery** supplies the legs; the **femoral vein** drains them.
- The **common iliac** (IL-ee-ak) **artery** supplies the legs and pelvic organs; the **common iliac vein** drains them.

Word Roots Related to Cardiovascular Circulation

Word Root	Pronunciation	Meaning
angi-	AN-jee	vessel
phleb-	FLUHB	vein
thromb-	THROMB	clot
valvul-	VALV-yool	valve
vasc-	VASC	vessel

Blood System

Blood serves many functions in the body. It delivers necessary nutrients and chemicals to the body's organs and carries waste products away from them. Blood protects the body by carrying immune cells, such as white blood cells and antibodies. These cells help fight infections and recognize foreign invaders; they also play a role in allergies. Blood also clots (solidifies) to seal off wounds and prevent people from bleeding to death. Blood has a homeostatic role as well. It helps maintain the body's optimal pH and regulate body temperature. Blood also contains hormones, which act as messengers between different organs and organ systems.

Blood consists of red blood cells, white blood cells, platelets, plasma, albumin, and other immune cells. Blood is created in bone marrow in a process called **hematopoiesis** (hi-mat-*uh*-poh-EE-*suhs*, hi-mat-*uh*-POH-uh-*suhs*). Production of red blood cells is called **erythropoiesis** (ih-RITH-*ruh*-poh-EE-*suhs*, ih-RITH-ruh-POH-*uh*-*suhs*). Production of white blood cells and platelets is called **myelopoiesis** (MEYE-*uhl-uh*-poh-EE-*suhs*, MEYE-*uhl-uh*-POH-uh-*suhs*).

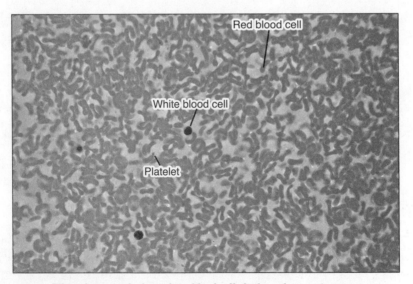

This photograph shows how blood cells look under a microscope.
M.I. Walker © Dorling Kindersley

Blood Terms and Word Parts

Term or Word Part	Pronunciation	Meaning
eryth-	ih-RITH-	red
-cyte	-seyet	cell
erythrocyte	ih-RITH-*ruh*-seyet	red blood cell that carries oxygen
hemat-, hem-	hi-MAT-, HEEM-	blood
hemoglobin	HEE-*muh*-gloh-bin	a chemical compound in red blood cells that enables them to carry oxygen
immunoglobulin	im-*yuh*-noh-GLOB-*yuh*-lin	antibody
platelet (thrombocyte)	PLEYT-lit (THROM-*buh*-seyet)	blood cell that functions in blood clotting
plasma	PLAZ-*muh*	liquid part of blood, which includes proteins, electrolytes, hormones, nutrients, and waste
albumin	al-BYOO-*muhn*	blood proteins
serum	SEER-*uhm*	liquid part of the blood from which the proteins have been removed
-crasia	-KREY-*zhuh*, -ZHEE-*uh*	mixture, blending; example: plasma cell dyscrasia
isch-	ISK-	to hold back, as in ischemia (a holding back of blood that causes tissues to die from lack of oxygen)

Lymphatic System

The **lymphatic** (lim-FAT-ik) system is often considered part of the circulatory system. This is because the lymphatic system returns extra **lymph** (LIMF) to the blood vessels for recycling, which replaces the fluid lost in the blood during normal circulation.

Lymph is basically made up of extra blood plasma that returns to the lymphatic system when it is no longer needed in the **interstitial** (*in-ter-STISH-uhl*) **fluid**. Interstitial fluid surrounds cells, delivering nutrients to the tissues and getting rid of waste products. Blood plasma is the liquid part of the blood. It is straw-colored (yellowish) in appearance and contains sugars, proteins, hormones, clotting factors, carbon dioxide, and other elements that are essential for life, like sodium and calcium. Lymph also transports fats from the digestive system.

The lymphatic system also plays a role in the immune system, and is a major route by which cancer **metastasizes** (*muh*-TAS-*tuh*-seyez-ez), or spreads, throughout the body.

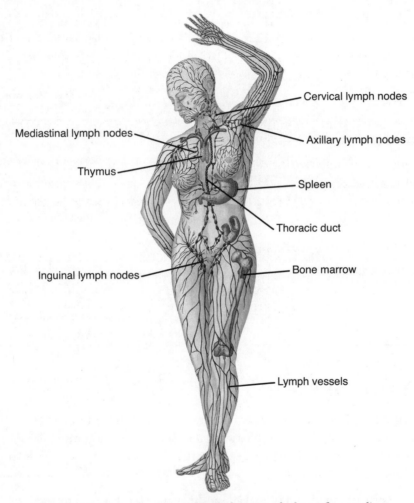

The lymphatic system returns blood plasma to the heart for recycling.
Joanna Cameron © Dorling Kindersley

The major organs in the lymphatic system are found throughout the body. **Lymph nodes** (LIMF NOHDS) are a collections of lymph tissue through which lymph passes when returning to the blood; they also function in the immune system. The **spleen** is like a large lymph node and helps create and store red blood cells; the spleen also helps with immunity.

Located near the breastbone, the **thymus** (THEYE-*muhs*) is an organ in which certain white blood cells develop into their mature forms. Located inside bone, **bone marrow** (BOHN MAR-oh) is where red and white blood cells are made.

Tonsils (TON-*suhlz*) contain lymphoid follicles and are immune tissue located at the back of the mouth. **Adenoids** (AD-n-oidz) also contain lymphoid follicles and are immune tissue located at the back of the nose.

Peyer patches (PEYE-er PACH-*ez*) are special collections of lymph tissue located in the small intestine. They provide extra protection against harmful organisms that may have entered the body through ingestion.

Right and left **thoracic ducts** (thaw-RAS-ik, thoh-RAS-ik DUHKTZ) are the largest lymphatic vessels, and they collect most of the lymph. They are located on either side of the vertebrae and run from the lumbar vertebrae to the bottom of the neck.

Lymphatic System Terms and Word Parts

Term or Word Part	Pronunciation	Meaning
duct	DUHKT	tube or canal
follicle	FOL-i-*kuhl*	sac or small collection of tissue
node	NOHD	gland or collection of tissue
nodule	NOJ-ool	small collection of tissue
lymphaden-	limf-AD-*uhn*	lymph node
lymph-	LIMF	lymph
lymphang-	limf-ANJ	lymph vessel
splen-	SPLEN	spleen
thym-	THEYEM	thymus

The Least You Need to Know

- The pulmonary system consists of the upper and lower respiratory tracts and functions to oxygenate the blood and remove waste products from the body.
- The cardiovascular system delivers nutrients to the body and gets rid of waste products.
- The cardiovascular system consists of: pulmonary circulation, systemic circulation, cardiac circulation, and related organs.
- Blood flows throughout the body, delivers nutrients and elements necessary for life, provides protection, and helps maintain body temperature.
- The lymphatic system helps recycle extra fluid found in the blood and functions in the immune system.

The Digestive System

In This Chapter

- Functions of the alimentary canal
- Upper gastrointestinal organs from the mouth to the duodenum
- Lower gastrointestinal organs from the jejunum to the anus
- The four layers of the gastrointestinal tract
- Digestive organs outside the GI tract

The digestive system is made up of various organs that are all interconnected and serve an overarching purpose: to keep the body well nourished and healthy. If the digestive system is confronted with challenges, such as digesting a double hot fudge sundae, it goes into overdrive. Normally it steps up to the task of digesting whatever people throw at it. It also functions quite well in eliminating substances that could cause illness or injury.

The digestive system is like a sports team, with each team member providing one or several functions and all members being dedicated to achieving the major goal of digesting the foods that enter through the mouth. Chapter 13 describes more about how these team members support metabolism and elimination. Before learning about the physiology of digestion, it helps to learn the names and roles of each team member in the process.

This chapter provides an overview of the anatomy of the gastrointestinal system. It explains how to identify, pronounce, and spell terms for the major organs of the digestive system. This chapter also describes terms for the cell layers that make up the digestive system. Learning the basic terminology for normal digestive anatomy helps develop the groundwork for learning clinical terms for digestive disorders and their treatment in Chapter 16 and Part 5.

The Alimentary Canal

Another term for the gastrointestinal tract is **alimentary canal** (al-*uh*-MEN-*tuh*-ree *kuh*-NAL). *Alimentary* comes from the Latin word *alimentum*, which means nutrient. A canal is a structure through which things (like water and digestive products) flow.

The alimentary canal is basically a nutrient highway. It is open to the outside world on both ends, starting with the mouth and ending with the **anus** (EY-*nuhs*). The alimentary canal forms a hollow space inside the body, which is called a **lumen** (LOO-*muhn*). All along its path everything found inside the lumen of the alimentary canal is considered outside the body. Basically, the alimentary canal can be thought of as a conduit through which matter passes without ever entering the interior of the body. Food and other substances are broken down inside the alimentary canal and absorbed through the layers of the alimentary canal into the body's interior.

The alimentary canal is sealed. Unless the seal is broken, such as by injury or infection, the alimentary canal protects the body from whatever is ingested—food, gum, pennies, bacteria, whatever. In combination with other organs in the digestive system, cells that line the alimentary canal also serve an immune function and make hormones for the body. Chapter 10 covers hormones in more detail, and Chapter 15 describes the immune system.

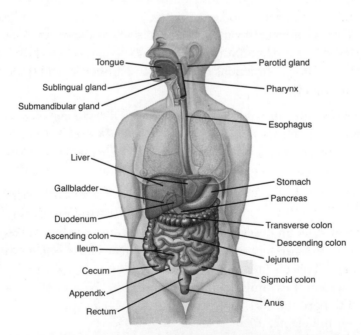

The alimentary canal starts with the mouth and ends with the anus.
Tony Graham © Dorling Kindersley

Upper Gastrointestinal Tract

When food is placed in the mouth, it embarks on quite a journey. It enters the **upper gastrointestinal tract** (UHP-er gas-troh-in-TES-*tuh*-nl trakt). This tract starts at the mouth and ends at the **duodenum** (doo-*uh*-DEE-*nuhm* or doo-OD-n-*uhm*), which is the first section of the small intestine.

Healthcare professionals use the following word roots to refer to the different parts of the upper gastrointestinal tract:

- Mouth, Oral Cavity: or-, oro-; stomat-, stomato-
- Pharynx: pharyng-, pharyngo-
- Esophagus: esophag-, esophago-
- Stomach: gastr-, gastro-
- Duodenum: duoden-, duodeno-

WORD ORIGINS

Gastro means stomach. *Intestinal* refers to the intestines. So *gastrointestinal* means "stomach and intestines." Healthcare professionals usually shorten *gastrointestinal* to *GI*. They often use *GI* to refer to all parts of the gastrointestinal system, from the mouth to the anus, and all associated organs.

The oral cavity (mouth cavity) contains the tongue, teeth, and gums. The oral cavity is bounded in the front by the lips, in the back by the **pharynx** (FAR-*ingks*), on the top and bottom by the palates (floor and roof of the mouth), and on the sides by the cheeks.

Most foods need to be chewed before swallowing. Chewing is essential for digestion. It breaks down food and mixes it with saliva, which begins the digestive process. The tongue also aids in the process. It helps mix the food with saliva, and helps transfer food to the back of the mouth for swallowing.

Food passes out of the oral cavity through the pharynx, which is part of the respiratory and digestive systems. The pharynx seals off the windpipe during swallowing so that food doesn't back up into the nose or go down into the lungs. People choke when the pharynx isn't sealed while they swallow, and some of the food enters the respiratory system.

WORDS OF WARNING

Don't confuse **pharynx**, which is part of the digestive and respiratory systems, with **larynx**, which is the voice box (see Chapter 6). Here is a saying to help you keep them straight: the *larynx* lets you *laugh loudly*, but it's not *phunny* when the *pharynx* mal*ph*unctions.

After the pharynx, food travels into the **esophagus** (ih-SOF-*uh-guhs*), which is a muscular tube that contracts rhythmically. With the help of gravity, the muscular contractions of the esophagus push food where it needs to go. The upper part of the esophagus has nerve endings that can feel pain when swallowing items that are too hot, too cold, too sharp, or too big. This response serves a protective function because it causes harmful materials to be coughed up before they go too far in the digestive system.

From the esophagus, food enters the **stomach** (STUHM-*uhk*). This very muscular organ churns food into bits, which is an essential process for tough or fibrous foods like meat or celery. The stomach also mixes the food with various digestive enzymes. Food stays in the stomach until it's ready to move onto the next stage of digestion. Food can take 6 to 8 hours to pass through the stomach. If the food is difficult to digest, like fatty steak, it may hang around for even longer.

From the stomach, food passes through the **pylorus** (pi-LOHR-*uhs*), which is a thick, muscular valve that lies where the stomach meets the duodenum. The pylorus controls the amount and speed of food that is dumped from the stomach. The **duodenum** is the first part of the small intestine. Most of the enzymes needed for digestion are mixed with food in the duodenum. The duodenum also provides important hormones that help regulate digestion.

Lower Gastrointestinal Tract

From the upper gastrointestinal tract, food travels into the lower gastrointestinal tract. Experts disagree about exactly where the upper gastrointestinal tract ends and the lower gastrointestinal tract begins. The duodenum is made up of four parts, and sometimes it can be hard to tell where one part ends and the next part begins. The dilemma has to do with how the organs form during fetal development. The upper gastrointestinal tract forms differently from the lower gastrointestinal tract. The upper gastrointestinal tract also has a different blood supply from the lower one. Some experts use these criteria—how the upper and lower gastrointestinal tracts form and which blood vessels serve them—to separate the two.

No matter how you define upper and lower, though, in order for digestion to continue, food needs to travel from the upper to the lower gastrointestinal tract. Most healthcare professionals consider the lower gastrointestinal tract to start after the duodenum.

Healthcare professionals use the following word roots to refer to the different parts of the lower gastrointestinal tract:

- Jejunum: jejun-, jejuno-
- Ileum: ile-, ileo-
- Cecum: ceco-, cecal-
- Colon: col-, colo-
- Sigmoid colon: sigmoid-, sigmoido-
- Rectum: rect-, recto-; proct-, procto-
- Anus: an-, ano-; proct-, procto-

The **jejunum** (ji-JOO-*nuhm*) is the second part of the small intestine. Here, absorption of the nutrients from food really takes off. The jejunum absorbs carbohydrates, proteins, fats, sugars, vitamins, minerals, and other important things like salt.

Food next enters the third and final part of the small intestine, the **ileum** (IL-ee-*uhm*). It absorbs whatever nutrients have not been absorbed in the previous parts of the digestive system. The ileum also absorbs vitamin B_{12}, which is very important to the nervous system and for the proper formation of blood cells. The ileum also adds additional digestive enzymes. The body is never wasteful, so the ileum starts the process of recycling digestive products that can be used for digesting the next meal.

From the ileum, food travels into the **large intestine** (in-TES-tin). Food reaches the large intestine through the **cecum** (SEE-*kuhm*), which means "blind pouch" in Latin because that's exactly what it looked like to scientists centuries ago when it was first discovered. But don't let the name fool you. The cecum isn't a dead end at all (which is good news, or our species would have become extinct eons ago). The cecum connects to the large intestine through the **cecocolic** (SEE-*ko*-KOL-*ik*) **junction**.

From the cecum, food begins traversing the large intestine, where water resorption takes place. Food passes up the **ascending colon** (KOH-*luhn*), across the **transverse colon**, down the **descending colon**, and through the **sigmoid colon**. Finally, food exits the gastrointestinal system through the **rectum** (REK-*tuhm*) and **anus** (EY-*nuhs*), where food looks much less appetizing than when it began its trip in the mouth.

Layers of the Gastrointestinal Tract

Viewing the GI tract through the lens of a microscope reveals that it is composed of four layers. These layers are important for digesting food. They form a seal around the lumen through which food travels.

The layers of the gastrointestinal tract lie one on top of the other. Each layer can be considered to be encircling and hugging the lumen. These layers keep food, foreign objects, and many bacteria that enter from outside the body via the mouth inside the lumen of the gastrointestinal tract, where they can do the least harm. Certain cells in these layers also serve an immune function, make products that are important for digestion, and produce hormones.

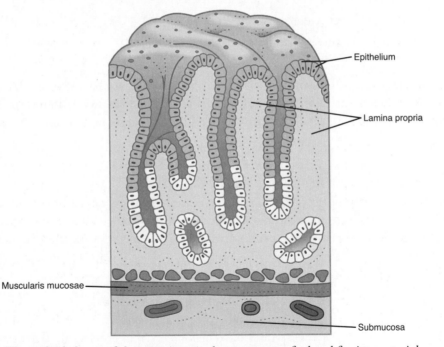

The multiple layers of the gastrointestinal tract separate food and foreign materials from the rest of the body.
Debbie Maizels © Dorling Kindersley

Mucosa

Mucosa (myoo-KOH-*suh*) refers to the layer of the gastrointestinal tract that lies closest to the lumen. The mucosa is specialized for different functions in different parts of the gastrointestinal tract. In the small intestine, the mucosa has **villi** (VIL-eye), which means fingers. Villi look just like the name suggests. They are tiny fingerlike structures that project from the mucosa into the lumen. They help increase the amount of surface area available for absorption.

The mucosa has three layers:

- **Epithelium** (ep-*uh*-THEE-lee-*uhm*)
- **Lamina propria** (LAM-*uh-nuh* PROH-*pree-uh*)
- **Muscularis mucosae** (mus-*kyoo*-LAYR-*is* myoo-KOH-*see*)

> **WORD ORIGINS**
>
> **Histology** comes from the Greek word *histo-*, which means tissue, and *-ology*, which means study. So *histology* means "the study of tissues." It explores how cells are organized and function together to form tissues that, in turn, are organized into body systems. Histology can be thought of as **microscopic anatomy** because it deals with structures that cannot be seen with the naked eye. The opposite of this is **macroscopic anatomy** or **gross anatomy**. In popular slang, *gross* usually means disgusting. But the medical term *gross* means big or whole. So gross anatomy is the study of the human body that is visible to the naked eye.

Submucosa

Submucosa (suhb-myoo-KOH-s*uh*) is the next layer of the gastrointestinal tract, and lies second closest to the lumen. Remember from Chapter 2 that *sub-* means below, so one way to remember the term *submucosa* is that it is the layer of the gastrointestinal tract that lies just below the mucosa. The submucosa consists of connective tissue, and that's basically its main function: it connects the mucosa to the other layers of the gastrointestinal tract. The submucosa also helps support the other gastrointestinal layers. It contains blood vessels, parts of the lymph system, and nerves, all of which help keep the other layers alive and healthy.

Muscularis Externa

The **muscularis externa** (mus-*kyoo*-LAYR-*is* EK-sturn-*uh)* comes next. It is made up of smooth muscle. Smooth muscle is also known as involuntary muscle because it is not under conscious control. It just works on autopilot. Think of how distracting it would be if every time you ate a meal you would have to remind your gastrointestinal tract to contract and push the food through. Smooth muscle allows you to truly rest and digest.

The thickness of the muscularis externa varies throughout the gastrointestinal tract. The muscularis externa is thinner in the small intestine and becomes thicker in the large intestine where digested matter becomes more solid, requiring more force to move it along. The muscularis externa also contains nerves called **Auerbach plexus** (OU-er-bahk PLEK-*suhs*). This network of nerves controls **peristalsis** (per-*uh*-STAWL-sis), which is the rhythmic contraction of the muscles of the gastrointestinal tract. Peristalsis pushes food along its path.

Adventitia and Serosa

The **adventitia** (ad-ven-TISH-*uh*) and **serosa** (si-ROH-s*uh*) form the fourth and last layer of the gastrointestinal tract. This layer is the part that lies closest to the interior of the body and farthest from the lumen. Both serosa and adventitia are connective tissue. The name used for this GI layer depends on where in the gastrointestinal tract you find it. Serosa is found on parts of the GI tract that are intraperitoneal; adventitia is found on parts of the GI tract that are retroperitoneal.

Intraperitoneal (in-*truh*-per-i-tn-EE-*uhl*) means "lying within the space of the abdominal cavity." Intraperitoneal parts of the gastrointestinal tract are covered with serosa and have a **mesentery** (MEZ-*uhn*-ter-ee). A mesentery is a tissue that connects one organ to another, but does not fix them in a set position. Intraperitoneal organs include the stomach, the first part of the duodenum, the jejunum, the ileum, the cecum, the appendix, the transverse colon, the sigmoid colon, and rectum.

Intraperitoneal organs are not fixed in place and sometimes move slightly in position, bringing their mesentery with them. When this happens, the mesentery can get looped around the organ, cutting off blood supply to it. This occurrence is termed **volvulus** (VOL-*vyuh-luhs*), and it is a surgical emergency. An organ that has its blood supply cut off for too long begins to die. People with this condition develop sudden, sharp abdominal pain. Of course, this type of pain could indicate other problems, too. Sometimes the only way to know what's going on is to perform an exploratory **laparotomy** (lap-*uh*-ROT-*uh*-mee). This procedure involves surgically opening the abdomen and searching for the cause of the problem.

Retroperitoneal (re-*troh*-per-i-tn-EE-*uhl*) means "lying behind the space of the abdominal cavity." Retroperitoneal parts of the gastrointestinal tract are covered with adventitia. Retroperitoneal organs cannot move freely and are fixed in place to the posterior abdominal wall. Retroperitoneal organs include parts of the oral cavity, the esophagus, the last part of the duodenum, the pylorus, the ascending colon, the descending colon, and the anus.

Accessory Organs of Digestion

The accessory organs of digestion produce enzymes and chemicals that help break down food so that it can be absorbed and properly nourish the body or be stored as fat. The accessory organs of digestion lie outside of the gastrointestinal tract. Some connect to it by **ducts** (duhkts), which are small tubes that bring the enzymes to the lumen where they can go to work.

Healthcare professionals use the following word roots to refer to the different accessory digestive organs:

- Teeth: dental-
- Tongue: lingual-
- Salivary glands: sialo-
- Liver: hepat-, hepato-
- Pancreas: pancreat-, pancreato-
- Gallbladder: cholecyst-, cholecysto-
- Appendix: append-, appendo-

The teeth break up food into bits that are small enough to be swallowed. The tongue helps mix the food with saliva and brings the food to the back of the mouth for swallowing.

Salivary (SAL-*uh*-ver-ee) **glands** produce saliva and are scattered around the oral cavity. Salivary glands have different names depending on where in the oral cavity they are located. Recall that *sub-* means below, and *-lingual* means tongue, so **sublingual** (suhb-LING-gw*uh*-l) **glands** are salivary glands that lie beneath the tongue. Likewise, **submandibular** (suhb-man-DIB-y*uh*-ler) **glands** are salivary glands that are found in the floor of the mouth, below the mandible. **Submaxillary** (suhb-MAK-*suh*-ler-ee) **glands** are salivary glands found on the lower jaw, below the maxilla. **Parotid** (*puh*-ROT-id) **glands** are salivary glands found on the upper jaw.

The **liver** (LIV-er) lies just under the right side of the diaphragm. It is made up of four lobes, each of which receives a rich blood supply. The liver is connected to the gallbladder, which in turn connects to the small intestine.

DID YOU KNOW?

Living donors who donate part of their livers to someone in need of a liver transplant can regrow the part of the liver that they donate. Regrowth is sometimes only partial, and liver donation is a major operation that requires recuperation. Organ donation is a personal and sometimes difficult decision, but it can also save a life.

The **pancreas** (PAN-kree-*uhs*) is located in the **hypogastrium** (heye-p*uh*-GAS-tree-*uhm*), an area of the body found below the stomach. This area usually corresponds to the belly button and below. The pancreas has four parts: the head, the neck, the body, and the tail. The pancreas is significant because it makes digestive enzymes as well as hormones. A duct carries these enzymes from the pancreas into the duodenum.

The **gallbladder** (GAWL-blad-er) is found next to the liver. The gallbladder is a round sac that stores **bile** (beyel) and has ducts that connect to both the liver, from which it receives bile, and to the duodenum, where the bile drains. The gallbladder also helps regulate secretion of bile. True to its ancient connection to the green-eyed monster of jealousy and anger, bile is green in color. But it doesn't function in emotion. Instead, it helps digest the fat in ingested food.

The **appendix** (*uh*-PEN-diks) is attached to the cecum in the lower right quadrant of the abdomen. Its usual position can be found by locating **McBurney point**. Surgeons coined this term for a common method of figuring out the most likely place of the appendix so that they know where to make their incision when performing an **appendectomy** (ap-uhn-*dek*-tuh-MEE). McBurney point is located midway on the diagonal line between the belly button and the right hip bone. However, the appendix is not always found exactly at McBurney point. Because the cecum is not fixed to the body wall, it has a certain degree of mobility, and it takes the appendix with it.

In rare cases of **situs inversus** (SEYE-*tuhs* in-VER-*suhs*), where the body organs form on the opposite side from where they're normally found, the appendix can be located on the left side of the abdomen. In addition, the abdomen has many nerves that sometimes cause the pain from an inflamed appendix, called **appendicitis**, to feel more diffuse or occur anywhere in the lower abdomen. So even though appendicitis is a common illness, diagnosing it can still be tricky!

The appendix is sometimes called the **vermiform appendix**. *Vermi* means worms in Latin, and that's exactly what the appendix looks like: a wiggly little worm that sometimes likes to act up when it gets infected.

The Least You Need to Know

- The digestive system is composed of the upper and lower gastrointestinal tracts and the accessory organs of digestion.
- The upper gastrointestinal tract starts in the outside world at the mouth and ends with the duodenum.
- The lower gastrointestinal tract starts at the jejunum and ends back in the outside world at the anus.
- The gastrointestinal tract has four layers that support digestion and help with hormonal, immunological, and homeostatic regulation. These layers are also protective.
- Digestion requires lots of chemicals and enzymes, which are provided by the upper gastrointestinal tract and the accessory organs of digestion.

Urinary, Reproductive, and Endocrine Systems

In This Chapter

- Organs that create and eliminate urine
- Female organs that produce sex characteristics and eggs
- Male organs that create sex characteristics and sperm
- Glands, organs, and other structures that secrete hormones

The urinary, reproductive, and endocrine systems all play important roles in keeping the body in balance. The endocrine system is primarily responsible for the secretion of hormones, which are chemical messengers that help regulate the body. The urinary and reproductive systems also secrete hormones that play roles in regulatory processes.

In addition, the urinary system helps the body rid itself of potentially dangerous wastes. The female and male reproductive systems are responsible for the creation of sexual characteristics. These systems also promote development of eggs and sperm, whose union becomes capable of creating another human being during pregnancy and gestation.

Reproduction consists of several processes and stages; the terms related to these processes and stages will be covered in Chapter 14. Chapter 10 introduces and explains the names and functions of the many different hormones in the human body.

Kidneys, Ureters, Bladder, and Urethra

The **urinary** (YOOR-*uh*-ner-ee) **system** is also called the **renal** (REEN-l) **system**. As the name suggests, this system deals mainly with generating and eliminating urine.

This is one of the main ways the body gets rid of potentially dangerous wastes left over from cellular metabolism in other organs.

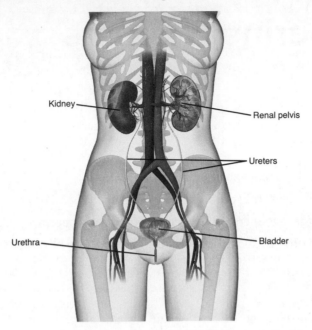

The organs in the urinary system help the body eliminate liquid waste.
Raj Dashi © Dorling Kindersley

Kidneys and Ureters

The kidneys are two bean-shaped organs that lie **retroperitoneally** (RE-troh-per-i-tn-EE-*uhl*-ee) behind the digestive organs in the upper abdomen. Waste products are filtered out of the blood in the kidneys. They also form **urine**, the fluid medium in which these waste products are excreted. The kidneys are major players in maintaining homeostasis, which is the proper balance of water and other important elements in the body. During the formation of urine, the kidneys reabsorb water, sugars, and proteins. They also help maintain the proper chemical (acid–base) balance in the blood. The kidneys also produce several hormones that play important roles in blood pressure control, red blood cell and platelet production, and calcium balance.

A cushion of fat surrounds the kidneys. Beneath the fat lies the **renal capsule** (KAP-*suhl*), the kidney's leathery, protective covering. Within the renal capsule is the functioning part of the kidney, which is called the **renal parenchyma** (*puh*-RENG-*kuh-muh*). The parenchyma consists of the **outer renal cortex** (KOHR-teks) and the **inner renal medulla** (*muh*-DUHL-*uh*). The outer renal cortex filters blood and makes hormones that affect red blood cell production. The inner renal medulla handles salt and water homeostasis.

The **renal pelvis** funnels urine from the kidney into the ureters. The **ureters** (yoo-REE-terz, YOOR-uh-terz) are muscular tubes—one for each kidney—that lead from the kidneys and carry urine away from them. The ureters' smooth muscle contracts and relaxes to help propel urine along its course. After exiting the kidneys, the ureters run downward along either side of the posterior abdominal cavity toward the pelvis.

> **DID YOU KNOW?**
>
> Kidney stones, or **renal calculi** (KAL-ky*uh-leye*), are crystals that form from minerals in the diet. Sometimes a kidney stone breaks free from the kidney and moves along the urinary tract. Many of these stones are small and pass out of the body unnoticed. If the stone is big enough, it can get caught along the way and cause pain, which is known as **renal colic** (KOL-ik). The most common area where this pain occurs is the side of lower back between the ribs and pelvis, also known as flank pain. Pain can also occur in the lower abdomen, continuing down into the groin area.

Bladder and Urethra

The ureters lead to the **bladder** (BLAD-er), which is a hollow, round organ in the pelvis. The bladder's muscular wall allows it to expel urine during urination, or **micturition** (MIK-*chuhr*-i-*shuhn*). The bladder's wall is very elastic, which means that it can stretch quite a lot to accommodate and collect urine. The average bladder can hold 350 to 550 milliliters of urine, although the urge to urinate usually occurs when the volume reaches 200 milliliters.

The **urethra** (yoo-REE-*thruh*) is a single tube that leads from the bladder to the external opening in the genitals, where urine is expelled. Two muscles, called **urethral sphincters** (SFINGK-terz), help control urination. They are made of striated muscle, which enables voluntary control of urination. Urination is also assisted by contracting the lower abdominal muscles.

Urinary System Terms and Word Roots

Term or Word Root	Pronunciation	Meaning
ammonium	*uh*-MOH-nee-*uhm*	metabolic waste product excreted by the kidneys to maintain acid-base balance in the blood
thrombopoetin	throm-boh-poi-ET-n	hormone excreted by the kidneys, liver, and muscles that stimulates platelet production
nephr-	nehfr	kidney
nephrology	*nuh*-FROL-*uh*-jee, neh-FROL-*uh*-jee	study and treatment of kidney diseases
ur-	yoor	urine
diuresis	deye-*uh*-REE-sis	heavy urination
urothelium	yoo-roh-THEE-lee-*uhm*	tissue that lines most of the urinary tract
detrusor muscle	duh-TROO-zer MUHS-*uhl*	type of smooth muscle found in the bladder
rugae	ROO-gey	folds, or ridges, in an organ (such as the bladder) that increase the area, allowing the organ to expand
cyst-	sist	bladder
vesic-	veh-SIK	bladder
pyel-	peye-EL	renal pelvis
ureter-	y*oo*-REE-ter, YOOR-e-ter	ureter

Female Reproductive Organs

The female reproductive system creates female sexual characteristics and helps form a human egg that is capable of being fertilized. Fertilization is the union of egg and sperm. If fertilization occurs, the female reproductive system supports and nourishes the **fetus** (FEE-*tuhs*), which is the developing human. Most of the female reproductive system lies internally in the pelvis, with the exception of the last part of the vagina and the external genitalia.

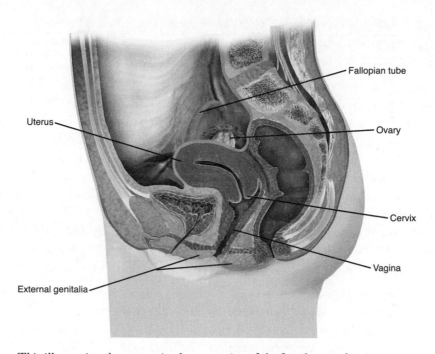

This illustration shows a sagittal cross-section of the female reproductive system.
Zygote Media Group © Dorling Kindersley

Ovaries and Fallopian Tubes

The **ovaries** (OH-*vuh*-reez) are two small organs that lie on either side of the uterus. The ovaries produce eggs and the female hormones **estrogen** (ES-tr*uh*-*juhn*) and **progesterone** (proh-JES-*tuh*-rohn), which create female sexual characteristics, support egg development, and maintain pregnancy should it occur.

Also known as the **oviducts** (OH-vi-duhkts), the **fallopian tubes** connect the ovaries to the uterus. Once the egg matures and is released in the ovaries, it travels along the fallopian tubes. The fallopian tubes are also the usual site of fertilization between egg and sperm.

Uterus and Cervix

The **uterus** (YOO-ter-*uhs*) is a thick, muscular organ that lies in the middle of the pelvis and is supported by three strong ligaments. The uterus functions in **gestation** (je-STEY-*shuhn*) to protect and support the developing fetus. The uterus is highly

vascularized (VAS-ky*uh-luh*-reyezd) and contains many blood vessels, especially during pregnancy. During pregnancy, blood vessels within the walls of the uterus develop specifically to support development of the fetus.

The uterus has three layers: the **endometrium** (en-doh-MEE-tree-*uhm*), the **myometrium** (meye-oh-MEE-tree-*uhm*), and the **parametrium** (PAH-rah-MEE-tree-*uhm*, PAHR-ah-MEE-tree-*uhm*). The endometrium is the inner layer in which a fertilized egg implants after it has traveled from the fallopian tubes to the uterus. During a woman's monthly cycle, the endometrium builds up to prepare for a fertilized egg. If fertilization does not occur, the endometrial lining sloughs off, causing **menstruation** (men-stroo-EY-*shuhn*), or monthly blood flow. The myometrium consists of a thick layer of strong, smooth (involuntary) muscle. The powerful contractions of the myometrium during birth move the baby along the birth canal. Myometrial contractions also cause menstrual cramps and play a role in sexual response. The parametrium is the loose tissue surrounding the uterus.

The **fundus** (FUHN-*duhs*) is the top part of the uterus. The **cervix** (SUR-viks), or "neck" of the uterus, is the lower part of the uterus that extends downward into the vagina. The cervix has an opening that enlarges during childbirth to allow the baby to pass through. The part of the opening that lies in the vagina is called the **external cervical os** (SUR-vi-*kuhl* os); the **internal cervical os** lies where the cervix opens into the uterus.

Vagina and External Genitalia

The **vagina** (*vuh*-JEYE-*nuh*) is a muscular passageway that leads from the cervix to the external genitalia. The vagina is elastic, which allows it to stretch during sexual intercourse and childbirth. Located near the vagina, **Bartholin** (BAHRT-*uh*-lin) **glands** and **Skene** (SKEEN) **glands** secrete fluid and mucous for lubrication.

The external genitalia are also called the **vulva** (VUHL-*vuh*). The **labia majora** (LEY-bee-*uh* muh-JAWR-uh) and **labia minora** (LEY-bee-*uh* mi-NAWR-*uh*) are folds of skin that protect the vagina and urethral opening. The **clitoris** (KLIT-er-is) is a collection of tissue that functions in sexual stimulation and lies at the anterior part of the external genitalia. The **mons pubis** (monz PYOO-bis) is a fat pad that lies at the front of the external genitalia and cushions the pubic bone.

Breasts

Even though men also possess breasts, which puts them at risk for many of the same breast diseases as women, breasts are often included in descriptions of only the female reproductive system. The structures in male and female breasts are basically the same, except that female breasts contain more fat tissue and a more elaborate milk duct system than male breasts. Breasts consist of the following structures:

- The **mammary papilla** (MAM-*uh*-ree pa-PIL-*uh*) is the raised part of the nipple, where milk exits the breast.
- The **areola** (uh-REE-uh-*luh*, air-ee-OH-*luh*) is the colored area around the papilla.
- **Mammary glands** produce milk, which is why they are also known as milk glands.
- **Lactiferous** (lak-TIF-er-*uhs*) **ducts** are small tubes that bring the milk to the nipple. They also are known as mammary ducts.

Female Reproductive Tract Word Roots

Word Root	Pronunciation	Meaning
cervic-	SUR-vik	cervix
colp-	KOLP-	vagina
hyster-	hi-STER-	uterus
mamm-	MAMM-	breast
mast-	MAST	breast
metri-	MEE-tree	uterus
oo-	OH-uh	egg
oophor-	oh-uh-FAWR	ovary
ovari-	OH-v*uh*-ree	ovary
salping-	sal-PINJ, sal-PING	fallopian tube
vagin-	vuh-JAYN-	vagina

STUDY TIP

Words that start with *oo-*, like *oocyte,* can be tricky to pronounce. You might be tempted to pronounce the double-O in the usual way, as in the word *shoot*. But the correct pronunciation gives emphasis to both letters. So *oocyte* is pronounced OH-*uh*-seyet. Once you learn this rule, you can apply it to most other words that begin with the word root *oo-*.

Male Reproductive Organs

The male reproductive system creates male sexual characteristics and produces sperm and semen, which are capable of fertilizing an egg. Most of the male reproductive system lies outside the body.

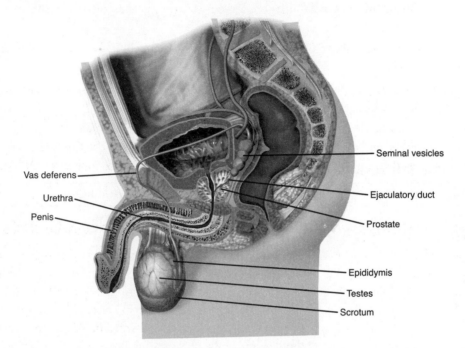

Vas deferens

Urethra

Penis

Seminal vesicles

Ejaculatory duct

Prostate

Epididymis

Testes

Scrotum

This illustration shows a sagittal cross-section of the male reproductive system.
Zygote Media Group © Dorling Kindersley

Penis, Scrotum, and Testes

The **penis** (PEE-nis) functions in sexual reproduction and serves as the evacuation route for urine. Both urine and semen exit the body via the urethra, which runs through the middle of the penis and ends at the **penile meatus** (PEE-neyel mee-EY-*tuhs*). The enlarged tip of the penis is called the **glans penis** (glanz PEE-nis), which is covered by the **foreskin** (FAWR-skin) in uncircumcised males.

The **scrotum** (SKROH-tuhm) is the sac that contains the testes. The **testes** (TES-teez) make sperm and male hormones, especially **testosterone** (tes-TOS-*tuh*-rohn). On top of the testes and within the scrotal sac is the epididymis. The **epididymis** (ep-i-DID-*uh*-mis) is a network of tubes where sperm mature and are stored.

DID YOU KNOW?

One reason why testes may be located outside the body is for temperature control. Sperm production is affected by temperature, especially temperatures on the higher and lower end of the spectrum. A muscle called the **cremaster** (kri-MAS-ter) **muscle** can contract to pull the testes closer to the body or relax to allow them to fall farther from the body for optimal temperature control during sperm production.

Vas Deferens

The **vas deferens** (vas DEF-er-*uhnz*) runs from each testis, and then heads internally into the pelvic cavity. Each vas deferens becomes an **ejaculatory** (ih-JAK-*yuh-luh*-tawr-ee) duct inside the prostate, and then joins the urethra so that fluids can exit the body via the penis. Smooth muscles in the vas deferens contract to push semen along its route. Muscles at the base of the penis also contract during orgasm and help expel the **ejaculate** (ih-JAK-y*uh*-lit), or sperm and semen, from the penis.

Prostate Gland, Seminal Vesicles, and Associated Glands

The prostate gland lies internally between the bladder and rectum. It secretes a large part of the fluid found in semen. The **seminal vesicles** (SEM-*uh*-nl VES-i-*kuhlz*) secrete the majority of the fluid found in semen. This fluid is high in **fructose** (FRUHK-tohs), a form of sugar. The fructose gives sperm energy and helps them navigate the female reproductive tract. The **bulbourethral** (BUHLB-oh- *yoo*-REE-*thruhl*) **glands**, or **Cowper** (kou-pur) **glands**, also contribute products to seminal fluid.

Male Reproductive Tract Terms and Word Roots

Term or Word Root	Pronunciation	Meaning
gonad	GOH-nad	gland that produces egg or sperm, used to refer to both ovaries and testes
semen	SEE-*muhn*	the liquid part of the ejaculate
balan-	BAL-*uhn*	penis
orch-	ORK	testis
orchid-	OR-kid	testis
prostate-	PROS-tat	prostate
scrot-	SKROHT-	scrotum
urethra-	*yoo*-REETHR-	urethra
vas-	VAS	vas deferens

Orch- is a word root that refers to the testes. It comes from the Greek word *orchis,* or flower. On cross-section, the convolutions of the seminiferous tubules in a testis give it the appearance of a many-petaled flower. The word root *orch-* is used in many terms referring to the testes, such as orchiectomy (removal of a testicle) and cryptorchidism (undescended testicle).

Endocrine Organs

The endocrine system is composed of various structures, most of which are glands, that lie in different parts of the body and secrete **hormones** (HAWR-mohnz) into the blood system. Hormones are chemicals that act as messengers, transmitting signals to other organs to help regulate the body and keep it in balance. Some of the processes that hormones help regulate include emotions, reproduction, growth, blood pressure, fluid and electrolyte homeostasis, and metabolism of nutrients. Some endocrine glands are sequenced together in an **axis** (AK-sis). The major axes include the hypothalamic-pituitary-adrenal axis, the hypothalamic-pituitary-gonadal axis, and the hypothalamic-pituitary-thyroid axis.

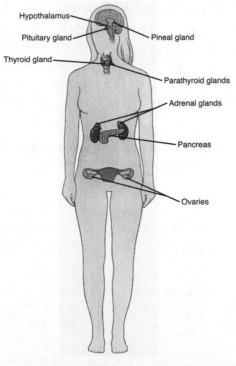

Several glands are included in the female endocrine system.
Michael Courtney © Dorling Kindersley

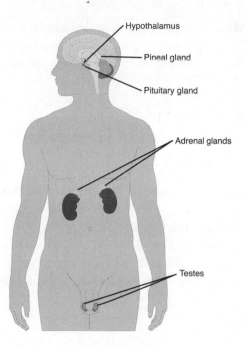

The male endocrine system includes structures throughout the body.
© Dorling Kindersley

Hypothalamus, Pineal Gland, and Pituitary Gland

The **hypothalamus** (heye-p*uh*-THAL-*am*-us) is not a gland; it is part of the brain. You can think of it as the regulator of the pituitary gland because it secretes hormones that either stimulate or inhibit the pituitary's release of hormones. The hypothalamus also produces hormones that act on the thyroid and the gonads (ovaries and testes). Regulation of hunger and thirst is also handled in part by the hypothalamus.

The brain also contains the **pineal** (PIN-ee-*uhl*, PEYE-nee-*uhl*) **gland**. This gland produces **melatonin** (mel-*uh*-TOH-nin), which controls **circadian** (sur-KEY-dee-*uhn*) **rhythms**, or sleep–wake cycles. The hypothalamus plays a part in this process, too.

The **pituitary** (pi-TOO-i-ter-ee) **gland** sticks out from the bottom of the hypothalamus. It looks like a small pea, and although it lies near the brain, it is not considered part of the brain. The pituitary gland secretes hormones that play important roles in growth, blood pressure control, fluid balance, reproduction, childbirth, and lactation. It releases hormones that stimulate the thyroid and gonads to release their own hormones. The pituitary also releases a hormone that signals cells in the skin to produce **melanin** (MEL-*uh*-nin), a pigment that gives the skin its color and allows for tanning.

Adrenal Glands

There are two **adrenal** (*uh*-DREEN-l, *uh*-DREN-l) glands, each of which lie on top of either kidney. The adrenal glands secrete hormones that help regulate energy production, cellular metabolism, and immune responses. They also release hormones that act on the kidney to regulate fluid and electrolyte balance. The adrenal glands also release **adrenaline** (*uh*-DREN-*uh*-lin)/**epinephrine** (ep-*uh*-NEF-rin) and **noradrenaline** (nawr-*uh*-DREN-*uh*-lin)/**norepinephrine** (nawr-ep-*uh*-NEF-rin). Both of these hormones increase heart and breathing rate, blood pressure, skeletal muscle responsiveness, and the amount of glucose released into the bloodstream. These hormones also increase alertness, dilate pupils, and shut down noncritical processes (like digestion) so that blood can go to critical areas, like the brain and heart.

DID YOU KNOW?

During stressful situations, the adrenal glands release adrenaline and noradrenaline. These hormones are primarily responsible for producing the fight-or-flight stress response. During evolution, this response may have been adaptive because the effects of these hormones would have enabled a quick escape from predators or a fighting stance when required. However, the stresses of modern life can cause this response to become chronically activated. Sustained high levels of adrenaline and noradrenaline can have harmful effects on health. Heart disease and diabetes are two diseases that are related to an overactive, or chronic, fight-or-flight response.

Organs in Other Systems That Release Hormones

Organs in various other organ systems play double roles, performing their roles in their respective organs systems as well as releasing hormones. As you learned earlier in this chapter in the section about the urinary system, the kidneys secrete hormones important in red blood cell and platelet production, calcium balance, and blood pressure control. In addition to being part of the circulatory system, the heart also secretes hormones important in blood pressure control and fluid and electrolyte balance.

In the reproductive system, the ovaries and testes secrete hormones primarily responsible for reproduction. These hormones also affect bone, muscles, skin, teeth, hair, the immune system, the digestive tract, blood clotting, and fluid and electrolyte balance.

In the digestive system, the pancreas produces and releases **insulin** (IN-*suh*-lin), which regulates blood sugar. The liver secretes hormones important in cell growth, blood vessel constriction, salt and fluid balance, and blood clotting. The stomach and duodenum secrete hormones important in digestion.

In addition, **adipose** (AD-*uh*-pohs), or fat, tissue secretes hormones that play a role in metabolism and appetite control. And bone marrow secretes a hormone that affects blood clotting.

Endocrine System Word Roots

Word Root	Pronunciation	Meaning	Example
adren-	*uh*-DREEN, *uh*-DREN	adrenal glands	adrenocortical hormones
adrenal-	*uh*-DREEN-l, *uh*-DREN-l	adrenal glands	adrenaline
hypophys-	heye-POF-*uh*s	pituitary gland	hypophysis
pancreat-	PAN-kree-at, PANG-kree-at	pancreas	pancreaticobiliary
parathyroid-	par-*uh*-THEYE-roid	parathyroid glands	parathyroidectomy
pituitar-	pi-TOO-i-ter	pituitary gland	pituitary adenoma
thyroadeno-	THEYE-roh-AD-noh	thyroid gland	thyroadenitis
thyroid-	THEYE-roid	thyroid gland	thyroiditis

The Least You Need to Know

- The urinary system produces and disposes of urine, ridding the body of waste products that could be harmful.
- The female reproductive system produces female sexual characteristics, creates an egg that is capable of fertilization, and supports the gestation of a fetus during pregnancy.
- The male reproductive system creates male sexual characteristics and produces sperm and semen.
- The endocrine system is made up of various structures scattered throughout the body. These organs secrete hormones, which are chemical messengers that keep the body in balance.

Brain, Nervous System, and Sense Organs

In This Chapter

- Names for parts of the brain and spinal cord
- Subdivisions of the nervous system
- Spinal nerves and other nerve terms
- Structures in the eyes, ears, nose, and mouth

Nerves play a role in almost every bodily process, so it's not surprising that numerous medical terms are associated with the nervous system. The main player in this system is, of course, the central nervous system. It controls vital bodily processes, as well as behavior and emotions. The peripheral nervous system lies outside the brain and spinal cord, and serves as a relay system between the central nervous system and the body's muscles and organs. The special organs for sight, hearing, smell, taste, and touch connect with both the central and peripheral nervous systems. Learning the basic word roots will keep these terms from getting on your nerves.

Central Nervous System

The **central nervous system** (CNS) serves as mission control for the entire human body. It receives information sent from other areas of the body, processes this information, and sends back commands for how to keep the body alive. The central nervous system is also responsible for the regulation of emotions and behavior. The two main organs of the CNS are the brain and the spinal cord.

Blood–Brain Barrier

Unlike many organ systems in the body, the central nervous system is separated from the bloodstream by the blood–brain barrier, which protects sensitive nerve tissue from possible infections or toxins in the blood. In the blood–brain barrier, cells that line capillaries are packed together in tight junctions that block materials that could harm the central nervous system. Necessary substances, like oxygen and glucose, move across the blood–brain barrier.

The brain and spinal cord are protected by an outer covering called the **meninges** (mi-NIN-jeez). The meninges have three layers: the outer **dura mater** (DOOR-*uh* MAH-*ter*), the middle **arachnoid mater** (*uh*-RAK-noid MAH-*ter*), and the inner **pia mater** (PEE-*uh* MAH-*ter*), which lies closest to the brain and spinal cord.

 WORD ORIGINS

In Latin, *mater* means mother and refers to all three layers of the meninges, perhaps because the meninges protect and nourish the brain and spinal cord the way a mother does her young. *Dura mater* means "tough mother," referring to the fact that the dura mater is the protective outer layer of the meninges. *Arachnoid* comes from the Greek word part *arachne*, which means spider, and the suffix *-oid*, which means "in the image of." The arachnoid mater is a network of fine spider weblike fibers that extend through the subarachnoid space to the pia mater. *Pia mater* means "little mother," which is appropriate because the pia mater is thin and delicate.

The **epidural** (ep-i-DOOR-*uhl*) **space** lies between the vertebrae and the meninges of the spinal cord and extends only to the base of the skull. The epidural space is the site of epidural injections that ease the pain of childbirth. In the brain, the epidural space normally exists only as a potential space. If blood or some disease process (like a tumor) occupies the epidural space in the brain, the brain can shift in position, which can be life-threatening. The **subdural** (suhb-DOOR-*uhl*) **space** is also a potential space between the dura mater and the arachnoid mater. Bleeding that occurs in this space is called a **subdural hematoma** (suhb-DOOR-*uhl* hee-ma-TOH-m*uh*). The **subarachnoid** (suhb-*uh*-RAK-noid) **space** lies between the arachnoid and pia mater.

Cerebrospinal (s*uh*-ree-broh-SPEYEN-l) **fluid** or CSF is a colorless fluid that circulates inside the subarachnoid space. CSF protects the brain and spinal cord by providing cushioning, carrying white blood cells to fight infection, and disposing of waste products produced by cells in the central nervous system. CSF also helps control the rate of blood flow in the brain. CSF circulates in **ventricles** (VEN-tri-kuhlz) inside the brain.

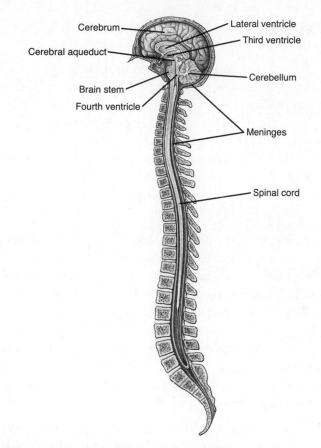

Cerebrum

Lateral ventricle

Third ventricle

Cerebral aqueduct

Cerebellum

Brain stem

Fourth ventricle

Meninges

Spinal cord

The central nervous system consists of the brain and spinal cord.
Halli Verrinder © Dorling Kindersley

WORD ORIGINS

Hydrocephalus (heye-dr*uh*-SEF-*uh-luh-*s) is a disorder characterized by too much CSF around the brain. The common name for this problem is "water on the brain." This term comes from a nearly direct translation of the word parts. In Greek, *hydro-* means water, and *cephalus* means head. Hydrocephalus can cause an enlarged head (especially in infants), behavior changes, brain damage, seizures, and sometimes death.

Cerebral Cortex Divisions

The brain lies in the cranial cavity and is protected by the skull and CSF. The brain is responsible for generating and controlling emotion and behavior; integrating movement; integrating and understanding sensory information; and regulating and controlling vital bodily processes, such as breathing.

The top layer of the brain consists of the **cerebral cortex** (*suh*-REE-*bruhl* KAWR-teks). The cerebral cortex is basically what makes us human. The human cerebral cortex is much larger than that of other animals, which is the reason why humans have the largest brain in relation to body size of any creature. The cerebral cortex is responsible for many of our thinking and emotional processes, such as language, **cognition** (kog-NISH-*uhn*)—a term for complex thought and intellectual abilities, decision-making processes, interpretation of sensory signals, and voluntary control of our limbs. The cerebral cortex contains many folds, which increases the surface area and accounts for the large size of human brains.

The cerebral cortex is divided into two halves, called **cerebral hemispheres** (*suh*-REE-*bruhl* HEM-is-feerz). These halves communicate with each other through a bundle of nerves called the **corpus callosum** (KAWR-*puhs kuh*-LOH-*suhm*). In addition, the cerebral cortex has four paired lobes or divisions. The lobe in each half has a corresponding lobe in the other half, which for the most part are mirror images of each other. However, for some processes, like language and spacial skills, the brain exhibits **lateralization** (lat-er-*uh*-*luh*-ZEY-*shuhn*), which means that one half dominates control of that activity. For example, language is most often controlled by the left side of the brain. Different parts of the cortex are dedicated to different tasks, such as movement and sensation.

The four cortical lobes are named after the skull bones nearest to them. At the front of the cerebral hemispheres, the right and left **frontal** (FRUHN-tl) **lobes** are responsible for self-awareness and executive functioning, which controls other thought processes, inhibits socially unacceptable behavior, guides attention and planning, initiates intentional movement, performs verbal reasoning, forms certain types of memories, and controls some types of emotion. Located behind the frontal lobes, the right and left **parietal** (*puh*-REYE-i-tl) **lobes** process spatial and sensory information, especially touch, and certain language tasks.

The right and left **temporal** (TEM-per-*uhl*, TEM-*pruhl*) **lobes** lie on the lateral sides of the cerebral hemispheres and beneath the frontal and parietal lobes. They form and store visual and long-term memories, generate emotions associated with memories, process hearing input, and enable language comprehension.

Right and left **occipital** (ok-SIP-i-tl) **lobes** lie at the back of the brain. They are also known as the visual cortex because they process visual information.

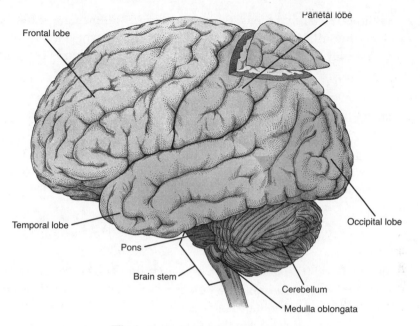

Frontal lobe

Parietal lobe

Temporal lobe

Occipital lobe

Pons

Brain stem

Cerebellum

Medulla oblongata

The brain is divided into several parts.
Halli Verrinder © Dorling Kindersley

Cerebellum and Brain Stem

The **cerebellum** (ser-*uh*-BEL-*uhm*) lies beneath the occipital lobes at the bottom and back of the brain. It controls and fine-tunes movement, especially coordination and balance. However, except for certain reflexes, the cerebellum does not initiate movement—the frontal lobes do.

The **brain stem** lies in the posterior part of the brain, beneath the cortex. Most of the **cranial** (KREY-nee-*uhl*) **nerves** emerge from the brain stem. (You will learn more about cranial nerves later in this chapter.) Motor and sensory nerve impulses cross over from the left brain hemisphere to the right side of the body, and from the right hemisphere to the left side of the body. These nerve impulses cross over in the medulla of the brain stem. The brain stem also regulates vital functions such as breathing, heart rate, and consciousness.

The brain stem has three subdivisions. The **midbrain** (MID-breyn) lies at the top of the brain stem. It transmits messages about hearing, vision, skeletal muscle movement, and wakefulness. It also regulates body temperature. The **pons** (PONZ) lies in the middle of the brain stem. It transmits messages between the cerebrum and the cerebellum and medulla oblongata. It also transmits signals about eye movement, facial expressions, facial sensations, sleep, breathing, swallowing, posture, and bladder function. The **medulla oblongata** (*muh*-DUHL-*uh* ob-lawng-GAH-*tuh*) lies at the bottom of the brain stem. It controls breathing; heart rate; blood vessel tone; and reflexes for vomiting, coughing, sneezing, and swallowing.

WORD ORIGINS

The word *pons* comes from the Latin word meaning bridge. Because one of the main functions of the pons is to serve as a bridge to relay nerve impulses from the cerebrum to other areas of the body, this name makes sense. One way to remember it is to think of the Pont Neuf, which is a famous bridge in Paris.

Spinal Cord

The spinal cord lies in the spinal cavity. It is surrounded by cerebrospinal fluid and is protected by the vertebrae and spinal meninges. The spinal cord does not run the full length of the vertebral column, but ends at about the level of the first and second lumbar vertebrae. The **central canal** of the spinal cord is like the fourth ventricle in the brain and contains CSF.

The spinal cord transmits nerve signals from the brain to lower parts of the body. Sensory connections travel up the spinal cord to the brain, which interprets them and generates a motor signal. This signal travels down from the brain to the spinal cord, which transmits the signal to the appropriate part of the peripheral nervous system via spinal nerves. These nerves exit at different levels of the spinal cord.

The spinal cord is also responsible for many reflexes. The nerve signals for reflexes stay at the level of the spinal cord without having to travel up to the brain for interpretation. Reflexes are protective because they allow for quicker skeletal muscle responses in dangerous situations.

Peripheral Nervous System

The nerves outside the brain and spinal cord make up the **peripheral nervous system** (PNS). The PNS has 12 paired cranial nerves and 31 paired spinal nerves. The PNS is at risk for injury from infections, toxins, and trauma because it is not protected by the meninges, blood–brain barrier, or any bony structures. Divisions of the PNS include the autonomic, somatic, and sensory nervous systems.

Autonomic Nervous System

The **autonomic** (aw-*tuh*-NOM-ik) **nervous system** (ANS) transmits nerve signals that maintain functioning of the body's organs, or **visceral** (VIS-er-*uhl*) functions. The activities of the ANS occur mostly outside of conscious control. They consist of breathing, digestion, heart rate, urination, reproductive processes, and other bodily processes necessary for life. Cranial and spinal nerves both carry nerve fibers that belong to the autonomic nervous system.

The ANS has two divisions whose functions often oppose, but sometimes complement, each other. The **sympathetic** (sim-*puh*-THET-ik) **division** deals with responses that promote an active/vigilant state and inhibit digestion. The **parasympathetic** (PAHR-ah-sim-*puh*-THET-ik) **division** deals with responses that promote a restive state. It stimulates digestion and calms the sympathetic response.

Sympathetic Responses	Parasympathetic Responses
Increased heart rate	Decreased heart rate
Increased blood flow to muscles	Gastrointestinal blood vessel dilation
Increased blood flow to lungs	Increased salivary gland secretion
Bronchiole dilation	Bronchiole constriction
Pupil dilation	Pupil constriction
Sexual orgasm	Increased sexual arousal

STUDY TIP

The sympathetic division is often linked to the fight-or-flight response because it often produces responses to stimuli that require immediate attention. For example, an attacking tiger would really wake up the sympathetic division. The parasympathetic division is often linked to the rest-and-digest phenomenon because it helps control bodily functions in nonemergency/nonstressful situations. The distinction between the two often holds true, but not always. For example, both the sympathetic and parasympathetic divisions play a role in sexual response.

Somatic and Sensory Nervous Systems

The somatic nervous system generates muscular contraction, often in response to signals about the environment, such as pain and temperature from the sensory system. The cranial and spinal nerves carry information for the somatic and sensory nervous systems, or **somatosensory system**.

Ten of the twelve cranial nerves emerge from the brain stem. The cranial nerves carry sensory and motor information for the face and neck, and a few shoulder muscles. The spinal nerves carry sensory information from the rest of the body to the spinal cord, where they are either interpreted as reflexes or relayed up to the brain. Motor information is relayed from the spinal cord via the spinal nerves to the rest of the body in order to generate movement.

Spinal nerves exit the spinal cord at the following sections:

- **Cervical** (SUR-vi-*kuhl*) **nerves:** Eight paired nerves that relay signals to and from the neck, diaphragm, shoulder, elbow, wrist, and hand
- **Thoracic** (thaw-RAS-ik, thoh-RAS-ik) **nerves:** Twelve paired nerves that relay signals to and from the intercostal muscles, chest, and some abdominal muscles
- **Lumbar** (LUHM-bahr) **nerves:** Five paired nerves that relay signals to and from most abdominal muscles, and parts of the hip, thigh, leg, and foot
- **Sacral** (SEY-*kruhl*, SAK-*ruhl*) **nerves:** Five paired nerves that relay signals to and from the hip, thigh, leg, and foot and to and from the bladder, descending colon, rectum, and genitals
- **Coccygeal** (KOK-si-jee-*uhl*) **nerve:** One paired nerve that relays signals to and from the **coccyx** (KOK-siks), or tailbone

Central and Peripheral Nervous System Terms and Word Roots

Term or Word Root	Pronunciation	Meaning
axon	AK-son	"tail" of a nerve cell that carries nerve impulses away from the cell body
ganglia	GANG-glee-*uh*	group/collection of nerves
gray matter	GREY MAT-er	area in the brain and spinal cord that contains the cell bodies of neurons

Term or Word Root	Pronunciation	Meaning
myelin	MEYE-*uh*-lin	material that surrounds nerve cells and increases the rate of nerve transmission
neur-	NOOR, NYOOR	nerves
neuroglia	NOO-roh-glee-uh	cells that support nerve cells
neuron	NOOR-on, NYOOR-on	nerve cell
neurotransmitter	noor-oh-TRANZ-mit-er	a chemical that carries a nerve transmission between cells and across a synapse
oligodendrocyte	OL-i-goh-DEN-droh-seyet	nerve cell that supports the axons in the central nervous system
soma	SOH-*muh*	nerve cell body
sulcus	SUHL-kuhs	bottom part, or valley, of a fold in the cerebral cortex
synapse	SIN-aps	space between two nerve cells, through which the neural signal travels
white matter	WEYET MAT-er	area in the brain and spinal cord that contains the tails, or axons, of nerves
cephalus-	SEF-*uh*-luhs	head
cerebell-	SER-*uh*-bel	cerebellum
cerebr-	suh-REE-br	cerebrum
encephal-	en-SEF	brain
glio-	GLEE-oh	glial cells; Latin for "glue"
medull-	muh-DUHL-uh	medulla oblongata
menin-	ME-nin	meninges
myel-	MEYE-uhl, meye-EL	spinal cord

Sensory Organs

Several organs are specialized to perform sensory functions. These organs include eyes, ears, nose, mouth, and skin.

Eyes

The eyes provide visual information about the environment. Two eyeballs located on the upper front of the face enable **binocular** (b*uh*-NOK-*yuh*-ler, beye-NOK-*yuh*-ler), or three-dimensional vision. The main parts of the eyes include the following:

- The **conjunctiva** (kon-juhngk-TEYE-v*uh*) is the outer layer of the eyeball and the inner layer of the eyelids.
- The **sclera** (SKLEER-*uh*, SKLAIR-uh) is the white outer covering of the eyeball.
- The **cornea** (KAWR-nee-*uh*) is the clear front part of the eye.
- The **lens** (LENZ) is the clear area at the front of the eye that helps focus light on the retina.
- The **iris** (EYE-ris) is the colored area at the front of the eyeball that helps to control the amount of light that enters the eye.
- The **pupil** (PYOO-*puhl*) is the dark area at the front part of the eye that controls the amount of light entering the eye by getting bigger and smaller.
- The **ciliary** (SIL-ee-er-ee) **muscle** controls the focus of light on the retina by changing the shape of the lens.
- The **retina** (RET-n-*uh*) is the area at the back of the eyeball that is capable of sensing light signals.
- **Rods** are cells in the retina that function in peripheral vision.
- **Cones** are cells in the retina that function in color vision.
- The **macula** (MAK-y*uh*-*luh*) is an area of the retina that functions in visual acuity.
- The **fovea** (FOH-vee-*uh*) is an area of the retina that functions in visual acuity and central vision, which is important in activities such as reading, hunting, and painting.
- The **optic** (OP-tik) **nerve** transmits visual stimuli from the retina to the brain.

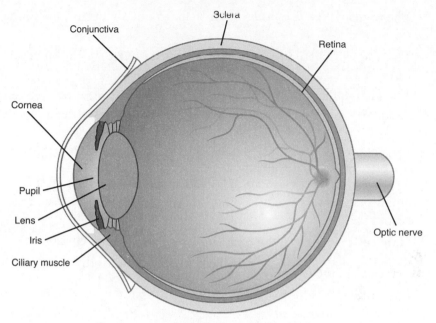

Eye structures help to collect visual information.
© Dorling Kindersley

Ears

The ears are located on either side of the head and are specialized for **auditory** (AW-di-tawr-ee), or hearing, perception. The ears also play a role in balance. The ear has three divisions: outer, middle, and inner.

The **outer ear** includes the following structures:

- The **pinna** (PIN-*uh*) is the external flap of the ear on the head.
- The **external auditory meatus** (mee-EY-*tuhs*) is the opening of the ear canal.
- The **external auditory canal** is the tube that runs from the outer ear to the middle ear and is a common site of ear infections.
- The **tympanic** (tim-PAN-ik) **membrane**, or eardrum, receives sound vibrations and transmits them to the middle ear.

The **middle ear** lies inside the tympanic membrane and includes the following structures:

- The **malleus** (MAL-ee-*uhs*) is a hammer-shaped bone that transmits sound vibrations.

- The **incus** (ING-*kuh*s) is an anvil-shaped bone that transmits sound vibrations.
- The **stapes** (STEY-peez)is a stirrup-shaped bone that transmits sound vibrations.
- The **eustachian** (yoo-STEY-*shuhn*) **tube** joins the nasal passage to the middle ear and functions in equalizing pressure and draining mucus.

The **inner ear** is the innermost part of the ear and includes the following:

- The **cochlea (KOK-lee-*uh*, KOH-klee-*uh*)** is a spiral, snail shell-shaped organ that converts sound vibrations into nerve impulses that are sent to the brain.
- **Hair cells** are cells in the cochlea that amplify sound vibrations.
- **Semicircular** (SEM-i-sur-*kuh*-lur) **canals** are tubes that sense bodily rotation.

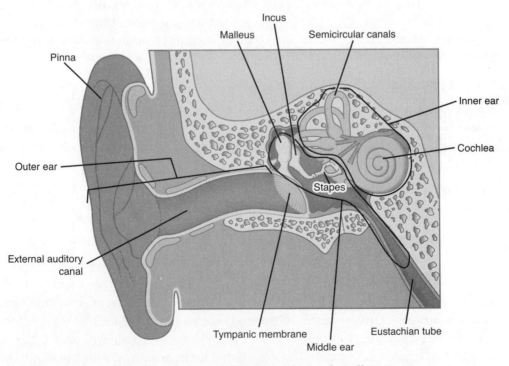

The ear has three main divisions and several smaller parts.
© Dorling Kindersley

Nose

The nose is specialized for **olfactory** (ol-FAK-*tuh*-ree) functions, or smelling. The nose also warms and humidifies air before it reaches the lungs. Hairs and mucous in the nose provide protection by trapping objects or bacteria that could harm the lungs.

The main structures of the nose include the following:

- **Nostrils** (NOS-*truhlz*): nasal openings
- **Olfactory receptors:** cells in the nose that bind odor molecules
- **Olfactory nerve:** nerve that transmits odor information to the brain
- **Olfactory bulb:** area in the brain that interprets odor information

Mouth

The mouth is the main site for **gustatory** (GUHS-*tuh*-tawr-ee), or taste, organs. Humans are capable of tasting sweet, sour, salty, bitter, and **umami** (oo-MAH-mee), or savory, tastes. Distinctions in flavor, such as citrus or bacon flavors, are primarily a function of smell. Taste occurs as a result of chemical reactions within taste buds in the mouth.

The main organs of taste include the following:

- **Tongue:** muscle in the mouth that functions in chewing and contains taste buds
- **Taste buds:** chemical receptors on the tongue that sense taste
- **Papillae** (*puh*-PIL-ee): bumps on the tongue where taste buds are found
- **Taste receptors:** cells that bind molecules and contribute to the sensation of taste

Skin

Skin is responsible for the sensation of touch. Receptors in the skin sense pressure, pain, temperature, and gradients of touch. These receptors help relay touch information to the spinal cord and brain. Small hairs on the skin also contribute to the sensation of touch. Skin sensation is distributed in dermatomes, which were covered in Chapter 5.

The Least You Need to Know

- The central nervous system consists of the brain and spinal cord, which receives information sent from other areas of the body, processes this information, and sends back commands on how to keep the body alive.
- The cerebral cortex makes us human and enables us to use language and engage in complex thought processes.
- The peripheral nervous system is made up of the autonomic nervous system and the somatosensory system.
- The autonomic nervous system control subconscious activities that keep the body's organs functioning.
- The somatosensory system transmits sensory information to the brain and spinal cord and motor information to the muscles.
- Special organs for sight, hearing, smell, taste, and touch are found in the eyes, ears, nose, mouth, and skin (respectively).

Physiology: How the Body Works

Part 3 is dedicated to physiology, which describes the processes and functions that keep the body alive. Many bodily processes rely on chemical, electrical, and physical processes, so some of these terms also stem from basic science.

Chapter 10 covers communication and regulation within the body. **Homeostasis** describes how the body maintains an optimal environment for bodily processes. Homeostasis is necessary for life, and much of Chapter 10 presents terms associated with how the various body systems stay in balance.

The remainder of Part 3 is divided according to the functions that various body systems provide. Chapter 11 describes terms related to the process of muscular contraction in the musculoskeletal system and includes a discussion about tendons, ligaments, and fascia. Chapter 12 explains the process of circulation and breathing provided by the heart and lungs, and presents terms associated with these processes. Chapter 13 covers metabolism, absorption, and elimination, which is how the body gets the nutrients it needs and gets rid of waste products that could be harmful. General biochemical terms associated with these processes are introduced. Key body systems covered in Chapter 13 include the digestive and urinary systems.

Chapter 14 covers reproduction, from the earliest stages of gamete production to pregnancy, childbirth, and lactation. Chapter 15 is dedicated to how the body protects itself from infectious pathogens like bacteria and viruses. Structures, processes, terms, and the different divisions of the immune system are explained.

Regulation and Communication

Chapter 10

In This Chapter

- Controlling body temperature
- Regulating blood clots
- Managing fluids
- Balancing blood composition
- Communicating with hormone feedback loops

The Greek word *homo* means same, and *stasis* means stable, so **homeostasis** (hoh-mee-*uh*-STEY-sis) refers to maintaining stability, or balance, in the body. This idea of maintaining balance goes back as far as Hippocrates, who theorized that an imbalance in the four bodily humors (black bile, yellow bile, phlegm, and blood) produced disease. The idea of bodily humors is now discredited, but the concept of maintaining balance within the body is still important. Because disease often causes dysregulation of bodily processes, many medical terms are associated with homeostasis.

In this chapter, you learn about several vital processes that need to be in balance in order to sustain life. These processes include thermoregulation, hemostasis, osmoregulation, and regulation of blood composition and iron levels.

Various organs and organ systems play a role in keeping the body in balance. Certain organs like the brain, kidneys, and liver play a big role. The nervous and endocrine systems also are key players in this process. This chapter explains how hormones serve as chemical messengers that help keep the body in balance. The several major hormonal axes in the body interact with each other through feedback systems, which are important ways that body systems communicate with each other to remain in balance.

Thermoregulation

The regulation of body temperature is called **thermoregulation** (thur-moh-reg-*yuh*-LEY-*shuhn*). Bodily processes function optimally within a narrow temperature range.

Core temperature is the temperature of vital organs, such as the liver and kidneys. A core temperature that falls below the normal range is called **hypothermia** (heye-*puh*-THUR-mee-*uh*). A core temperature above the normal range is called **hyperthermia** (heye-per-THUR-mee-*uh*). A core temperature in the normal range is called **normo-thermia** (NAWR-*muh*-THUR-mee-*uh*) or **euthermia** (yoo-THUR-mee-*uh*). **Basal body temperature** refers to the temperature measured at rest.

The main temperature regulatory center lies in the **hypothalamus** (heye-*puh*-THAL-*uh-muhs*) in the brain. It receives signals from throughout the body and sends back signals for how to increase or dissipate heat.

Processes important in temperature regulation include **vasoconstriction** (vas-oh-*kuhn*-STRIK-*shuhn*, vey-zoh-*kuhn*-STRIK-*shuhn*) and **vasodilation** (vas-oh-deye-LEY-*shuhn*, vey-zoh-deye-LEY-*shuhn*). In vasoconstriction, capillaries in the skin become smaller, which redirects blood away from the skin, where heat is lost, to vital organs like the brain and heart. In vasodilation, capillaries in the skin become larger, which causes more blood to flow to skin, where heat is dissipated.

As you learned in Chapter 5, the skin contains several structures that help with thermoregulation. When the body is cold, the **arrector pili** (uh-REK-ter peye-leye) muscles in the skin contract to make hairs stand on end, which traps air close to the skin and reduces heat loss. This process causes "goose bumps" and is called **piloerection** (peye-loh-ih-REK-*shuhn*). When the body is hot, **eccrine** (EK-rin, EK-reen) glands in the skin release sweat, which cools the body as the fluid evaporates.

Cellular metabolism is another process for regulating temperature. For example, the contractions of shivering muscles produce heat through cellular metabolism. Brown fat also can generate heat through cellular metabolism. Brown fat is found in infants and in small amounts in some adults. Unlike brown fat, white fat can only provide insulation against cold.

Hemostasis

Hemostasis (hee-*muh*-STEY-sis) refers to the regulation of blood clotting. Forming a blood clot helps control bleeding following trauma. On the other hand, keeping blood sufficiently fluid is important to avoid life-threatening clots within blood vessels and vital organs.

Hemostasis is tightly controlled via the **coagulation** (koh-AG-*yuh*-ley-*shuhn*) **cascade**. **Endothelial** (en-doh-THEE-lee-*uhl*) **cells** line blood vessels and secrete coagulation factors and other substances that either inhibit or promote coagulation. **Blood platelets** (PLEYT-lits) are key players in this process. One of the first steps in the coagulation cascade is the formation of a "platelet plug."

Other substances that play major roles in coagulation include the following:

- **Von Willebrand factor** (von WIL-*uh*-brand FAK-ter) is a substance that helps to form the platelet plug.
- **Clotting factors** (KLOT-ing FAK-terz) are 12 substances that act on each other to regulate the coagulation cascade.
- **Prothrombin** (proh-THROM-bin) and **thrombin** (THROM-bin) promote the formation of a clot.
- **Fibrinogen** (feye-BRIN-*uh*-*juhn*) and **fibrin** (FEYE-brin) promote the formation of a tight seal around the clot.
- **Plasminogen** (plaz-MIN-*uh*-*juhn*) and **plasmin** (PLAZ-min) dissolve the clot after healing is completed.

WORD ORIGINS

In 1924, a Finnish doctor named Erik von Willebrand described a familial bleeding disorder that was usually milder than hemophilia and differed from it several other ways. This disorder thus became known as von Willebrand disease. In the 1950s, the cause of the disease was found to a particular blood-clotting protein, von Willebrand factor, which also was named in honor of the doctor. Since then, several variants of von Willebrand disease have been discovered.

Three substances on endothelial cells prevent blood from clotting:

- **Thrombomodulin** (THROM-boh-MOJ-*uh*-lin)
- **Nitric oxide** (NEYE-trik OK-seyed)
- **Prostacyclin** (pros-*tuh*-SEYE-klin)

Osmoregulation

The body monitors **osmoregulation** (oz-moh-reg-yuh-LEY-*shuhn*), or control of fluid balance, through various mechanisms.

Osmosis (oz-MOH-sis) and active transport are important processes that help balance body fluid levels. Osmosis refers to the tendency for fluids to flow from areas where there are a lot of dissolved substances to areas where there are fewer dissolved substances. During active transport, cells expend energy to transport substances across a membrane.

Hypertonic (heye-per-TON-ik) solutions have many dissolved particles in comparison to a reference solution. Water tends to flow into hypertonic solutions in order to make them more diluted. **Hypotonic** (heye-p*uh*-TON-ik) solutions have few dissolved particles in comparison to a reference solution. Water tends to flow out of hypotonic solutions to make them more concentrated. **Isotonic** (eye-s*uh*-TON-ik) solutions have the same amount of dissolved particles as compared to a reference solution. Water does not flow into or out of solutions that are isotonic to each other.

Extracellular (ek-*struh*-SEL-*yuh*-ler) fluid refers to the fluid outside cells, which includes **extravascular** (ek-*struh*-VAS-*kyuh*-ler) **fluid** and **intravascular** (in-*truh*-VAS-*kyuh*-ler) **fluid**.

Extravascular Fluid

Extravascular fluid is the fluid outside of blood vessels. Another term for this fluid is **interstitial** (in-ter-STISH-*uhl*) **fluid**, which refers to the fluid in the spaces between tissues, or the **interstitium** (in-ter-STISH-*uhm*). Interstitial fluid contains water, salts, fatty acids, enzymes, hormones, amino acids, neurotransmitters, and waste products.

When there is a lot of fluid in blood vessels, but relatively less fluid in the interstitium, fluid and certain solutes flow from the blood vessels into the interstitial fluid. This process is also affected by blood pressure. The lymphatic system removes extra fluid and solutes from the interstitium.

Intravascular Fluid

Regulating intravascular fluid, or blood volume, is one way in which the body regulates blood pressure. The kidneys, liver, lungs, adrenal glands, and hypothalamus play major roles in this process.

Blood osmolality (oz-mohl-AL-*uh*-tee) refers to the amount of substances dissolved in blood. In response to low blood osmolality, the kidneys increase reabsorption of urea and uric acid into the blood. **Urea** (yoo-REE-*uh*, yoo-REY-*uh*) is a waste product resulting from protein breakdown, and **uric** (YOOR-ik) **acid** is a waste product resulting from the breakdown of nucleic acids (the chemicals that carry genetic information). As a result, water flows back into the blood vessels from the kidney tubules. This causes blood volume to expand and blood pressure to increase. The kidney also controls blood volume through the renin-angiotensin-aldosterone system, a feedback system that is covered later in this chapter.

Blood Composition

Keeping the proper balance of nutrients; minerals; and **electrolytes** (ih-LEK-*truh*-leyets), which are substances like sodium and potassium, in the blood is vital to maintaining homeostasis.

Blood Glucose

Blood glucose (GLOO-kohs), or blood sugar, is regulated by the pancreatic hormones **insulin** (IN-*suh*-lin) and **glucagon** (GLOO-*kuh*-gon). Insulin is released in response to high blood sugar levels. It lowers blood sugar levels by causing cells to take up more glucose. Glucagon is released in response to low blood sugar levels. It increases blood sugar by increasing the rate of **glycogenolysis** (GLEYE-*kuh-juhn*-awl-*uh*-sis). Glycogenolysis is the breakdown of sugar stores in the liver. The kidneys also play a role by increasing the amount of glucose reabsorbed from the urine.

Acid–Base Balance

Acid–base balance, or blood pH, refers to the amount of dissolved carbon dioxide and hydrogen ions found in the blood. The kidneys are the main organs that regulate acid–base balance. **Buffers** (BUHF-erz) are chemicals that help to maintain proper pH balance. The main buffers of blood pH are **bicarbonate** (beye-KAHR-*buh*-neyt) and **ammonium** (*uh*-MOH-nee-*uhm*). The kidney can increase or decrease the reabsorption of bicarbonate and excretion of hydrogen ions and ammonium to maintain acid–base balance.

The lungs and the respiratory center in the brain also play a role through respiratory compensation. The respiratory center senses the amount of carbon dioxide in the blood and changes the respiratory rate to affect how much carbon dioxide the lungs release into the air. This is one way the body compensates for too much acid in the blood.

Electrolytes

The main electrolytes in the blood are sodium, chloride, potassium, and phosphate. Electrolytes are ions, or charged particles, that are necessary elements in many vital processes. For example, potassium is required for proper conduction of the electrical impulses in the heart that produce the heartbeat. The kidney handles most of the regulation of blood electrolytes.

The kidney has specialized transporter proteins that help regulate the amount of electrolytes that are reabsorbed or excreted. Absorption of sodium and hydrogen are linked via a special transporter protein. Reabsorption of chloride is also linked to sodium reabsorption. Chloride is either actively reabsorbed via a special transporter protein, or passively follows the reabsorption of sodium. Phosphate is also absorbed along with sodium.

Fats

The medical term for fat is **lipid** (LIP-id, LEYE-pid). Fats from the diet are processed in the digestive tract, cross the intestinal wall, and are then taken up into the blood and lymphatics. Fats in the blood are transported in the form of **cholesterol** (*kuh*-les-*tuh*-rawl), fatty acids, and **triglycerides** (treye-glis-*uh*-reyedz). Most fats in the diet are triglycerides, which are large fat molecules. Triglycerides are too large to be transported across the intestinal wall. They are broken down in the intestine into smaller fat molecules, and then reformed as triglycerides once they cross the intestinal wall. The liver plays the main role in metabolizing and processing fats in the bloodstream and controls the amount of cholesterol in the blood. **Adipose** (ad-*uh*-pohs), or fat, **tissue** stores fat. The hormones insulin and glucagon also help regulate blood lipid levels.

DID YOU KNOW?

High-density lipoprotein (HDL), or "good" cholesterol, carries cholesterol to the liver for disposal. **Low-density lipoprotein (LDL)**, or "bad" cholesterol, is the form of cholesterol that circulates around the body, sometimes clogging up arteries.

Calcium

When blood calcium levels are too low, the **parathyroid** (par-*uh*-THEYE-roid) **glands** release parathyroid hormone. This hormone causes bones to release calcium and the intestines to increase their absorption of calcium, both of which raise blood calcium levels.

When blood calcium levels are too high, the thyroid releases **calcitonin** (kal-si-TOH-nin). This hormone causes bone cells to increase uptake of calcium, which lowers blood calcium levels.

The kidney also plays a part. When blood calcium levels are too high, the kidney reduces the amount of magnesium it reabsorbs. As a result, calcium reabsorption by the kidney decreases, which lowers blood calcium levels.

STUDY TIP

One way to remember what calcitonin does is to look at the word parts. *Calci-* refers to calcium, so you know calcitonin does something related to calcium. *Ton-* comes from the Greek *tonos,* which means tone. So calcitonin tones down calcium in the blood.

Iron Stores

Iron is important for proper red blood cell functioning. The **hemoglobin** (HEE-*muh*-gloh-bin) molecules in red blood cells contain iron that binds oxygen. Without enough iron, red blood cells cannot function properly in carrying out their task of transporting oxygen for use in vital processes. Conversely, too much iron can be toxic to many organs, especially the liver, heart, and digestive tract. Iron is stored in the form of **ferritin** (FER-i-tn) in the bone marrow, liver, and spleen. When iron stores are too low, iron absorption from the duodenum increases. Individual cells can also increase production of **transferrin** (trans-FER-in), which transports iron and increases the amount of iron taken into cells.

Hormones: Chemical Messengers

Hormones are chemical messengers that are released by one organ and travel via the bloodstream to act on another organ. Hormones released by organs in different parts of the body often work together in an axis.

Major endocrine axes in the body include the following:

- Hypothalamus-pituitary-adrenal axis
- Hypothalamic-pituitary-gonadal axis

• Hypothalamic-pituitary-thyroid axis
• Renin-angiotensin system

Hormonal axes often interact with each other via feedback loops or systems. Some feedback loops are positive feedback loops, meaning that the release of a certain hormone in the loop causes an increase in the release of other hormones in the loop. Other feedback loops are negative feedback loops, meaning that the release of a certain hormone in a loop causes a decrease in the release of other hormones in the loop.

An example of a feedback loop is the renin-angiotensin-aldosterone axis. When blood pressure is too low, certain cells in the kidney release **renin** (REE-nin, REH-nin), which activates the hormone **angiotensin** (an-jee-oh-TEN-sin). Angiotensin does several things:

• It constricts blood vessels to raise blood pressure.
• It causes the hypothalamus to increase the release of corticotropin-releasing hormone, which in turn causes the anterior pituitary gland to increase the release of ACTH (see following table).
• It induces the release of **antidiuretic** (an-tee-deye-*uh*-RET-ik) hormone (ADH), or **vasopressin** (vas-oh-PRES-in), from the posterior pituitary gland.

ACTH causes the adrenals to release **aldosterone** (al-DOS-*tuh*-rohn), which causes the kidneys to increase sodium reabsorption. ADH causes blood vessels to contract and the kidneys to reabsorb water. Increased water reabsorption and sodium reabsorption in the kidney consequently increase blood volume and blood pressure.

Hormones and Other Substances Involved in Homeostasis

Term	Pronunciation	Tissue Released From	Role
adrenocorticotropic hormone (ACTH)	*uh*-DREE-noh-cohr-ti-coh-TROH-pic HAWR-mohn	anterior pituitary gland	increases the release of cortisol from the adrenal glands, increases fat breakdown
atrial natriuretic peptide (ANP)	EY-tree-*uhl* ney-tree-*yoo*-REE-tic PEP-teyed	heart	reduces blood pressure
calcitriol	kal-SI-tree-awl	kidneys	active form of vitamin D, promotes intestinal absorption of calcium and renal absorption of phosphate

Term	Pronunciation	Tissue Released From	Role
cortisol	KAWR-t*uh*-sawl	adrenal glands	increases **gluconeo-genesis** (production of sugar), raises blood sugar, suppresses the immune system
epinephrine/ adrenaline	ep-*uh*-NEF-rin/ *uh*-DREN-l-in	adrenal glands	involved in fight-or-flight response; increases heart rate, blood pressure, oxygen supply to brain and muscles, blood glucose, fat breakdown, pupil dilation, sexual orgasm; inhibits digestion; suppresses immune system
erythropoietin	*uh*-rith-roh-poh-EE-tin	kidney	increases production of red blood cells in the bone marrow
growth hormone	GROHTH HAWR-mohn	anterior pituitary	promotes cell growth, raises blood sugar
norepinephrine (noradrenaline)	nawr-ep-*uh*-NEF-rin/ nawr-*uh*-DREN-l-in	adrenal glands	involved in fight-or-flight response: increases heart rate, blood pressure, oxygen supply to brain and muscles, blood glucose, fat breakdown, suppresses immune system
somatostatin	*soh*-mat-*uh*-STAT-n	pancreas, small intestine, hypothalamus	decreases release of insulin, glucagon, and digestive hormones; lowers blood sugar; slows digestion
thyroid hormone	THEYE-roid HAWR-mohn	thyroid	increases basal metabolic rate, increases body's response to stress hormones
thyroid-stimulating hormone	THEYE-roid STIM-y*uh*-leyt-ing HAWR-mohn	anterior pituitary	stimulates the thyroid to release thyroid hormones

The Least You Need to Know

- Homeostasis is the way the body stays in balance.
- Major processes that the body needs to keep in homoeostasis are body temperature, fluid volume, blood composition, calcium levels, iron levels, and blood clotting.
- Hormones are chemical messengers that help maintain homeostasis.
- Hormones work together in hormonal axes and interact with each other via negative and positive feedback loops.

Locomotion

In This Chapter

- Why we move the way we do
- How muscles contract
- What tendons, ligaments, and fascia do
- How the brain directs the body to respond to the environment

Life is full of movement made possible by different kinds of muscles. There are many types of muscles, and they all have different names. Skeletal muscle enables conscious control of the body. Cardiac muscle has amazing endurance and keeps the heartbeat going for a lifetime. Smooth muscle keeps vital processes like digestion and the circulation of the blood moving along.

Muscular contraction is an electrochemical process that occurs slightly differently in different types of muscle. Tendons, ligaments, and fascia are connective tissues that help muscles perform their jobs. The brain integrates many types of sensory information and tells the muscles what to do. At each step along the way, many medical terms describe what's going on.

Stance and Gait

Humans are **bipedal** (beye-PED-l), meaning that we stand upright and walk on two feet. Special adaptations in our skeleton help us do this. A curved lower spine; angled femur; and a short, broad pelvis all help support an upright posture and make bipedalism possible.

A disadvantage of bipedalism is that the shape of the pelvic bones provide a narrow birth canal relative to the size of the human baby's head. This mismatch is one of the main reasons for obstetrical difficulties that some women encounter during childbirth.

As a result of our upright, bipedal stance, humans have a striding gait. Each leg alternates between a swinging phase and a standing phase. The center of gravity shifts from one leg to the other during these phases. The **gluteus maximus** (GLOO-tee-*uhs* MAX-*uh-muhs*), butt muscle, on the side that happens to be in the standing phase provides stabilization.

> **DID YOU KNOW?**
>
> Variations from normal gait are sometimes used as clues in diagnosing certain illnesses. For example, a sign of Parkinson disease is a characteristic shuffling gait. In fact, this type of walking is called a **parkinsonian gait**. Sometimes it is also called **festination** (fes-*tuh*-NEY-*shuhn*), which comes from the Latin word *festinare*, meaning "to hurry." People with a parkinsonian gait look like they are hurrying because they have short stride lengths and tend to walk flat-footed. They also commonly walk with their upper bodies bent slightly forward. The parkinsonian gait is due to loss of brain cells in the midbrain that produce the neurotransmitter dopamine.

Skeletal Muscle Contractions

Muscles are made of the proteins **actin** (AK-tin), or thin filaments, and **myosin** (MEYE-*uh*-sin), or thick filaments. Muscular contraction happens when these two proteins make cross-bridges with each other. This process happens differently in different types of muscle.

As Chapter 5 explained, skeletal muscle is also called voluntary muscle. The contractions of skeletal muscle are under voluntary control and produce movements such as walking and running. The following sections describe the skeletal muscle structures and processes that produce these movements.

Skeletal Muscle Cells and Fibers

Skeletal muscle is made up of individual muscle cells called **myocytes** (MEYE-*uh*-seyets). During development, skeletal muscle myocytes fuse together to become

myofibers (MEYE-uh-FEYE-bers), which in turn are grouped together as **myofibrils** (MEYE-uh-FEYE-*bruhls*).

In myofibrils, the myosin and actin are grouped into regular patterns called **sarcomeres** (SAHR-*kuh*-meerz). The regular alternating pattern of myosin and actin give skeletal muscle a **striated** (STREYE-ey-tid), or striped, appearance under the microscope. Another term for skeletal muscle is striated muscle.

Though differences of opinion exist, there are at least two types of myosin. Type I, or slow-twitch, muscle fibers have **myoglobin** (MEYE-*uh*-gloh-bin), which makes these fibers appear red. Myoglobin binds oxygen, which is required for **aerobic** (ai-roh-bik, *uh*-roh-bik) metabolism. Type I muscle fibers are capable of generating sustained contractions because of aerobic metabolism. This type of muscle fiber does not fatigue easily. For this reason, endurance activities such as long-distance running use slow-twitch muscle fibers.

Type II, or fast-twitch, muscle fibers are white because they do not have myoglobin. They rely on both aerobic and **anaerobic** (an-*uh*-ROH-bik) metabolism. Anaerobic metabolism uses enzymatic reactions rather than oxygen to generate energy. Lactic acid, a by-product of anaerobic metabolism, builds up in type II muscle fibers and contributes to muscle fatigue. Because type II muscle fibers can generate quick bursts of energy, they are best suited for tasks demanding speed and power that is not sustained for long periods of time, such as sprinting. People are born with different proportions of fast-twitch and slow-twitch muscle fibers, which is why some people are natural-born sprinters while others are natural distance runners. To a certain extent, athletic training can change the proportion of fast-twitch to slow-twitch muscle fibers.

Types of Skeletal Muscles

Muscle fibers are arranged in parallel **fascicles** (FAS-i-*kuhlz*). These fascicles are arranged in different patterns to create different types of muscles. In **parallel muscles**, for example, fascicles run parallel to each other and function as one big muscle fiber. They can generate powerful, linear contractions, as in the biceps muscles of the arms.

In **convergent muscles**, fascicles have a common attachment and are arrayed in different directions. They can produce contractions in different directions, but they are not as powerful as parallel muscles. The pectoralis major muscle of the chest is an example of a convergent muscle.

Pennate (PEN-eyt) **muscles** have one or more tendons that run through the muscle and fan off at angles like feathers—pennate means feathered—from the tendon. Like parallel muscles, they can generate a lot of force. The quadriceps muscle of the thigh is an example of a pennate muscle.

Circular muscles are also called sphincter muscles because they lie around an opening. When they contract, they make the opening smaller, as in the external anal sphincter.

Steps from Action Potential to Muscle Contraction

In order for skeletal muscle to contract, the brain must generate an **action potential**, which is an electrical impulse that travels along nerve cells until it reaches a motor neuron. The motor neuron initiates a series of interactions involving sodium, calcium, potassium, and **acetylcholine** (*uh*-seet-l-KOH-leen), which is a neurotransmitter found between the motor neuron and the muscle cell. This neurotransmitter causes the action potential to spread throughout the skeletal muscle.

Calcium is vital to muscular contraction. Calcium released from the **sarcoplasmic reticulum** (SAHR-*kuh*-plaz-mik ri-TIK-*yuh*-*luhm*), where calcium is stored inside of skeletal muscle cells, causes the protein **troponin** (TROH-*puh*-nin) to change shape. This causes the protein **tropomyosin** (troh-poh-MEYE-sin) to move from the myosin binding site on actin. When this happens, myosin can form cross-bridges with actin. These cross-bridges shorten the muscles and produce a muscular contraction.

The muscular contraction lasts until the bridges between myosin and actin are broken. A molecule called **adenosine triphosphate** (*uh*-DEN-*uh*-seen treye-FOS-feyt), or ATP, stores energy for use in cellular processes. When ATP binds to myosin, it causes myosin to release actin. At the same time, calcium is pumped back into muscle cells, ready to be released again when the next action potential hits.

 WORD ORIGINS

In Latin, the word *rigor* means stiffness, and the word *mortis* means death. In medical terminology, the term **rigor mortis** (RIG-er MAWR-tis) refers to the stiffening of muscles after death. The calcium needed for muscles to contract must be pumped back into the cells to end the muscle contraction. Energy is required for this process, and oxygen is required to generate this energy. After death, cells lack the necessary oxygen to fuel the energy to pump calcium back into the cells to end the contraction. As a result, the muscles stiffen and stay in the contracted position.

Terms for Skeletal Muscle Contractions

Several medical terms describe skeletal muscle contractions. For example, **fasciculation** (*fuh*-sik-*yuh*-LEY-*shuhn*) is a minor involuntary twitch in part of a muscle. This type of twitch is mostly benign, but it can be an indication of a muscular disorder.

Myoclonus (meye-oh-KLOH-*nuhs*) refers to sudden, involuntary contractions or relaxations of an entire muscle or group of muscles. It is usually benign, as in the body jerks many people feel before falling sleep. Sometimes, it can indicate underlying disease, such as epilepsy or Huntington disease. A hiccup is a myoclonic contraction affecting only the diaphragm.

A **tic** is a nonrhythmic contraction of a single, or a few, muscle groups. It can be motor, involving movement only, or phonic, involving the production of sound. Tics are sometimes common in psychiatric disorders, such as Tourette syndrome. A **spasm** is a sudden contraction of a muscle or group of voluntary or involuntary muscles, usually accompanied by pain. It is also called a cramp. Examples include spasm in the calf muscle (charley horse) or spasms in the bile ducts (biliary colic).

A **tremor** is an involuntary, rhythmic contraction and relaxation of a single muscle. Tremors are common and can be benign—teeth chattering and shivering are examples of tremors. Tremors also can indicate underlying disease, such as hyperthyroidism or Graves disease.

Rapid contraction and relaxation of most of the muscles in the body is called a **convulsion** (*kuhn*-VUHL-*shuhn*). Convulsions are seen in epileptic seizures.

Dystonia (dis-TOH-nee-*uh*) is abnormal muscle tone due to sustained muscular contraction. It causes painful, twisting movements and postures. Dystonia is seen only in illness, disease, or as a reaction to certain medications such seizure medications.

Hypotonia (heyep-*uh*-TOH-nee-*uh*) is decreased muscle tone. Hypotonia is seen in genetic disorders like Down syndrome and acquired disorders like paralysis resulting from spinal cord trauma.

Tetanus (TET-n-*uhs*) is sustained contraction of a muscle fiber due to action potentials arriving so rapidly that the muscle cannot relax; it is the maximal amount of contraction of which a muscle is capable. This type of contraction is seen, as you might expect, in the disease tetanus (also known as lockjaw) or as a response to toxins or an overdose of some antipsychotic medications.

Dyskinesia (dis-ki-NEE-*zhuh*) refers to abnormal movements, difficulty initiating voluntary movements, and the presence of involuntary movements. It usually indicates an underlying medical condition such as the permanent side effects of long-term use of certain antipsychotic medications. **Chorea** (KAW-ree-*uh*) is a form of dyskinesia characterized by involuntary writhing dancelike movements (*chorea* means "to dance" in Greek). Chorea is commonly seen in Huntington disease.

Akathisia (ak-*uh*-THEEZH-*uh*) is a feeling of inner restlessness that produces an irresistible urge to move, as in pacing. This feeling is sometimes a side effect of certain seizure and psychiatric medications.

Ataxia (ey-TAK-see-*uh*) is a lack of coordination. Ataxia is characterized by disordered voluntary movements, often accompanied by poor balance. It is sometimes seen in neurological disorders and vitamin B$_{12}$ deficiency resulting from alcoholism.

Cardiac Muscle Contractions

Cardiac muscle is a special type of striated muscle found only in the heart muscle, or **myocardium** (meye-*uh*-KAHR-dee-*uhm*). Heart muscle is made up of muscle cells called **cardiomyocytes** (KAHR-dee-oh-meye-*uh*-seyets). Like skeletal muscle, heart muscle is made up of alternating actin and myosin, which gives cardiac muscle a striated appearance. Unlike skeletal muscle, the actin and myosin in cardiac muscle are not arranged in regular, parallel patterns.

Heart muscle is a type of involuntary muscle, meaning that it is not under conscious control. It does not need voluntary stimulation by the nervous system in order to contract, but instead relies on its own pacemaker (more about this in Chapter 12). The synchronized spread of action potentials generates the heartbeat.

Heart muscle has specializations that make it capable of generating the coordinated contractions necessary for the heartbeat. **Intercalated** (in-TUR-*kuh*-leyt-ed) discs connect cardiac muscle cells and enable rapid spread of the action potential throughout the myocardium. Gap junctions in intercalated discs allow **ions** (EYE-onz), or charged particles, to pass between cardiomyocytes. This is how the action potential spreads quickly throughout the myocardium.

Unlike skeletal muscle, which relies on the release of stores of intracellular calcium for contraction, cardiac muscle relies on extracellular calcium. Like skeletal muscle, the spread of the action potential throughout cardiac muscle cells involves the movement of sodium, potassium, and calcium across the cardiac muscle cell membranes. In cardiac muscle cells, calcium binds troponin, which enables actin–myosin cross-bridges to form and causes muscular contraction. Cardiac muscle has special membrane channels that prolong the movement of extracellular calcium stores across the cell membrane. The reliance on extracellular calcium extends the **refractory** (ri-FRAK-*tuh*-ree) period during which muscle cells are not able to contract. This protects the heart muscle from going into tetanus, or sustained, maximal contraction. It also gives the heart chamber enough time to fill with blood before the next heartbeat starts.

Heart muscle is a distinctive kind of tissue that is highly adapted to resist fatigue. Cardiomyocytes contain many **mitochondria** (meye-*tuh*-KON-dree-*uh*), which are the energy-generating structures inside cells. Mitochondria generate energy by producing ATP through aerobic metabolism. Cardiomyocytes also contain large amounts of myoglobin, which makes them reliant on oxygen for metabolism and helps them resist fatigue. The high concentrations of mitochondria and myoglobin in cardiac cells make them highly dependent on oxygen for proper functioning. This is the main vulnerability of the cardiac muscle: during **ischemic** (ih-SKEE-mik) conditions, when the oxygen supply to the heart is reduced, cardiac tissue is susceptible to damage.

Smooth Muscle

Smooth muscle is found in many of the body's visceral organs, such as the stomach, intestines, uterus, bladder, and the linings of the blood vessels. Smooth muscle is also called involuntary muscle because it is not under conscious control. Because smooth muscle does not appear striated under the microscope, it is also called nonstriated muscle.

Smooth muscle is classified as either single-unit or multiunit smooth muscle. Most smooth muscle found in the body is single unit. It exists as a **syncytium** (sin-SISH-*uhm*), which is like a bunch of cells fused together to create one continuous cell that is not separated by cell membranes and contains many nuclei. Because of this, single-unit smooth muscle cells contract and relax as one big unit. Examples of organs containing single-unit smooth muscles include the bladder and intestines. In multiunit smooth muscle, cells are not fused and can function separately. Examples of multiunit smooth muscle include the muscle lining the airways and blood vessels.

More than skeletal or cardiac muscle, smooth muscle is able to maintain elasticity while still being able to contract. This property is important for organs like the intestines and the lining of the urinary tract. An **extracellular matrix** (ek-*struh*-SEL-*yuh*-ler MEY-triks) is composed of **collagen** (KOL-*uh*-*juhn*), **elastin** (ih-LAS-tin),

proteoglycans (proh-tee-oh-GLEYE-kanz), and **glycoproteins** (gleye-koh-PROH-teenz) and contributes to the elasticity of smooth muscle.

As in cardiac muscle, the action potential spreads via gap junctions between smooth muscle cells. Contraction occurs as a result of the formation of cross-bridges between actin and myosin filaments. However, the mechanism is a little different in smooth muscle. Smooth muscle contractions use **calmodulin** (kal-MOJ-*uh*-lin) instead of the troponin. Calcium binds to calmodulin, which initiates a series of chemical reactions that enables myosin to bind actin. Contraction is maintained until ATP use and calcium levels drop.

Slower formation and breakage of cross-bridges between myosin and actin account for the long, sustained contractions of smooth muscle. Some smooth muscle contractions are termed **tonic** (TON-ik), or continuous, contractions. More rapid, powerful contractions are called **phasic** (FEYZ-ik), or rhythmic, contractions. Vascular smooth muscle produces tonic contractions in order to maintain the tone of the blood vessels. Peristalsis in the intestines is an example of phasic contractions.

The Role of Tendons, Ligaments, Fascia

Tendons (TEN-*duhnz*) attach muscle to bone, and **ligaments** (LIG-*uh-muhnts*) attach bone to bone or hold internal organs in place. **Fascia** (FA-*shuh*) connects muscle to muscle. All three are considered connective tissue, which provides support and protection to organs and tissues.

Tendons, ligaments, and fascia are made mostly of collagen. This extracellular protein provides strength and resilience. **Fibroblasts** (FEYE-*bruh*-blasts) make collagen, which is one of the most abundant proteins in the human body. It is also found in skin, bones, cartilage, some blood vessels, the cornea of the eye, and connective tissue of the internal organs. Tendons, ligaments, and fascia also contain elastin, which is a protein that allows them to stretch. Various other types of proteins provide nourishment, support, and strength to these tissues.

DID YOU KNOW?

Osteogenesis imperfecta (os-tee-*uh*-JEN-*uh*-sis im-pur-FEKT-*uh*) is a genetic disease that causes abnormal collagen synthesis. It is an autosomal-dominant disorder, meaning that it is passed from mother or father to offspring. People who receive at least one copy of the damaged gene inevitably develop the disorder. The disorder is characterized by deformed bones that break easily, weak muscles, loose joints, and sometimes hearing or breathing problems.

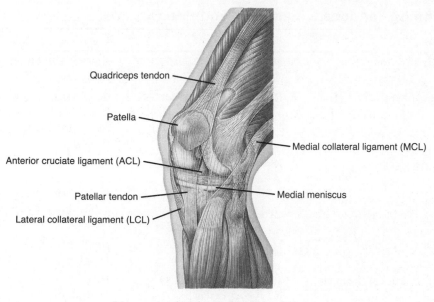

Ligaments and tendons help the knee function.
© Dorling Kindersley

An **aponeurosis** (ap-*uh*-noo-ROH-sis) is a broad sheet of connective tissue that is similar to a tendon. Aponeuroses are found in the ventral abdomen, the lower back, the palms of the hands, the soles of the feet, and the scalp.

In general, ligaments connect bone to bone and are capable of withstanding a large degree of tension or stress. Exceptions to this rule include **peritoneal** (per-i-tn-EE-*uhl*) ligaments, which are made of one layer of peritoneum that folds onto another layer of peritoneum. Peritoneal ligaments help support internal organs, such as the broad ligament of the uterus and many of the ligaments that support the intestines. **Periodontal** (per-ee-*uh*-DON-tl) ligaments are another exception: they connect teeth to bone.

Fetuses contain structures that are important for fetal development but that disappear in later life. During later development, these fetal structures close up and become ligamentous structures. These fetal remnant ligaments include the round ligament of the liver and medial umbilical ligaments.

Fascia is connective tissue that supports and wraps around muscles, blood vessels, and nerves. Fascia allows muscles to slide past each other. It provides a supportive wrapping to many internal organs and a flexible, movable environment for blood vessels and nerves.

Common Tendons, Ligaments, and Fascia

Name	Pronunciation	Location/Function
Achilles tendon	*uh*-KIL-eez TEN-*duhn*	attaches the calf muscles to the heel bone
iliotibial band	IL-ee-oh-TIB-ee-*uhl* BAND	tendon that runs from the lateral hip to the lateral knee, rotates the hip and stabilizes the knee
quadriceps tendon	KWOD-*ruh*-seps TEN-*duhn*	common tendon made up of the fusion of the four quadriceps muscle tendons, connects the quadriceps muscles to the lower leg
hamstring tendons	HAM-string TEN-*duhnz*	connect the three hamstring muscles to the back of the knee
anterior cruciate ligament (ACL)	an-TEER-ee-er KROO-shee-it LIG-*uh-muhnt*	front of the knee, stabilizes knee joint
posterior cruciate ligament (PCL)	po-STEER-ee-er KROO-shee-it LIG-*uh-muhnt*	back of the knee, stabilizes knee joint
medial collateral ligament (MCL) of the knee	MEE-dee-*uhl kuh*-LAT-er-*uhl* LIG-*uh-muhnt*	medial side of the knee, stabilizes knee joint
lateral collateral ligament (LCL) of the knee	LAT-er-*uhl kuh*-LAT-er-uhl LIG-uh-muhnt	lateral side of the knee, stabilizes knee joint
patellar ligament	p*uh*-TEL-er LIG-*uh-muhnt*	connects the kneecap to the tibia; holds the kneecap in place; sometimes called the patellar tendon because it lies within the quadriceps tendon
ulnar collateral ligament	UHL-ner *kuh*-LAT-er-*uhl* LIG-*uh-muhnt*	medial elbow; stabilizes elbow joint
radial collateral ligament	REY-dee-*uhl kuh*-LAT-er-*uhl* LIG-*uh-muhnt*	lateral elbow; stabilizes elbow joint
rotator cuff	ROH-tey-ter KUHF	group of four tendons that stabilize and move the shoulder joint
lateral collateral ligament of the ankle	LAT-er-*uh l kuh*-LAT-er-*uhl* LIG-*uh-muhnt*	group of three ligaments that support the lateral part of the ankle
deltoid ligament	DEL-toid	supports medial part of ankle

Name	Pronunciation	Location/Function
inguinal ligament	ING-*gwuh*-nl	runs from pubic bone to top of the hip bone; provides space through which nerve, blood vessels, and muscles run from the pelvis to the lower extremities; common area for hernias
broad ligament of the uterus	brawd	connects sides of uterus to pelvic wall
suspensory ligaments of the breast	*suh*-SPEN-*suh*-ree	run from clavicle to the breast, also called Cooper ligaments
pericardium	per-i-KAHR-dee-*uhm*	fascia that surrounds the heart
fascia lata	FASH-*uh* LAH-*tuh*	fascia that surrounds the thigh muscles

WORDS OF WARNING

Many knee injuries are the result of a torn medial or lateral **meniscus** (mi-NIS-*kuhs*). The **menisci** (mi-NIS-eye, mi-NIS-keye) of the knee lie on the medial (inside) and lateral (outside) of the knee. *Meniscus* means crescent in Greek, which refers to the crescent shape of these structures. Knee menisci are cartilaginous structures that lie between the tibia and the femur. The menisci provide cushioning and decrease friction between these two bones.

Sensorimotor Integration

Sensorimotor (sen-*suh*-ree-MOH-ter) **integration** refers to how the brain integrates various sensory inputs into a coherent whole and directs the body's response to these inputs. Chapter 9 highlighted the organs involved in the basic senses: hearing, taste, sight, touch, and smell. The brain also receives signals regarding **proprioception** (proh-pree-*uh*-SEP-*shuhn*), or the sense of one's body position in space, and **vestibular** (ve-STIB-*yuh*-ler) sense, or the sense of movement and balance. An example of sensorimotor integration is hand–eye coordination.

Sensorimotor integration starts with the activation of sensory nerves by some kind of stimulus in the environment. The sensory nerves send signals to the brain, which integrates them and sends signals via an upper motor neuron in the central nervous system. The signals are passed to the muscles via lower motor neurons in the peripheral nervous system.

The Least You Need to Know

- Special adaptations in the human skeleton make human bipedal locomotion possible.
- Muscle contraction occurs when cross-bridges form between actin and myosin.
- Striated, cardiac, and smooth muscle have different ways of contracting that make them suited for the tasks they perform.
- Tendons, ligaments, and fascia are all types of connective tissue that provide support and structure to muscles and bones.
- Sensorimotor integration is how the brain integrates sensory signals from the environment and tells the body how to respond.

Circulation and Breathing

In This Chapter

- Understanding the role of heart valves in pumping blood
- Learning how the heart beats
- Inhaling, exhaling, and gas exchange in the lungs
- Measuring lung volumes and estimating lung capacity

The heart and lungs work together to get oxygen and vital substances to the tissues, and carry waste products away from them. The heart pumps the blood where it needs to go. The lungs make sure there is enough oxygen in the blood to keep the body going.

The heart is an endurance athlete that can keep going on its own steam, independent of the brain, because it has its own electrical pacemaker. There are many medical terms that describe the structures and processes that make the heartbeat possible.

The lungs are like bellows inside the chest. Air flows in and out due to pressure gradients. Measuring the amount of air that flows into and out of the lungs, and how much air the lungs can hold, is an important way that medical professionals estimate the health of the lungs. For this reason, many medical terms are associated with lung measurements.

The Heart as a Pump

The heart is one of the first organs to form. The heartbeat can usually be detected at about 21 days after conception and continues throughout life. The heart generates almost all the force necessary to push the blood through the body's blood vessels.

The blood vessels contribute their part by maintaining or changing their tone in response to the force generated by the heartbeat and changes in blood volume.

Recall from Chapter 6 that the heart has four chambers: the right and left atria and the right and left ventricles. The right and left sides of the heart are separated by a thick **septum** (SEP-*tuhm*). Blood flows from the right side of the heart to the lungs (cardiopulmonary circulation), and from the left side of the heart to the rest of the body (systemic circulation). Blood flows from the lungs through the pulmonary vein to the heart, then through the left atrium, through the left ventricle, and finally out the aorta to the rest of the body. Blood from the body returns to the heart through the superior and inferior vena cavae, and then flows through the right atrium into the right ventricle. From there blood flows through the pulmonary arteries back to the lungs.

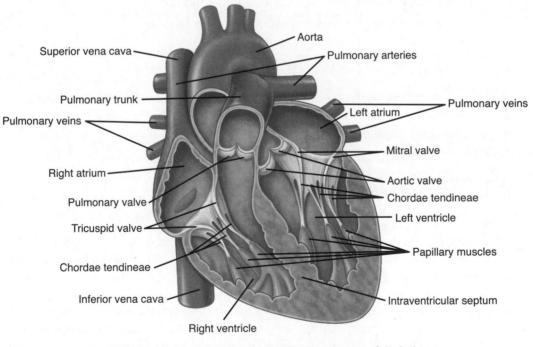

The heart's valves help it to pump blood to the rest of the body.
© Dorling Kindersley

The heart's main role in the body is to act as a pump. Various structures contribute to this role by enabling the heart to build up force across pressure gradients.

The **tricuspid** (treye-KUHS-pid) **valve** lies between the right atrium and right ventricle. The **mitral** (MEYE-*truhl*) **valve** lies between the left atrium and left ventricle. It is also called the **bicuspid** (beye-CUSP-*id*) valve. Together these valves are called **atrioventricular** (EY-tree-oh-ven-TRIK-*yuh*-ler) **valves** or **AV valves** because they both lie between the atria and ventricles.

Papillary (PAP-*uh*-ler-ee) **muscles** attach the mitral and tricuspid valves to the side of the ventricles. These muscles contract to keep the valves closed and prevent **prolapse** (PROH-laps), or collapse, of the valves. **Chordae tendineae** (kawr-dee TEN-*duhn*-ee-uh, KAWR-dey TEN-*duhn*-ey-uh) connect the papillary muscles to the tricuspid and mitral valves. These are also called heartstrings.

The **aortic** (ey-AWR-tik) **valve** lies between the left ventricle and the aorta. The **pulmonary** (PUHL-*muh*-ner-ee) **valve** lies between the right ventricle and pulmonary artery. These valves are commonly called **semilunar** (sem-ee-LOO-ner, sem-eye-LOO-ner) **valves** because both have **cusps** (kuhsps), or valve leaflets, that are shaped like half-moons.

STUDY TIP

Knowing the meaning of word parts can help you understand the heart valves. *Cusp* means point and refers to the leaflets of the valves. *Tri-* means three, so *tricuspid* valve means a valve with three points, or three leaflets. Similarly, *bicuspid* valve means a valve with two points, or two leaflets. Because the hat worn by a church bishop, a miter, looks similar to the bicuspid valve (both have two pointed leaflets joined front to back), the bicuspid valve is also called the mitral valve. *Atrio-* refers to the atrium, and *ventricular* refers to the ventricles, so the atrioventricular valves lie between the atria and ventricles. *Semi-* means half, and *lunar* means moon. So *semilunar* valves look like half-moons.

The Cardiac Cycle

The term **cardiac cycle** refers to the sequence of events that must occur to produce the heartbeat. The cardiac cycle has different phases. During **diastole** (deye-AS-tl-ee), the heart is relaxed. Blood flows into and fills the heart during diastole. During **systole** (SIS-*tuh*-lee), the heart muscle is actively contracting and pushing blood into the systemic circulation. Diastole and systole are separated into different phases during which specific electrical impulses are transmitted to different parts of the heart to coordinate contraction. The closing of the valves during certain parts of these phases correspond to the familiar "lub-dub" sound of the heart.

Electrical Stimulation of the Heart

Heart muscle is **myogenic** (meye-*uh*-JEN-ik), which means that it can generate its own electrical impulses needed for contraction without being dependent on the brain for stimulation. Input from the sympathetic and parasympathetic nervous systems and from various hormones, emotions, and physical activity can affect the heart rate. But the heart is not dependent on these factors in order to keep going.

The heart has its own pacemaker, called the **sinoatrial** (SEYE-noh-EY-tree-*uhl*) **node**, or SA node. The SA node lies at the top of the right atrium, near the superior vena cava. It generates sinus rhythm, or the pattern exhibited by a normal heartbeat. The SA node also receives parasympathetic innervation from the **vagus** (VEY-*guhs*) **nerve**, which can slow down the heartbeat. But the SA node is not dependent on the vagus nerve for the initiation of electrical impulses that cause the heartbeat.

WORD ORIGINS

The term *vagus nerve* comes from the Latin term *vagus*, which means wandering. Similar terms in English, like *vagabond* and *vague*, also share this Latin root. This name is appropriate for the vagus nerve because it basically wanders all over the body and relays information to the brain about what's going on with the internal organs. In addition to carrying sensory information from many of the body's internal organs, the vagus nerve carries some motor, sympathetic, and parasympathetic nerve fibers. The vagus nerve provides neural input for controlling many activities, such as the heart rate, intestinal peristalsis, sweating, talking, and keeping the airway open during breathing.

Electrical signals initiated in the SA node spread from cell to cell throughout the right and left atria until they reach the AV node. The AV node lies between the atria and ventricles. It serves as a backup pacemaker of the heart in case the SA node stops functioning properly. The AV node slows down the electrical impulses received from the atria, allowing the atria time to fill with blood before contracting and filling the ventricles with blood. This node also helps coordinate ventricular contraction so that the ventricles contract in synchrony.

The electrical impulses travel from the AV node through various conducting tissues to initiate ventricular contraction. First, the impulses travel through the **bundle of His** (HISS), then through the left and right bundle branches, and finally ending in **Purkinje** (pur-KIN-jee) **fibers**, which stimulate the right and left ventricles to contract at the same time. Carefully coordinated contraction is important for the heart to properly and efficiently carry out its role of pumping blood throughout the body.

Atrial Systole

Atrial systole refers to the time during which the atria are contracting but the ventricles have not yet begun to do so. The time during which the atria contract slightly before the ventricles appears as the P wave on the electrocardiogram (ECG). Ventricular filling is mostly due to passive flow down pressure gradients from the atria to the ventricles. The earlier contraction of the atria wrings the last bits of blood from the atria into the ventricles and is called the **atrial kick**.

When the pressure in the ventricles exceeds the pressure in the atria, the AV valves close. This corresponds to the first heart sound, or the "lub," which is also called S1. Closure of the AV valves causes pressure to build even more in the ventricles. At about the same time, the ventricles begin to contract, which causes yet more pressure to build.

Ventricular Systole

The period during which the ventricles contract and the AV valves close is called **ventricular systole**. Contraction of the ventricles is due to spread of electrical impulses throughout the ventricles and corresponds to the QRS complex on the ECG.

The period when the ventricles are contracting and the aortic valve and AV valves are closed is called **isovolumetric** (EYE-soh-vol-*yuh*-ME-trik) **ventricular contraction time**. Recall that *iso-* means "the same," so **isovolumetric** refers to maintaining the same volume.

When pressure in the ventricles exceeds pressure in the aorta and pulmonary vein, the semilunar valves open and blood flows from the ventricles to the lungs and the rest of the body. This phase of ventricular systole is called the ejection phase.

Several terms refer to the amount of blood pumped by the ventricles during the ejection phase. These measurements are used to assess and monitor the severity and progression of various cardiac conditions. For example, **cardiac output** refers to the volume of blood ejected in 1 minute. **Ejection fraction** refers to the fractional volume of blood pumped out of the ventricles during the ejection phase of the cardiac cycle. Diseased hearts are not able to efficiently pump out blood, which leaves some pooled in the ventricle and decreases the ejection fraction. **Stroke volume** refers to the volume of blood pumped out of each ventricle during the ejection phase.

At the end of ventricular systole when there is little blood left in the ventricles, pressure in the ventricles drops. When pressure in the aorta and pulmonary vein exceed pressure in the ventricles, the semilunar valves close. This action corresponds to the second heart sound, or the "dub," which is also called S2.

DID YOU KNOW?

Unlike the first heart sound, the second heart sound often occurs asynchronously, which can make it sound like there are three heart sounds (think "lub-dub-dub, three men in a tub"). This is called a **split S2**. It happens because the aortic valve closes slightly earlier than the pulmonary valve. A split S2 is often completely normal. It can be heard only during inhalation, and is most common in young, physically fit people. Sometimes, however, a split S2 indicates underlying cardiac disease. The electrical conducting system in the heart may be damaged, causing the pulmonary valve to close before the aortic valve. This condition is called a **paradoxically split S2**.

During the last part of systole, the ventricles **repolarize** (ree-POH-*luh*-reyez), which is the recovery period during which the ventricles prepare for generating the next heartbeat. During this time, the ventricular muscles are **refractory** (ri-FRAK-*tuh*-ree) and are not able to contract. The time during which the ventricles repolarize corresponds to the T wave on the ECG.

Diastole

During early diastole the entire heart is relaxed. The term **isovolumetric ventricular relaxation time** refers to the time when the ventricle is relaxed and both the AV valves and the semilunar valves are closed. When pressure from buildup of blood in the atria exceeds the pressure in the ventricles, the AV valves open. When this happens, blood flows passively from the atria and fills the ventricles. The pulmonary and aortic valves are both closed at this point, allowing for the buildup of pressure as the ventricles fill.

More Terms Associated with the Heartbeat

Several medical terms describe what happens when the heart beats abnormally. These terms include the following:

- **Asystole** (ey-SIS-*tuh*-lee) is when the cardiac muscle can no longer generate electrical activity and stops contracting. This corresponds to a flat line on the ECG.

- **Arrhythmia** (ey-RITII-mee-*uh*) is an irregular heartbeat.
- **Tachycardia** (tak-ee-KAHR-dee-*uh*) is an abnormally fast heartbeat.
- **Bradycardia** (brad-ee-KAHR-dee-*uh*) is an abnormally slow heartbeat.
- **Fibrillation** (feye-*bruh*-LEY-*shuhn*) is uncontrolled, irregular contractions in the atria or ventricles caused by electrical impulses that don't originate in the normal cardiac pacemakers.
- **Flutter** is a fast heartbeat resulting from prematurely generated, self-perpetuating electrical impulses. It can occur in the atria or ventricles.
- **Heart block**, also known as AV nodal block, occurs when electrical impulses are slowed or cannot conduct through the AV node.

Respiratory Physiology

Human respiration involves breathing air into the lungs, where oxygen moves into the bloodstream for distribution to tissues. Carbon dioxide and other waste products move from the blood into the lungs, where they are exhaled into the environment. Respiration consists of two main processes: gas transport and breathing control.

Gas Transport

Recall from Chapter 6 that air usually enters the body through the nose, goes down the pharynx and trachea, and then flows through the bronchi and bronchioles until it reaches the alveoli. The alveoli are small sacs in the lung specialized for gas exchange.

A rich network of capillary beds surround the alveoli. Both the capillaries and alveoli have very thin walls that directly abut each other. This arrangement allows for simple gas diffusion between the alveoli and pulmonary capillaries.

Gas flows into and out of the alveoli across pressure gradients. During inhalation, pressure is greater in the alveoli than in the capillaries, so gas flows from the alveoli into the capillaries. During exhalation, pressure is greater in the capillaries than in the alveoli, so gas flows from the capillaries into the alveoli.

Surfactant (ser-FAK-*tuhnt*) is a substance that increases surface tension and helps alveoli stay inflated. If there is insufficient surfactant, the alveoli collapse and cannot properly function in air exchange. This condition is called **atelectasis** (at-l-EK-*tuh*-sis). It can occur for various reasons, including trauma, infection, or scarring resulting from illnesses like pneumonia.

The respiratory system also contains various immune cells and lymphoid tissue that produces mucus, which lubricates the airways and traps foreign particles. **Cilia** (SIL-ee-*uh*), or small hairlike projections, line the trachea and sweep foreign objects, mucus, and bacteria away from the lungs. Cilia can be damaged by certain activities, such as smoking, which can put the lungs at risk for infection. Stopping the damaging activity gives the cilia a chance to grow back.

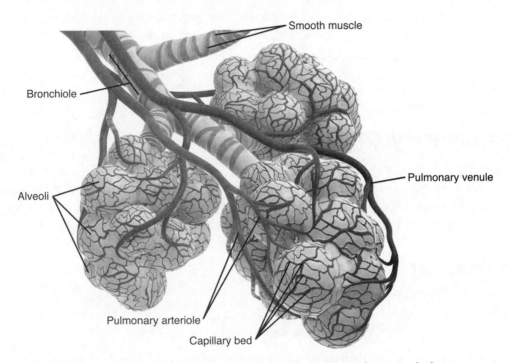

The alveoli have a rich blood supply and specialize in gas exchange in the lung.
© Dorling Kindersley

Medical terms that refer to the gas exchange involved in respiration include the following:

- **Ventilation** is the movement of gases into and out of the lungs.
- **Pulmonary gas exchange** is the transfer of waste gases from the pulmonary capillaries into the alveoli, and the transfer of oxygen from the alveoli to the pulmonary capillaries.
- **Gas transport** is the movement of gases from the lungs to the tissues and the movement of gases from the tissues back to the lungs.

- **Peripheral gas exchange** is the transfer of waste gases from the tissues into the peripheral capillaries, and the transfer of oxygen from the peripheral capillaries to the tissues.

Breathing Control

Human respiration is a semivoluntary process. Respiration can be consciously controlled by activation of various accessory muscles of respiration. Involuntary respiration is controlled by the respiratory center located in the medulla and pons of the brain stem. Carbon dioxide, oxygen, and acid concentrations in the blood are sensed by chemoreceptors in the aorta and carotid arteries. The respiratory center in the brain interprets these signals and changes the respiratory rate accordingly.

For example, when the carbon dioxide concentration is too high, the respiratory rate increases so that the lungs can blow off the excess carbon dioxide. Exercise, increased body temperature, and stress-related hormones like adrenaline also increase respiratory rate. Irritant and stretch receptors in the lungs signal to the brain when involuntary exhalation should occur. This often occurs in response to inhaled irritants and results in coughing.

Inhalation (in-*huh*-LEY-*shuhn*), or breathing in air, begins when the diaphragm contracts. Inhalation is also sometimes called **inspiration** (in-sp*uh*-REY-*shuhn*). The diaphragm is innervated by the **phrenic** (FREN-ik) **nerve**, which carries nerve fibers for the sensory, motor, and sympathetic nervous systems. The presence of sympathetic nerve fibers means that the diaphragm can be stimulated to contract in response to signals from the sympathetic nervous system, like the fight-or-flight response that causes the respiratory rate to increase.

The contraction of the diaphragm expands the rib cage, which pushes down the abdominal organs. This movement creates more space in the thoracic cavity and increases the volume of the lungs. When the lung volume increases, pressure inside the lungs is lower than atmospheric pressure. Air flows into the lungs as a consequence of this pressure difference, from the high pressure outside the body to the low pressure inside the body.

Voluntary inhalation is called forced inhalation. Several accessory muscles of inhalation contract and further expand the rib cage. These include the external intercostal muscles, several muscles in the neck, and sometimes the pectoralis muscles of the chest.

Exhalation (eks-*huh*-LEY-*shuhn*), or the movement of air out of the lungs, occurs passively as a result of the lungs' normal elastic recoil. During inhalation, the lungs are stretched, which causes elastic energy to build up. When the diaphragm stops contracting at the end of inhalation, the abdominal organs return to their previous positions, and the size of the thoracic cavity decreases. In turn, the lungs spring back to their previous size, forcing air out of the lungs.

Forced, or voluntary, exhalation occurs as a result of contracting the internal inter-costal muscles and some of the abdominal muscles, which pushes air out of the lungs. Voluntary control over exhalation is important for many activities. Speech can occur only during exhalation. Changing the rate of exhalation modulates tone, pitch, and volume of speech.

> **DID YOU KNOW?**
>
> The word *yawn* comes from an Old English word *geonian*, which means "to open the mouth wide." Yawning is considered to be a reflex that is nonrespiratory, even though it involves the respiratory system. Although many theories exist, no one really knows why we yawn. There is wide agreement that yawning can be contagious and often occurs in response to fatigue or boredom. More recent theories hold that yawning may occur in response to high carbon dioxide levels in the blood, as a way to control brain temperature, or in response to stress or emotions. Yawning while stretching is called **pandiculation** (pan-dik-yuh-LEY-*shuhn*), which comes from the Latin word *pandere*, meaning "to stretch."

Lung Volumes and Capacity

Lung volumes refer to how much air enters, leaves, and stays in the lungs during inhalation and exhalation. Lung volumes can be directly measured using **spirometry** (speye-ROM-i-tree). Lung capacity, however, cannot be measured directly. It is inferred from lung volumes and refers to the amount of air the lungs are capable of holding.

Humans only use a small proportion of their total lung volume, about 4 to 6 liters during normal respiration. Lung volumes and capacities are affected by many factors, including body type, geographical location, and lifestyle. Men and people who are tall, thin, or physically active, or who live at high altitudes, tend to have larger lung volumes. Women and people who are short or overweight, or who smoke or live at low altitudes, tend to have smaller lung volumes.

Several terms describe respiratory ventilation:

- **Minute ventilation** is the amount of gas inhaled or exhaled in 1 minute, also called respiratory minute volume.

- **Alveolar** (al-VEE-*uh*-ler) **ventilation** is the amount of gas exchanged at the level of the alveolus.

- **Dead space ventilation** is the amount of gas that remains in the airways (dead space) and does not participate in gas exchange.

Lung Volume and Capacity Terms

Term	Abbreviation	Meaning
total lung capacity	TLC	total volume of air the lungs are capable of holding at maximal inhalation
tidal volume	TV	amount of air that moves into and out of the lungs during normal breathing
residual volume	RV	amount of air left in the lungs after maximal exhalation
expiratory reserve volume	ERV	amount of additional air that can be forcibly expelled from the lungs at the end of the exhalation cycle
inspiratory reserve volume	IRV	amount of additional air that can be inhaled into the lungs at the end of the inhalation cycle
inspiratory capacity	IC	the total amount of air that the lung is capable of inhaling
inspiratory vital capacity	IVC	the total amount of air that can be inhaled after a maximal exhalation
vital capacity	VC	the total amount of air that can be exhaled from the lungs after maximal inhalation
functional residual capacity	FRC	amount of air left in the lungs after normal exhalation
forced vital capacity	FVC	estimation of vital capacity after maximal forcible exhalation
forced expiratory volume	FEV	amount of air that can be forcibly exhaled from the lungs in a certain amount of time

The Least You Need to Know

- The heart has its own pacemaker that allows it to independently create the electrical stimulus for the heartbeat.
- Force for the heartbeat is created by contractions of the cardiac muscle and across pressure gradients created by the opening and closing of heart valves.
- Respiratory inhalation is an active process created mostly by contracting the diaphragm.
- Respiratory exhalation is a passive process produced by the elastic recoil of the lungs.
- Lung volumes and capacities are ways to measure how much air the lungs can hold, as well as air movement into and out of the lungs.

Metabolism and Elimination

In This Chapter

- How food becomes energy
- What enzymes and hormones do to aid digestion
- Where nutrients are absorbed and how waste is eliminated
- How the liver and kidneys detoxify waste

The human body needs energy to carry out its tasks. This energy comes from metabolism, which either breaks down foods to release energy or stores energy in chemical bonds for later use. Digestion is the main process by which the body gets energy from food. Many medical terms are related to digestion. For example, the specific enzymes and hormones involved in this process are numerous.

Some substances can't be metabolized and must be eliminated from the body before they can build up and become toxic. The liver and kidney play major roles in detoxification and elimination. Many medical illnesses cause problems with detoxification and elimination, so it is important to know the medical terms associated with these processes.

Metabolism

Metabolism refers to the process by which energy is extracted from, or converted into, substances that the body can use. Chemical reactions within cells drive metabolism.

Metabolism is made of up two broad categories: catabolism and anabolism. **Catabolism** (*kuh*-TAB-*uh*-liz-*uhm*) is a process that uses energy to break down substances in order to use the energy stored in chemical bonds within these substances. One example of a catabolic process is **glycolysis** (gleye-KOL-*uh*-sis), which breaks down carbohydrates. Instead of breaking down substances, the processes in **anabolism** (*uh*-NAB-*uh*-liz-*uhm*) use energy to build substances in order to store energy in chemical bonds. For example, **gluconeogenesis** (gloo-koh-nee-*uh*-JEN-*uh*-sis) builds carbohydrates from the body's energy stores. **Lipogenesis** (leyp-*uh*-JEN-*uh*-sis) builds fat molecules.

The chemicals involved in metabolism are transformed via metabolic pathways into other chemicals. **Enzymes** (EN-zeyemz) are proteins that play a major role in metabolic pathways. Enzymes work as **catalysts** (KAT-*uh*-lists), which means that they speed up chemical reactions or cause chemical changes that make these reactions possible. Some of the chemical reactions in metabolism are common in many different types of organisms. The citric acid cycle is one of these common metabolic pathways. It is found in almost every living creature, from unicellular bacteria, to whales, to humans.

Biochemical Terms Used in Metabolic Processes

Term	Pronunciation	Meaning
adenosine triphosphate (ATP)	*uh*-den-*uh*-seen treye-FOS-feyt, *uh*-DEEN-*uh*-seen treye-FOS-feyt	main coenzyme used in metabolism, stores energy for use in metabolic reactions
amino acid	*uh*-MEE-noh AS-id	the building block of proteins
carbohydrate	kahr-boh-HEYE-dreyt, kahr-*buh*-HEYE-dreyt	the building block of sugars
coenzyme	koh-EN-zeyem	compound that is bound to an enzyme and helps it carry out its role of enabling chemical reactions; an example is ATP
DNA	DEE-EN-EY	double-stranded nucleic acid that contains genetic information
electron transport chain	ih-LEK-tron	group of cell membrane proteins that help form ATP
lipid	LIP-id, LEYE-pid	fat
macromolecule	MAK-roh-MOL-*uh*-kyool	large molecule

Term	Pronunciation	Meaning
mineral	MIN-er-*uhl*	charged electrical particle (electrolyte) that plays an important role in electrical impulse conduction, like nerve transmission and muscle contraction; examples are sodium, potassium, chloride, calcium, magnesium
monosaccharide	mon-*uh*-SAK-*uh*-reyed	simple carbohydrate unit, like glucose
polymer	POL-*uh*-mer	several different biochemical compounds joined together in repeating units
polysaccharide	pol-ee-SAK-*uh*-reyed	complex sugar made up of many repeating monosaccharides, like starch
RNA	AHR-EN-EY	single-stranded nucleic acid that contains the genetic information needed for making proteins
vitamin	VEYE-*tuh*-min	a compound that cells cannot make on their own; after modification, vitamins function as coenzymes to assist in metabolic reactions

The Digestive Process and the Role of Enzymes

Digestion (dih-JES-*chuhn*, deye-JES-*chuhn*) is an example of catabolism. Digestion breaks down large molecules into smaller ones through mechanical means, such as chewing, and chemical reactions. Enzymes secreted by digestive organs help break down large molecules in food into smaller molecules that can cross the lining of the digestive tract.

DID YOU KNOW?

Cooking is sometimes thought of as one of the initial steps in the digestive process. Cooking breaks down hard-to-digest foods, such as raw meat and tough, fibrous vegetables, so that the human body can extract more nutrients from them. Some cooking techniques even detoxify potentially harmful foods. For example, taro, a staple food in Southeast Asia and the Pacific Islands, is toxic when raw. Cooking destroys the toxin so that taro can be used as a source of nourishment.

Digestion involves at least four stages in humans. **Ingestion** (in-JEST-*chuhn*) occurs when food is taken into the mouth, where it enters the digestive system. The next stage is **mastication** (MAS-ti-key-*shuhn*) and **deglutition** (dee-gloo-TISH-*uhn*)—that is, chewing and swallowing. In the mouth, food is masticated and formed into a **bolus** (BOH-*luhs*), or ball, for deglutition and further chemical and mechanical digestion in the rest of the digestive tract. The third stage of digestion, **absorption** (ab-ZAWRP-*shuhn*), occurs when substances move via active transport, diffusion, or osmosis into the bloodstream and lymphatics.

In the final stage of digestion, **excretion** (ik-SKREE-*shuhn*), waste products leave the body. **Defecation** (DEF-i-key-*shuhn*), also rarely called **egestion** (ih-JES-*chuhn*), is the excretion of solid waste. **Urination** (YOOR-*uh*-ney-*shuhn*), also called **micturition** (mik-*chuh*-RISH-*uhn*), is the excretion of liquid waste.

Role of Enzymes in Digestion

Different categories of enzymes help break down different types of nutrients during digestion. These categories include the following:

- **Protease** (PROH-tee-eys) helps break down proteins.
- **Glycoside hydrolase** (GLEYE-*kuh*-seyed HEYE-*druh*-leys) helps break down carbohydrates.
- **Transaminase** (trans-AM-*uh*-neys) participates in the breakdown of proteins in the urea cycle.
- **Lipase** (LEYE-peys) helps digest fats.
- **Nucleosidase** (noo-klee-*uh*-SEYE-deys) helps digest nucleic acids, also called a **nuclease** (NOO-klee-eys).

STUDY TIP

Looking at the word parts will help you figure out whether a word is an enzyme. The suffix *-ase* is commonly used to refer to enzymes. Another suffix that is used for enzymes is *-in*. However, be aware that *–in* is used for other substances that are also made of proteins, such as hormones.

The chemical breakdown of carbohydrates and a certain amount of fats begins in the mouth, and protein digestion begins in the stomach. But the majority of the chemical breakdown of food takes place when stomach **chyme** (KEYEM) is released into the small intestine. Chyme is a semiliquid mass of partially digested food. At each step along the way, the organs of the digestive tract secrete different enzymes and other substances that help break down the different nutrients found in food.

Major Enzymes in Digestion

Term	Pronunciation	Secreted by	Function
salivary amylase	SAL-*uh*-ver-ee AM-*uh*-leys	salivary glands	enzyme that begins digestion of polysaccharides (complex carbohydrates)
lingual lipase	LING-*gwuhl* LEYE-peys, LIP-eys	salivary glands	enzyme that begins fat breakdown
hydrochloric acid (HCl)	heye-*druh*-KLOHR-ik AS-id	parietal cells in stomach	acid that lowers stomach pH and makes stomach juices acidic for better digestion
intrinsic factor	in-TRIN-zik FAK-ter	parietal cells of stomach	protein that helps vitamin B_{12} to be absorbed later in the GI tract
pepsin	PEP-sin	chief cells of the stomach	enzyme that breaks down proteins
pepsinogen	pep-SIN-*uh*-jen	chief cells of the stomach	precursor form of pepsin
bile	BEYEL	produced in the liver, stored in the gallbladder, released into the small intestine via the bile ducts	fluid that emulsifies (ih-muhl-*suh*-feyez) fats (makes fats easier to digest) and raises the acidity level of chyme released from the stomach
pancreatic amylase	PAN-kree-at-ik AM-*uh*-leys	pancreas	enzyme that digests carbohydrates
pancreatic lipase	PAN-kree-at-ik LEYE-peys, LIP-eys	pancreas	enzyme that digests fats
trypsin	TRIP-sin	pancreas	enzyme that breaks down proteins in the small intestine
trypsinogen	trip-SIN-*uh*-jen	pancreas	zymogen (enzyme precursor) that activates trypsin

continues

Major Enzymes in Digestion (continued)

Term	Pronunciation	Secreted by	Function
chymotrypsin	keye-moh-trip-SIN	pancreas	enzyme that breaks down proteins in the small intestine
chymotrypsinogen	keye-moh-trip-SIN-*uh*-jen	pancreas	enzyme precursor of chymotrypsin
enteropeptidase, also called enterokinase	en-teyr-oh-PEP-ti-deys, en-teyr-oh-KEYE-neys	duodenum of small intestine	enzyme that converts trypsinogen to trypsin
lactase	LAK-teys	small intestine	enzyme that converts lactose to simple sugars like glucose and galactose
maltase	MAWL-teys	small intestine	enzyme that converts maltose to simple sugars like glucose
sucrase	SOO-kreys	small intestine	enzyme that converts sucrose to simple sugars like glucose

WORD ORIGINS

Precursor (inactive) enzymes are called **zymogens** (ZEYE-muh-*juhnz*). The term derives from the word root for enzyme, *zyme*, and the suffix *-gen*. *Zyme* comes from the Greek word *enzymos,* which means leavened. An obsolete medical theory held that many infectious diseases were due to organisms that caused fermentation in the body, like the fermentation of yeast that leavens bread. The suffix *-gen* comes from the Greek word *genes*, which means born. So zymogen refers to a substance that causes an enzyme to be born, or produced.

Digestive Hormones

Like most processes in the human body, digestive enzymes need to be regulated so that they don't go to work when they're not needed. Hormones help regulate digestive enzymes.

Food in the stomach stimulates the stomach's G cells to secrete **gastrin** (GAS-trin). This hormone triggers parietal cells to produce gastric juice (HCl, potassium chloride) and the gastric glands to secrete pepsinogen. D cells in the stomach secrete

somatostatin (soh-mat-*uh*-STAT-n), a hormone that activates the stomach's G cells to stimulate parietal cells, which in turn produce gastric juices.

The duodenum secretes several digestive hormones as well. In response to the acid level of chyme, **secretin** (si-KREE-tin) activates and regulates stomach and pancreatic secretions and activates bile secretions. In response to fat, **cholecystokinin** (koh-lee-sis-*tuh*-KEYE-nin) stimulates the gallbladder to release bile and the pancreas to release pancreatic enzymes. It also decreases the feeling of hunger. **Gastric inhibitory peptide** (GAS-trik in-HIB-i-TAWR-ee PEP-teyed) or GIP, decreases production of HCl in the stomach and prompts the release of insulin. **Motilin** (moh-TIL-in) increases GI motility and stimulates the release of pepsin.

Absorption and Elimination

The main reason nutrients need to be broken down is for absorption into the body. Large compounds cannot be absorbed across the intestinal lining, so they need to be broken down into smaller ones. Absorption of different nutrients takes place at different locations in the digestive tract. After absorption, the body must get rid of substances that it cannot metabolize. The disposal of metabolic waste products is called elimination. Without this process, metabolic waste products can build up and become toxic.

Absorption

Most absorption occurs in the small intestine. The stomach reabsorbs water and some minerals. Ethyl alcohol, the intoxicant found in alcoholic beverages, is absorbed directly into the bloodstream from the stomach. Iron and many minerals are absorbed in the duodenum. Sugars, amino acids, fatty acids, and many minerals and vitamins are absorbed in the jejunum. The ileum absorbs vitamin B_{12} and folate, as well as bile salts and acids, which are recycled for later use.

Water and electrolytes like sodium, chloride, and potassium are reabsorbed in the colon, which also stores stool for **evacuation** (ih-vak-yoo-ey-shuhn) or defecation through the rectum and anus. The colon contains large numbers of benign gut bacteria called **microflora** (meye-kroh-flawr-uh). These bacteria are **commensal** (kuh-MEN-suhl), meaning that they hitch a ride on (or in) us, but do not produce disease. We benefit from them because they help us break down nutrients that we have trouble digesting. They benefit from us because they feed on the nutrients we have trouble digesting. Eating a lot of foods that cannot be entirely digested in the small intestine can increase the amount of **flatus** (fley-tuhs), or gas, because more material is available for fermentation by these bacteria.

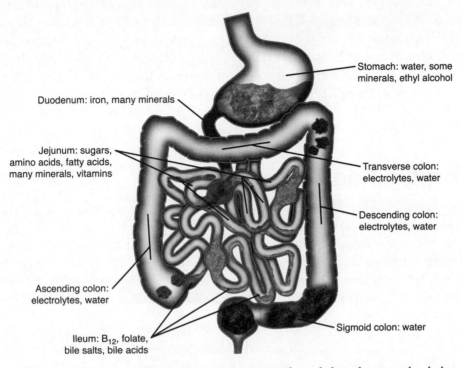

Protein, carbohydrates, fats, water, vitamins, minerals, and electrolytes are absorbed at different points in the digestive system.

Pilar Morales © Dorling Kindersley

Elimination

The **excretory** (ek-skri-TAWR-ee) system handles the **elimination** (ih-lim-*uh*-NEY-*shuhn*) process to rid the body of substances that cannot be used in metabolism. Various organ systems play a role in elimination:

- The urinary system eliminates liquid waste (urine).
- Skin eliminates excess water, urea (waste product of protein catabolism), and other substances.
- The lymphatic system eliminates excess interstitial fluid and waste products from cellular metabolism.

- The digestive system eliminates solid waste through defecation.
- The respiratory system eliminates waste gases like carbon dioxide.

WORD ORIGINS

The word *diarrhea* comes from the Greek words *dia-* (through) and *rheo* (flow). So the literal meaning of *diarrhea* is "flowing through," which is a pretty accurate description of the phenomenon. Common causes of diarrhea are illness or infection that affect the absorptive abilities of the intestines or cause excess water to flow into the intestines. Along with water, electrolytes and nutrients are also lost during diarrheal episodes.

Detoxification

The liver and kidneys provide detoxification of dangerous substances and the waste products of metabolism.

The liver has four lobes, and liver cells are called **hepatocytes** (hi-PAT-*uh*-seyets). The liver has many enzymes that help to detoxify chemical compounds. It breaks down toxic products left over from metabolism through a process called **methylation** (meth-*uh*-LEY-*shuhn*). It also processes the waste products of protein catabolism by converting **ammonia** (*uh*-MOHN-*yuh*, *uh*-MOH-nee-*uh*) to **urea** (yoo-REE-*uh*, yoo-REY-uh) in the urea cycle. The liver is the main site of **glucuronidation** (glookyoor-on-i-DEY-*shuhn*), which is a chemical reaction that adds an acid group to hormones, proteins, bile, and many toxins, making them more soluble in water and easier to excrete from the body.

The liver plays a major role in detoxifying alcohol and metabolizing drugs and medications, a process called **drug metabolism**. The liver produces alcohol **dehydrogenase** (dee-HEYE-dro-*juh*-neys), which detoxifies alcohol. The major drug detoxification system in the liver is called the **cytochrome** (SEYE-*tuh*-krohm) **P450 system**. Genetic differences exist in the cytochrome P450 system. These differences are the reason why some people metabolize drugs faster than others and why some people experience more side effects from drugs than other people do.

The kidneys filter the blood, removing extra water and wastes. The filtering unit of the kidney is called the **glomerulus** (gloh-MER-*yuh*-luhs, gluh-MER-*yuh*-luhs), which is a bundle of blood vessels that lies at the beginning of each **nephron** (NEF-ron). The nephron is the tubular loop that filters blood and forms urine.

The kidneys assist in elimination by performing the following functions:

- **Urea filtration:** Urea is a waste product that results from protein catabolism.
- **Ammonia filtration:** Ammonia is a waste product resulting from protein catabolism.
- **Uric acid** (YOOR-ik AS-id) **filtration:** Uric acid is a waste product resulting from nucleic acid metabolism.
- **Hydrogen ion (H+) excretion:** This process maintains proper blood pH (acid–base balance).
- **Water, electrolyte, and glucose excretion:** This process maintains proper blood volume and composition.
- **Drug metabolite excretion:** This process filters and eliminates drugs that have been metabolized elsewhere in the body.
- **Drug metabolism:** The kidneys glucuronidate toxins for excretion, though the liver remains the main organ for this process.

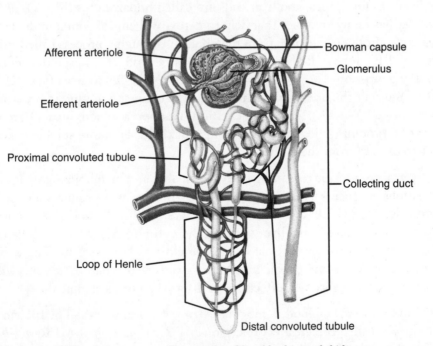

This nephron is one of many that filter blood in each kidney.
© Dorling Kindersley

The Least You Need to Know

- Metabolism is the process by which energy is released (catabolism) from or stored (anabolism) in chemical bonds.

- Many different kinds of enzymes and hormones are needed to break down the different chemical compounds in food.

- Once food is broken down, it is absorbed in different parts of the digestive tract.

- Waste products are eliminated through the urinary, digestive, skin, lymphatic, and respiratory systems.

- The liver plays the main role in detoxifying waste products; the kidneys filter toxins from the blood and eliminate them.

Reproduction

In This Chapter

- Formation of egg and sperm cells
- Union of egg and sperm cells
- The offspring's development
- The birth process
- Physical changes in the new mother and newborn

Human reproduction consists of several stages and processes. The first stage involves the production of cells that are capable of combining to produce an offspring. The second stage involves fertilization, which, if successful, is followed by pregnancy and childbirth. Many of these stages are subdivided into even more stages.

Human reproduction is highly dependent upon hormones, which interact with each other and guide the process almost every step of the way. Familiarizing yourself with medical terms associated with reproduction will help you learn about all the stages and processes involved.

Formation of Gametes

Gametes (GAM-eets) are cells that contain genetic information needed for the reproduction of an organism. The formation of gametes is called **gametogenesis** (*guh*-mee-*tuh*-JEN-*uh*-sis) and occurs through a process called **meiosis** (meye-OH-sis). Before meiosis, cells have two complementary pairs of **chromosomes** (KROH-*muh*-sohmz) that carry the genetic information for the organism. After the completion of meiosis, each gamete contains one copy of each chromosome. Both women and men produce gametes, but the names and processes are different for each sex.

During **fertilization** (fur-tl-*uh*-ZEY-*shuhn*), gametes from two different individuals fuse to produce a **zygote** (ZEYE-goht, ZIG-oht). During this process, the chromosomes from each gamete combine, resulting in a zygote with two copies of each chromosome. Humans have 23 pairs of chromosomes. Twenty-two of these are **autosomes** (AW-*tuh*-sohmz), meaning that they do not contain information for sexual characteristics. One pair, called the sex chromosomes, contains the information for sexual characteristics. The chromosome that contains information for making a female is called the X chromosome. The chromosome that contains the information for making a male is called the Y chromosome.

> **DID YOU KNOW?**
>
> The word **karyotype** (KAR-ee-*uh*-teyep) refers to the complete array of nuclear chromosomes that a particular individual possesses. *Karyo-* means nucleus or kernel in Greek. Scientists use a stain called **Giemsa** (GEE-em-*suh*, JEE-em-*suh*) to see the chromosomes in a karyotype under the microscope. When stained, the chromosomes show banding patterns. Scientists analyze the banding patterns and the lengths of the arms of the chromosomes for genetic mutations, as well as missing or extra chromosomes.

Oogenesis and Folliculogenesis

The ovum is the female gamete in humans. Immature eggs are called **oocytes** (OH-*uh*-seyets) and are housed within primary **follicles** (FOL-i-*kuhz*). The follicle supports the oocyte and provides hormones necessary for its maturation. Each month one follicle is selected to mature and release an **ovum** (OH-*vuhm*) through the process of **oogenesis** (oh-*uh*-JEN-*uh*-sis).

Folliculogenesis (*fuh*-li-kyoo-loh-JEN-*uh*-sis) refers to the maturation of an ovarian follicle from a primary follicle to a **tertiary** (TUR-shee-eyr-ee, TUR-*shuh*-ree) or dominant follicle. Both processes are tightly regulated by hormones in the hypothalamic-pituitary-gonadal axis (see Chapter 10).

Menstrual Cycle and Related Hormones

The menstrual cycle lasts about 28 days in most women. This cycle consists of three phases. At the beginning of the menstrual cycle, rising follicle-stimulating hormone (FSH) levels released from the anterior pituitary stimulate several primary follicles to develop into secondary follicles. This phase of the menstrual cycle is called the **follicular** (*fuh*-LIK-*yuh*-ler) **phase** or **proliferative phase** because it is the phase when several follicles grow and undergo further development.

At about day 9 or 10 of the menstrual cycle, most of these secondary follicles die off, with one dominant follicle remaining. The process of dying off is called **atresia** (*uh*-TREE-*zhuh*, *uh*-TREE-zhee-*uh*), and it results from **apoptosis** (ap-*uh*-TOH-sis, ap-awp-TOH-sis), or cell death.

In response to luteinizing hormone (LH) released from the anterior pituitary, the dominant follicle begins producing **estradiol** (es-*truh*-DEYE-awl), a form of estrogen. Estradiol has a negative feedback effect on FSH, whose levels fall during this time. This keeps too many follicles from developing. Only the dominant follicle continues to develop in the environment of lower FSH levels.

Estradiol has a positive feedback effect on LH. At about day 14, the rising levels of estradiol trigger a surge of LH release. The LH surge causes the dominant follicle to mature, culminating in the release of the ovum from the follicle at about 24 to 36 hours after the LH surge. This phase of the menstrual cycle is called **ovulation** (OV-*yuh*-ley-*shuhn*, OH-vyuh-ley-*shuhn*).

After ovulation, the empty follicle becomes the **corpus luteum** (KAWR-*puhs* LOO-tee-*uhm*), which secretes progesterone and causes the lining of the uterus to thicken in preparation for pregnancy. The corpus luteum also secretes **inhibin** (in-HIB-in), which keeps FSH levels low. This part of the menstrual cycle is called the **luteal** (LOO-tee-*uhl*) **phase**.

If fertilization does not occur, the corpus luteum begins to die. This causes progesterone and estrogen levels to fall. When these hormones decline, the lining of the uterus cannot be maintained and sloughs off, causing menstruation. The death of the corpus luteum also triggers release of FSH. This stimulates another round of follicular development, and the cycle repeats.

Spermatogenesis

Spermatozoa (spur-*muh-tuh*-ZOH-*uh*, spur-mat-*uh*-ZOH-uh), or sperm cells, are the male gamete in humans. **Spermatogenesis** (spur-mat-*uh*-JEN-*uh*-sis) refers to the formation of spermatozoa from **spermatocytes** (spur-MAT-*uh*-seyets) or immature sperm cells. Spermatogenesis is a continuous, noncyclical process and takes about 64 days.

Spermatogenesis occurs in the seminiferous tubules of the testes. Spermatocytes first develop into **spermatids** (SPUR-*muh*-tids), which initially lack tails. During maturation, DNA is tightly packaged into the head of the sperm. Mitochondria, which generate energy, are grouped together in a midsection called an **axoneme**

(AK-*suh*-neem), or body of the sperm. The spermatids also gain **acrosomes** (AK-*ruh*-sohm), which are like caps at the end of the heads. The acrosome contains enzymes that can dissolve the wall of the ovum so that the genetic material from the sperm can enter the egg during fertilization.

The immature spermatids travel to the epididymis, where they begin to grow tails, or **flagelli** (*fluh*-GEL-ey). The tails enable them to become motile.

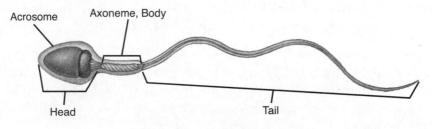

The tail makes up most of the sperm cell.
Debbie Maizels © Dorling Kindersley

☞ **DID YOU KNOW?**

Scientists used to think that sperm contained all the material necessary to create another human being. They even thought that sperm contained a microscopic, preformed human being called the **homunculus** (*huh-MUHNG-kyuh-luhs*), which means "little man" in Latin. This theory was called preformationism, or spermism, and has long been obsolete. These days it has widely been recognized that the female products contribute important roles in fertilization, including secreting key substances that promote sperm capacitation, the process by which sperm go through further maturation in the female reproductive tract, gaining hypermotility and enabling them to bind with the egg during fertilization.

Fertilization

Ejaculation (ih-jak-*yuh*-LEY-*shuhn*) is the discharge of semen. During sexual intercourse, ejaculation places the sperm in the vagina. The sperm then swim up the female reproductive tract. Fertilization, or joining of egg and sperm, normally occurs in the fallopian tubes. Several steps are required for fertilization to take place. These steps include capacitation, the acrosomal reaction, and the cortical reaction.

Capacitation (*kuh*-PAS-i-tey-*shuhn*) is the final process in sperm cell maturation and occurs once sperm reach the female reproductive tract. The uterus secretes certain enzymes that enable capacitation to occur. During capacitation, the cell membrane on the head of the sperm becomes more fluid, which allows it to fuse with the egg more easily. The increased fluidity of the membrane also allows calcium to flow into the sperm, which increases its motility.

The **acrosomal** (*ak*-ruh-SOHM-uhl) **reaction** is the next step of fertilization and consists of the following processes:

1. The head of the sperm meets the **corona radiata** (*kuh*-ROH-*nuh* rey-dee-AH-*tuh*), which is the outermost extracellular material of the egg.

2. The head of the sperm releases an enzyme called **hyaluronidase** (heye-*uh*-loo-RON-i-deys), which allows the sperm to dig through the corona radiata.

3. The sperm burrows through the corona radiata to reach the **zona pellucida** (ZON-*nuh* puh-LOO-si-*duh*), an extracellular layer lying just beneath the corona radiata.

4. The head of the sperm releases an enzyme called **acrosin** (AK-roh-sin) that eats through the zona pellucida and the cell membrane of the egg.

 WORD ORIGINS

The terms *corona radiata* and *zona pellucida* got their names directly from their appearance. In Latin, *corona* means crown, and *radiata* means shining. Under the microscope, the corona radiata appears as the outermost layer of cells that radiate out in all directions, like a crown surrounding the egg cell. In Latin, *zona* means zone, and *pellucida* means clear. Under the microscope, the zona pellucida looks like a clear belt of cells surrounding the egg and lies just beneath the corona radiata.

The **cortical** (KAWR-ti-*kuhl*) **reaction** is also called egg activation and occurs when the sperm cell membrane fuses with the egg cell membrane. This causes the release of **cortical granules** (GRAN-yoolz) from inside the egg. These granules contain enzymes that digest proteins on the egg cell membrane that act as receptors for sperm cell binding. Once these receptors are digested, further sperm binding is blocked. The cortical reaction spreads in a wavelike fashion around the egg cell membrane and prevents **polyspermy** (POL-ee-*spur*-mee), or the fertilization of one egg by several sperm. Polyspermy is a nonviable condition because it would result in multiple copies of genetic material within the same egg.

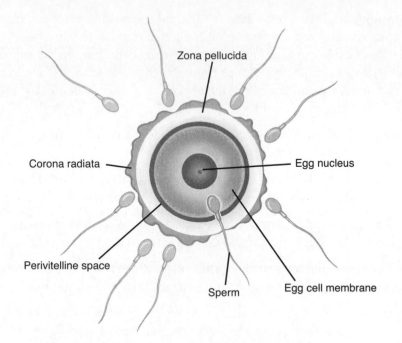

The egg has several layers that play a role in fertilization.
Michael Courtney © Dorling Kindersley

Pregnancy and Prenatal Development

Pregnancy, also called **gestation** (je-STEY-*shuhn*), is the sequence of biological events that occurs in the mother and the offspring during its development in the uterus. This time is also the stage of **prenatal** (pree-NEYT-l) development of the offspring.

The gestational period of a human pregnancy usually lasts about 40 weeks, or 9 months. Pregnancy is divided into the following time periods:

- The **first trimester** (treye-MES-ter, TREYE-mes-ter) starts from the date of the last menstrual period and ends at 13 weeks.

- The **second trimester** lasts from week 14 to week 27. This period is when **quickening,** or movement of the developing offspring, can be felt.

- The **third trimester** lasts from week 28 to week 42, unless birth occurs earlier.

Prenatal development consists of four progressive stages of development: zygote, blastocyst, embryonic, and fetal. The following sections describe each of these stages.

Zygote Stage

The earliest stage of prenatal development begins when the fertilized egg, which is now called a **zygote** (ZEYE-goht), starts migrating almost immediately from the fallopian tubes to the uterus. During migration, the zygote grows through a process called mitosis (meye-TOH-sis), a type of cell division that begins and ends with the same amount of genetic material in each cell.

Blastocyst Stage

The zygote divides rapidly to become a **blastocyst** (BLAS-*tuh*-sist). The blastocyst is surrounded by the **trophoblast** (TROH-*fuh*-blast), a layer of cells that provides nutritional support and eventually develops into the **placenta** (*pluh*-SEN-*tuh*). At around day 5 after fertilization, the blastocyst attaches to the uterine wall. This action is called **implantation** (im-plan-TEY-*shuhn*) and is the official start of pregnancy.

During the blastocyst stage, the offspring's basic body shape forms, a process called **morphogenesis** (mawr-*fuh*-JEN-*uh*-sis). The blastocyst has three layers, called germ cell layers:

- The **ectoderm** (EK-*tuh*-durm) is the outer layer. It provides components to the skin and nervous system.
- The **mesoderm** (MEZ-*uh*-durm) is the middle layer. It provides components to the muscle, skeletal, circulatory, and renal systems.
- The **endoderm** (EN-*uh*-durm) is the inner layer. It provides components to the digestive, respiratory, endocrine, auditory, and renal systems.

Embryonic Stage

After further cell division, the group of cells is called an **embryo** (EM-bree-oh) and enters the embryonic stage. The term *embryo* refers to the developing offspring from about the fifth week after the last menstrual period to about eight weeks of development.

During this time, **embryogenesis** (em-bree-oh-JEN-*uh*-sis) occurs, in which the cells begin to **differentiate** (dif-*uh*-REN-shee-eyt), or become specialized into cells that will form different organ systems. At this time, the brain, spinal cord, heart, and other internal organs begin to form.

At this stage, the placenta also begins to develop. The placenta connects the developing offspring to the uterine wall and allows for gas and nutrient exchange and waste elimination via the mother. The **umbilical** (*uhm*-BIL-i-*kuhl*, *uhm*-bi-LEY-*kuhl*) **cord** also develops at this time. The umbilical cord contains two arteries and a vein and connects the developing offspring to the placenta.

Fetal Stage

The final stage of development starts after the eighth week of development and is called the **fetal** (FEET-l) stage. After this point, the term **fetus** (FEE-*tuhs*) is used for the remainder of the pregnancy. During this stage, the body systems that began to develop during the embryonic stage continue to grow. The sex of the fetus can usually be determined by the third month of development. During the last few weeks before birth, the fetus lays down layers of fat in preparation for birth and grows markedly in size.

Hormones of Pregnancy

A number of hormones play important roles in the support of pregnancy and development of the offspring. For example, **human chorionic gonadotropin** (HYOO-*muhn* KAWR-ee-on-ik goh-nad-*uh*-TROH-pin) or **HCG** is an early sign of pregnancy that can be detected in the mother's urine and blood. This hormone is produced by the trophoblast and developing placenta.

The placenta also produces **progesterone** (proh-JES-*tuh*-rohn) and **estrogen** (ES-*truh-juhn*). Progesterone supports pregnancy by maintaining the uterine lining and causing an increase in uterine blood vessels in order to feed the fetus. Estrogen also helps to maintain the uterine lining and supports pregnancy in addition to increasing breast growth. **Prolactin** (proh-LAK-tin) is another hormone that increases growth of the breasts and mammary glands.

Lastly, **oxytocin** (ok-si-TOH-*suhn*) stimulates uterine contractions during childbirth, helps the placenta separate from the uterine wall after delivery, and causes the milk letdown effect during nursing.

WORDS OF WARNING

The terms *oxytocin* and *oxycodone* look similar, but they refer to two very different types of substances. In addition playing an important role during childbirth, oxytocin is sometimes called the "love hormone" because it is released during sexual orgasm and plays a role in pair bonding. It also decreases anxiety. Oxycodone, which has the trade name Oxycontin, is a pharmaceutical painkiller. Oxycodone is a narcotic that can be addictive (see Chapter 26).

Female Physiological Changes of Pregnancy

The female body goes through many physiological changes during pregnancy. Most prominently, the added weight of the fetus, placenta, enlarging uterus, amniotic fluid, and related tissues causes weight gain. Just about every system in the female body changes to accommodate the developing offspring.

In the hematological system, the liver produces more coagulation factors, making the woman's blood **hypercoagulable** (HEYE-per koh-AG-*yuh-luh-buhl*). This may be protective to stem the tide of bleeding during childbirth. Levels of erythropoietin increase, which increases the woman's production of red blood cells. Blood volume dramatically increases. In the cardiovascular system, progesterone causes a decrease in vascular tone to accommodate this increased blood volume. The increased blood volume also correlates with a large increase in cardiac output.

In the endocrine system, the size of the pituitary gland increases to produce prolactin and other pregnancy hormones. Progesterone and estrogen levels increase dramatically. In the reproductive system, progesterone causes the formation of a cervical mucous plug, which seals off the uterus. Progesterone also encourages growth of the myometrium, in order to increase its strength for labor and delivery. Estrogen causes the breasts and mammary glands to grow in preparation for lactation. In the immunological system, progesterone makes the woman's immune system less sensitive so that the woman's body doesn't reject the developing offspring.

In the gastrointestinal system, nausea often occurs during early pregnancy due to high levels of HCG. Decreased gastrointestinal smooth muscle tone can lead to constipation and stomach reflux.

In the metabolic system, protein and carbohydrate metabolism increase in order to nourish the fetus and uterus. The liver increases **gluconeogenesis** (gloo-koh-nee-*uh*-JEN-*uh*-sis) to increase blood glucose.

In the musculoskeletal system, the torso widens because the abdominal and pelvic muscles and ligaments stretch to accommodate growth of the fetus. For other systems, the accommodation is not so easy. In the respiratory system, the weight of the offspring can press on the lungs, making breathing difficult. In the urinary system, the weight of the offspring often presses on the bladder, increasing the urge to urinate. The kidneys also increase their filtration rate.

Labor and Delivery

Parturition (PAHRT-*uhr*-i-*shuhn*) refers to birth. The period immediately before and after birth is called the **peripartum** (pair-ee-PAHRT-*uhm*). The **perinatal**

(pair-ee-NEYT-l) **period** extends from a few months before birth to about one month after birth.

Labor is an example of a positive feedback cycle between various hormones and physiological processes. Growth of the fetus causes increased downward pressure against the cervix, which sends nerve signals to the brain. These signals cause oxytocin release, which promotes uterine smooth muscle contractions. Uterine contractions stimulate the release of more oxytocin, which stimulates more uterine contractions in a positive feedback loop.

At about the same time, the fetal adrenal glands increase production of cortisol, which inhibits production of progesterone. During most of the pregnancy, high progesterone levels discourage uterine contractions. When progesterone levels begin to drop in response to higher fetal cortisol levels, uterine contractions increase in preparation for birth. Levels of **prostaglandins** (pros-*tuh*-GLAN-dinz), fatty acids that cause the cervix to soften, also increase.

Stages of Labor

There are several stages of labor:

- In the **latent stage**, uterine contractions and cervical dilation begin. Cervical **effacement** (ih-FEYS-ment), or thinning, also occurs.
- The **first stage** is also called active labor. It begins when the cervix dilates to about 3 to 4 centimeters. Rupture of the membranes ("breaking the water") may occur.
- The **second stage** is also called descent and birth. The fetus enters the birth canal and does a series of movements that, combined with uterine contractions, complete birth.
- In the **third stage**, the placenta separates from the uterine wall.

Stages of Birth

During the stages of birth, the fetus executes a series of instinctual movements that facilitate birth. The stages of birth include the following:

- **Engagement:** The fetus changes position so that it lies transversely in the mother's abdomen.
- **Descent and flexion of the head:** The fetus turns so that its head is oriented downward and flexes its neck in order to descend toward the birth canal.

- **Internal rotation:** The fetus turns so that its face is oriented toward the mother's rectum.

- **Extension of the head and delivery:** The fetus' head passes out of the vagina, with the neck extended so that the crown of the head leads the way out of the vagina.

- **Restitution** (res-ti-TOO-*shuhn*): The fetus' head turns 45 degrees to its normal position in relation to the shoulders.

- **External rotation:** The shoulders repeat the corkscrew movements of the head so that they can clear the birth canal and the rest of the body can be delivered.

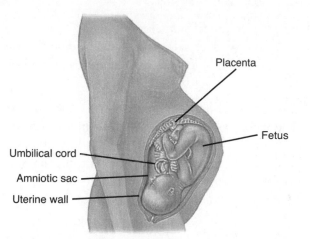

When the fetus is ready for birth, it turns so that its head faces downward.
Philip Wilson © Dorling Kindersley

Postpartum and Lactation

Postpartum (pohst-PAHR-*tuhm*) refers to the period following birth. **Postnatal** (pohst-NEYT-l) is a similar term that refers to the period up to 6 weeks after birth.

Immediately after birth, the newborn goes through a series of physiological changes. Aided by the presence of **surfactant** (ser-FAK-*tuhnt*), a substance which increases surface tension, the newborn's lungs inflate. In fetal life, blood does not flow through the lungs but is shunted to the rest of the body by the **ductus arteriosus** (DUHKT-*us ahr*-TEER-ee-oh-*suhs*), a vessel that connects the pulmonary artery to the aortic arch, and the **foramen ovale** (*fuh*-REY-*muhn* oh-VAL-ey), an opening in the septum between the right and left atria. With the inflation of the lungs, pressure increases in the respiratory system, causing closure of the ductus arteriosus and foramen ovale. This effectively separates the systemic and pulmonary circulations so that blood can flow through the lungs. Prostaglandins secreted during the birth process also cause the ductus arteriosus to close.

> **DID YOU KNOW?**
>
> In some people, the foramen ovale does not completely close. This is called a **patent foramen ovale** or, more commonly, a hole in the heart. If the hole is small enough, the person may not have any problems. A larger hole can be heard as a heart murmur and can cause heart and lung problems later in life.

Shortly after birth, the umbilical vein closes and becomes the round ligament of the liver. Parts of the umbilical artery also close and become the medial umbilical ligaments. Other parts of the umbilical artery remain open and become part of the iliac artery.

In the mother, the abrupt withdrawal of progesterone at birth stimulates high prolactin levels and milk production. High oxytocin levels in the mother also cause milk letdown and contribute to mother–infant bonding. The suckling stimulus also stimulates milk production and letdown. The first milk that's produced contains **colostrum** (*kuh*-LOS-*truhm*), which has high levels of maternal antibodies that are important for the infant's immature immune system.

The Least You Need to Know

- Human reproduction involves the formation of gametes through meiosis. This process is called oogenesis in females and spermatogenesis in males.
- After fertilization, the developing offspring goes through a series of stages involving cell division (mitosis) and differentiation (cell specialization).
- Pregnancy, or gestation, requires many hormones and is accompanied by many physical changes in the mother.
- Partition, or childbirth, also requires several hormones and is divided into stages during which the fetus executes instinctual movements to navigate the birth canal.
- The postpartum period is characterized by several physiological changes in the offspring and mother, including lactation.

Immunity

Chapter 15

In This Chapter

- Mechanical, physiological, and chemical defenses
- Immediate responses: inflammation and leukocytes
- Lymphocytes and long-term immunity
- The role of the lymphatic system

The immune system protects the body against foreign pathogens that can produce disease. The first line of defense is the innate immune system. The adaptive immune system is the second line of defense. These systems have a series of components, each of which has several associated medical terms.

White blood cells play important roles in immunity. There are several different types of white blood cells, and each one has a different name. The lymphoid tissue plays an important role in production and maturation of immune cells. Knowing the medical terms associated with the cells and tissues of the immune system can help you understand it better.

Protective Barriers

The human body has several protective barriers that provide defense against **pathogens** (PATH-*uh-juhnz*, PATH-uh-jenz). Common pathogenic invaders include the following:

- **Bacteria** (bak-TEER-ee-*uh*) are one-celled organisms that are capable of reproducing themselves.

- **Viruses** (VEYE-*ruhs*-ez) are infectious agents consisting of a protein coat and a strand of RNA or DNA. They can reproduce themselves only by using a host cell's machinery for replication.
- **Parasites** (PAR-*uh*-seyets) are organisms that live and feed off of other organisms.
- **Toxins** (TOK-sinz) are poisons that activate an immune response.
- **Fungi** (FUHN-jeye, FUHNG-geye) are primitive organisms that can reproduce by forming spores. This category includes yeasts and molds.

To produce illness, these organisms must breach the body's protective barriers and reach the interior of the body. The following sections describe the body's protective barriers.

Skin

Skin acts like a mechanical barrier against foreign invaders by walling off the body. The **epidermis** (ep-i-DUR-mis) is the outer layer of the skin. **Epithelial** (ep-*uh*-THEE-lee-*uhl*) cells are found in the upper layer of the epidermis, as well as the lining of the digestive, respiratory, reproductive, and urinary tracts. Epithelial cells have tight junctions that form a seal between cells and inhibit pathogens from crossing the epithelium into the interior of the body.

The skin also contains **Langerhans** (LANG-ur-hanz) **cells**. These immune cells pick up microbial antigens and present them to the adaptive immune system. The term *antigen* is a contraction of the words *antibody generator*, and that's exactly what an **antigen** (AN-ti-*juhn*, AN-ti-jen) does. It is a substance that induces antibody production. The mucosa of the mouth, lymph nodes, and tissue around some blood vessels also contain Langerhans cells.

Mucosa

The **mucosa** (myoo-KOH-s*uh*, myoo-KOH-z*uh*), also called mucous membranes, is covered with epithelium. Mucosae line the nasal passages, mouth, lips, eyes, ears, genitals, and anus. The reproductive, digestive, and respiratory tracts also are lined with mucosae. Areas in the body where the skin transitions to mucous membranes are called **mucocutaneous** (myoo-koh-kyoo-TEYN-ee-*uhs*) zones. Examples include the area around the mouth, eyes, nostrils, urethra, vagina, foreskin, and anus.

Mucosa contains lymphoid tissue called mucosa-associated lymphoid tissue, which contains a host of immune cells that can attack invading pathogens. **Goblet** (gob-lit) cells secrete mucus and are found in the mucosal epithelium of the respiratory, digestive, and reproductive tracts. Mucus traps pathogens and foreign particles before they can harm the body.

Cilia

Cilia (SIL-ee-*uh*) are hairlike projections that line the bronchi of the respiratory tract. Cilia are covered in mucus and sweep pathogens and foreign materials away from the lungs. This process is called **mucociliary** (myoo-koh-SIL-ee-er-ee) **clearance**.

Protective Physiological Responses

Many organ systems have responses that are protective against pathogens. These responses include the following:

- Coughing and sneezing propel pathogens and irritants from the respiratory tract.
- Tears wash pathogens from the eyes.
- Urination flushes pathogens from the urinary tract.

Chemical Barriers

Several body systems also produce chemicals that help in defense against pathogens:

- Acid is found in vaginal secretions and stomach fluid.
- Immune cells in the skin and male reproductive tract produce a protein called **defensin** (dih-FENS-in). It burrows through bacterial cell membranes, destroying the bacteria.
- **Lysozyme** (LEYE-*suh*-zeyem) is a protein found in saliva, tears, and mucus that destroys bacterial cell walls.
- **Mucin** (MYOO-sin) is a protein that can form gels and bind pathogens for protection. This protein is in mucus and saliva.

Innate Immune System

The innate immune system is the body's first line of defense against pathogens. This system is also called the **nonspecific immune system** because it responds in a similar manner to an array of pathogens. The response happens almost immediately, but it does not provide lasting immunity. The next time the pathogen is encountered the same response will need to be mounted again. Most of the protective barriers listed previously include elements of the innate immune system. Other elements of this system are inflammation, the complement system, and certain white blood cells.

Inflammation

Inflammation (in-*fluh*-MEY-*shuhn*) is a nonspecific immune response caused by injured cells. The characteristics of inflammation include the following:

- **Rubor** (ROOB-awr): redness
- **Calor** (KAL-awr): fever, heat
- **Tumor** (TOOM-awr): swelling
- **Dolor** (DAWL-awr): pain
- **Functio laesa** (FUNK-tee-oh LES-*uh*): loss of function

During inflammation, injured cells release **eicosanoids** (eye-koh-SAN-oh-idz) and **cytokines** (SEYET-*uh*-keyenz). Eicosanoids are a category of fatty acids. Two types of eicosanoids are involved in inflammation:

- **Prostaglandins** (pros-*tuh*-GLAN-dinz) cause fever and blood vessel dilation.
- **Leukotrienes** (loo-*kuh*-REYE-eenz) attract white blood vessels to the site.

Cytokines are a category of protein molecules that perform cell-to-cell communication. Types of cytokines involved in inflammation include the following:

- **Interleukins** (in-tur-LOO-kinz) help regulate inflammation and immune responses. They also help activate white blood cells.
- **Chemokines** (KEE-*muh*-keyenz) help with **chemotaxis** (kee-moh-TAX-is), which is the attraction of immune cells to the site of infection or injury.
- **Interferons** (in-ter-FEER-onz) help regulate inflammation and immune responses, especially the activation of the immune system in fighting viruses.

Complement System

The **complement** (KOM-*pluh*-ment) **system** is also called the **complement cascade** and consists of a group of proteins that circulate in the blood and help antibodies and other immune cells get rid of pathogens. Complement proteins bind to antigenic proteins or to antibodies that have already bound to and coated pathogens.

The complement cascade is an example of a positive feedback system. When one complement protein binds, it activates a **protease** (PROH-tee-ace, PROH-tee-aze) enzyme that activates other complement proteases, which activates others, and so on, amplifying the signal. The end product is **opsonization** (OP-*suh-nuh*-ZEY-*shuhn*), or coating the pathogen with complement proteins or antibodies to mark it for destruction and clearance. The complement cascade can also activate the membrane attack complex (MAC). The membrane attack complex **lyses** (LEYES-ez), or breaks up, bacterial cell walls.

White Blood Cells of Innate Immunity

Many types of white blood cells, or **leukocytes** (LOO-*kuh*-seyets), circulate in the blood and help the immune system do its job. There are two main categories of leukocytes: **granulocytes** (GRAN-*yuh-luh*-seyets) and **agranulocytes** (ey-GRAN-*yuh-luh*-seyets).

Granulocytes have granules that kill pathogens. This category includes the following:

- **Mast cells** play a major role in allergic and autoimmune responses.
- **Basophils** (BEY-*suh*-filz) play a role in allergic and parasitic reactions.
- **Eosinophils** (ee-*uh*-SIN-*uh*-filz) play a major role in allergic, autoimmune, and parasitic responses.
- **Neutrophils** (NOO-*truh*-filz) are one of the first to migrate to the site of infection or inflammation. They can engulf pathogens and are the main cells in pus.

Agranulocytes do not contain granules. Instead, agranulocytes kill pathogens by engulfing and digesting them. This category includes **monocytes** (MON-*uh*-seyets), which are immature circulating immune cells that travel to the site of infection or injury and transform into macrophages or dendritic cells.

Macrophages (MAK-*ruh*-feyj-ez) are phagocytes that function in both innate and adaptive immunity by eating pathogens and stimulating lymphocytes to respond to pathogens. Macrophages also are considered scavenger cells because they eat up and help the body get rid of cellular debris.

> **STUDY TIP**
>
> The term *phagocyte* comes from the Greek word roots *phagos-*, which means "to eat," and *-kyto*, which means body. So a phagocyte is a body, or cell, that eats. Lots of other medical terms use the word root *phago-*. A macrophage is a big (macro) cell that eats. The process of engulfing a pathogen is called **phagocytosis**. Once inside the immune cell, the pathogen is packaged into a **phagosome**, which fuses with a lysosome (a cell part that contains digestive enzymes) to form a **phagolysosome**. A **bacteriophage**, commonly called a phage, is a virus that eats bacteria.

Dendritic (den-DRIT-ik) **cells** are antigen-presenting cells (APC) that process antigens and present them on their cell surfaces to act as messages to the adaptive immune system. Dendritic cells are found in tissues in contact with the external environment (skin, GI tract, nose, lungs). For example, Langerhans cells are dendritic cells found in the skin.

The category of agranulocytes also includes **lymphocytes** (LIMF-*uh*-seyets). Lymphocytes mainly belong to the adaptive immune system, with the exception of natural killer cells, which are part of innate immunity. Natural killer cells are lymphocytes that release **cytotoxic** (seye-*tuh*-TOK-sik) cell-killing material when they recognize tumors or cells infected with viruses.

Adaptive Immune System

The innate immune system activates the adaptive immune system response. Adaptive immunity is the second line of defense against pathogens. The adaptive immune system is also called the specific immune system.

Characteristics of adaptive immunity include delayed response time upon pathogen exposure and the ability to create long-term immunological memory. Adaptive immunity relies upon antigen presentation and recognition.

Two categories of lymphocytes are involved in adaptive immunity. B lymphocytes are involved in humoral immunity. T lymphocytes are involved in cell-mediated immunity.

STUDY TIP

The terms *humoral immunity* and *cell-mediated immunity* apply to both the innate and adaptive immune responses. *Humoral* refers to body fluids and comes from the discredited theory of bodily humors that dominated Western medicine for more than 2,000 years, from the time of the Greeks. Referred to as humorism, this theory proposed that four bodily humors circulated in the body. So **humoral immunity** refers to immune molecules that circulate in body fluids, such as the complement system. **Cell-mediated immunity** refers to immune responses that are dependent on the activation of immune cells, such as cytotoxic T-lymphocyte activation.

B Lymphocytes and Antibodies

B lymphocytes (also called B cells) have **antibody** (AN-ti-bod-ee) molecules on their cell surfaces. Antibodies are proteins that either coat and tag a pathogen for recognition by other immune cells, activate the complement cascade, or directly interfere with pathogen functioning, effectively destroying the pathogen. Antibodies can circulate in bodily fluids, or they can be attached to the surface of B cells.

There are five different classes, or **isotypes** (EYE-*suh*-teyeps), of antibodies in humans:

- **Immunoglobulin A** (IgA) is found in mucosa and mucosal fluids. It prevents colonization by pathogens.

- **Immunoglobulin D** (IgD) is found in B cell membranes. It helps activate immune cells.

- **Immunoglobulin E** (IgE) binds to allergens and causes **histamine** (HIS-*tuh*-meen) release. It is a major player in allergic and parasitic responses.

- **Immunoglobulin M** (IgM) is found on B-cell surfaces and in bodily fluids. It appears early in the adaptive immune response and indicates recent infection.

- **Immunoglobulin G** (IgG) is the predominant antibody in bodily fluids. It binds bacteria, viruses, fungi, and toxins. It crosses the placenta to confer protection to the fetus. It appears later and provides longer-term immunity than IgM.

WORD ORIGINS

The *Ig* designation in antibody isotypes is short for the word **immunoglobulin** (ih-MYOON-OH-GLOB-*yuh*-lin). The word root *immuno-* refers to immunity. *Globulin* comes from the Latin word *globulus* and refers to spherical bodies. More commonly, globulins are groups of biological proteins. So an immunoglobulin is a protein that functions in the immune system.

T Lymphocytes

T lymphocytes are white blood cells of the adaptive immune system that are capable of antigen recognition, but require antigens to be processed before they can recognize them. Antigen processing and presentation requires antigen-presenting cells (APCs), which are immune cells that process and present antigen molecules on their cell surface and activate cells of the adaptive immune system. B cells, dendritic cells, and macrophages are specialized to be APCs. T cells recognize antigen proteins only when the latter are bound to molecules of the **major histocompatibility** (his-toh-*kuhm*-pat-*uh*-BIL-i-tee) **complex** (MHC), which is known as the **human leukocyte antigen** (HLA) system in humans. Different types of T cells are specialized to recognize different types of pathogens.

STUDY TIP

The adaptive immune system depends on the body's ability to distinguish between self and nonself. *Self* refers to molecules that the immune system does not recognize as being different from the body's own molecules. *Nonself* refers to molecules that the immune system recognizes as being foreign.

White Blood Cells of the Adaptive Immune System

Term	Meaning
plasma cells	B lymphocyte that produces antibodies
CD4+ helper T cells	T lymphocyte that produces cytokines and regulates the immune system, not capable of killing pathogens
CD8+ cytotoxic T cells	T lymphocyte that is activated by antigens presented by APCs and is capable of killing pathogens or infected cells
memory cells	B or T lymphocytes that stay in the bloodstream and can be mobilized to fight future infections by the same organism

Immunological Memory

Immunological memory is the primary way in which the body produces immunity against various organisms. **Immunity** (ih-MYOO-ni-tee) means that the immune system remembers and recognizes pathogens that it has seen in the past. The immune system then can mount a stronger and quicker response each time the pathogen is seen.

The immune system forms immunological memory in two ways. Passive memory confers short-term immunity that lasts several days to months because it involves only premade antibodies, not the activation of immune cells. Active memory confers long-term immunity because it involves B and T cell activation. Some B and T lymphocytes become memory cells after they have been activated. Memory cells can circulate in bodily fluids for months, years, and sometimes an entire lifetime.

DID YOU KNOW?

Immunization (im-*yuh-nuh*-ZEY-*shuhn*) is the practice of artificially inducing immunity. It relies both on passive and active immunological memory. Immunoglobulins can be injected and confer passive immunity and short-term protection against pathogens. An example is an immunoglobulin injection for the prevention of hepatitis A, which is often given to people who are traveling to areas of the world where this infection is common. Other vaccines rely on active immunity and the formation of memory cells. Most of these types of vaccines are **attenuated** (*uh*-TEN-yoo-eyt-ed), meaning that they contain the part of a pathogen that activates the immune system but have been weakened so that they do not produce disease. An example is the polio virus vaccine.

Lymphatics and Lymphoid Tissue

Recall from Chapter 6 that the lymphatic system is composed of a network of vessels that return interstitial fluid to the blood vessels for recycling. The lymphatic system is also a major route by which many cells of the immune system travel throughout the body. **Lymphoid** (LIMF-foid) tissue is part of the lymphatic system and serves as a production site for lymphocytes. Lymphoid tissue is aggregated into **lymph nodes** (NOHDZ) and **lymph follicles** (FOL-i-*kuhlz*).

Certain lymphoid structures have special roles in the formation and maturation of lymphocytes:

- The **spleen** filters blood, stores lymphocytes, makes antibodies, and clears opsonized pathogens. It is capable of producing lymphocytes, but it doesn't normally do so.
- The **thymus** (THEYE-*muhs*) is where immature **thymocytes** (THEYE-*muh*-seyets) mature into T lymphocytes.
- Bone marrow produces different types of white blood cells.

The GI tract has its own specialized type of immune system called **gut-associated lymphoid tissue** (GALT). The gut has a huge surface area that is exposed to the environment, so it's no surprise that GALT is the largest network of lymphoid tissue in the body. GALT stores various immune cells and is found in various parts of the digestive tract, including the tonsils, adenoids, esophagus, stomach, and the small and large intestines.

Lymphoid nodules in the small intestine are called **Peyer** (PEY-erz) **patches.** Peyer patches have special antigen-presenting cells that can activate cells of the immune system.

The Least You Need to Know

- Protective barriers against pathogens include the skin, mucosa, and cilia, as well as chemical and physiological responses.
- The innate immune system involves nonspecific responses and is the body's first line of defense against pathogens.
- The adaptive immune system requires activation of immune cells and is the body's second line of defense against pathogens.
- Activation of the adaptive immune system results in immunological memory.
- Immune cells are produced and mature in lymphoid tissue.

Pathophysiology: Disease and Injury

Part 4 covers pathophysiology, which is the study of abnormal physiology. Disease processes and injury are presented according to medical specialty, which is generally divided by body system. Because the body is one big, interrelated machine, with one system affecting another, there is often overlap between body systems in pathophysiology. When medical specialties overlap substantially with each other, they are grouped together in the same chapter.

Because internal medicine is a vast field that includes many subfields, it is separated into two chapters. Chapter 16 presents terms related to disease processes in the heart, lungs, digestive organs, kidneys, and endocrine glands. Chapter 17 presents blood, rheumatic, immunologic, neurological, and psychiatric diseases. Neurological and psychiatric diseases traditionally are grouped in their own section, but because there is so much overlap between neurology, psychiatry, and internal medicine, they are also included in Chapter 17. As I learned in medical school, disease processes affecting other organ systems can produce neurological and psychiatric symptoms, so it's important not to make snap judgments about psychiatric and neurological symptoms. Including them in the internal medicine section is one way of making this important connection.

Chapter 18 covers pediatrics, from preterm birth to diseases of childhood and adolescence. Chapter 19 presents surgery, which is divided into various surgical subfields dedicated to different body systems. Because surgical subfields share many terms, the chapter begins with an overview of general surgical terms before presenting terms specific to the major surgical subfields. Chapter 20 is dedicated to emergency medicine and trauma, and includes medical, surgical, and psychiatric emergencies. Chapter 21 describes genetic disorders. Because many genetic terms come from basic biology, the chapter provides an overview of basic genetic terms before presenting specific genetic diseases. Chapter 22 covers cancer and is arranged according to the major cancers found in each body system. It was a difficult chapter to write and is one of the longest chapters in the book. After completing it, I realized that all I needed to write were two words: smoking kills. The primary risk factor for many of the most widespread and deadliest cancers is cigarette smoking.

Internal Medicine, Part 1

In This Chapter

- Heart and lung diseases
- Digestive disorders
- Kidney diseases
- Disorders related to hormones and endocrine glands

Internal medicine is a broad-ranging branch of medicine dedicated to the pharmaco-logic treatment of human disease. Internists specialize in subfields organized by body system or organ. Because this field is so broad, diseases and disorders associated with internal medicine will be covered in two chapters.

This chapter covers five internal medicine subfields:

- **Cardiology** (kahr-dee-OL-*uh*-jee) refers to the treatment of diseases and conditions related to the heart.
- **Pulmonology** (PUHL-*muh*-nawl-*uh*-gee) refers to the treatment of diseases and conditions related to the respiratory tract.
- **Gastroenterology** (gas-troh-en-*tuh*-ROL-*uh*-jee) refers to the treatment of gastrointestinal conditions.
- **Nephrology** (*nuh*-FROL-*uh*-jee) refers to the treatment of kidney conditions.
- **Endocrinology** (en-doh-kr*uh*-NOL-*uh*-jee)refers to the treatment of endo-crine disorders.

Cardiac and Pulmonary Diseases

Cardiac (KAR-dee-AK) **disease** refers to a condition that predominantly affects the heart. Because the heart and lungs are intimately connected, diseases of the heart often affect the lungs, and vice versa.

Diseases of the heart and lungs can cause a variety of symptoms. Difficulty breathing is called **dyspnea** (disp-NEE-*uh*). Fast breathing is called **tachypnea** (*tuh*-kip-NEE-*uh*). Some lung diseases cause **hemoptysis** (hi-MOP-*tuh*-sis), or coughing up bloody **sputum** (SPYOO-*tuhm*), which is a mixture of saliva, mucus, and sometimes pus.

Chest pain that happens when the heart muscle doesn't receive enough oxygen is called **angina pectoris** (an-JEYE-*nuh* PEK-tuh-rus, AN-*juh-nuh* PEK-tuh-rus). **Ischemia** (ih-SKEE-mee-*uh*) results when a tissue has insufficient oxygen and can cause angina. If ischemia goes on for too long, it can cause an **infarct** (IN-fahrkt), or dead tissue.

Many physiological abnormalities accompany cardiovascular and pulmonary disease. **Valvular regurgitation** (VAL-*vyuh*-ler ri-gur-ji-TEY-*shuhn*) or **valvular insufficiency** (in-*suh*-FISH-*uhn*-see) is backflow of blood caused by failure of a heart valve to properly close. **Prolapse** (PROH-laps) is the collapse of a tissue or valve, causing incomplete closure and backflow of blood.

Stenosis (sti-NOH-sis) is a narrowing that restricts blood flow through an opening, like a blood vessel or heart valve. Stenosis can also occur in the coronary and systemic arteries, often due to **atherosclerosis** (ath-*uh*-roh-*skluh*-ROH-sis), or hardening of the arteries.

An **aneurism** (AN-*yuh*-riz-*uhm*) is weakening in the wall of a blood vessel, causing dilation which can result in rupture of the vessel. **Dissection** (dih-SEK-*shuhn*, deye-SEK-*shuhn*) is separation of the walls of a blood vessel, which causes bleeding into the vessel wall.

There are many general terms associated with disorders of the heart and lungs. **Cardiovascular** (kahr-dee-oh-VAS-*kyuh*-ler) **disease** refers to a condition that affects the heart as well as the blood vessels. According to the World Health Organization, cardiovascular disease is the leading cause of death worldwide. People with cardiovascular disease often have high blood pressure, which means that the heart is working overtime. Eventually, this extra work makes the muscle of the left ventricle **hypertrophy** (heye-PUR-*truh*-fee) or grow thick and stiff. Hypertrophied hearts cannot properly perform their functions of pumping blood.

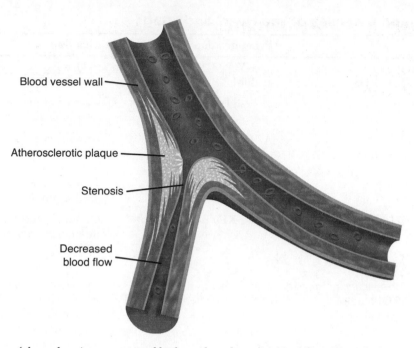

Atherosclerosis can narrow blood vessels and restrict blood flow through them.
© Dorling Kindersley

Congestive heart failure is the inability of the heart to pump enough blood to meet the body's metabolic requirements. Heart failure can be caused by a **cardiomyopathy** (kahr-dee-oh-meye-OP-*uh*-thee), which is a disease or disorder of the heart muscle; **congenital** (*kuhn*-JEN-i-tl) heart defects, which are present at birth; or a lifetime of accumulated damage to the heart muscle.

Heart failure often is accompanied one or more of the following conditions:

- **Pulmonary edema** (ih-DEE-*muh*) is extra water in the lungs.
- **Peripheral edema** is extra water in the extremities, which causes them to swell.
- **Pleural effusion** (ih-FYOO-*zhuhn*) is water in the tissue around the lungs.
- **Pulmonary hypertension** is excess pressure in the blood vessels of the lungs.

Chronic pulmonary hypertension can cause **cor pulmonale** (KAWR PUHL-*muh*-nawl-ee), or pulmonary heart disease, in which the right ventricular enlarges.

Common Diseases of the Heart and Lungs

Term	Pronunciation	Meaning
acute respiratory distress syndrome (ARDS)	*uh*-KYOOT RES-per-*uh*-tawr-ee dih-STRES SIN-drohm	sudden failure of lung function
asbestosis	az-be-STOH-sis	scarring of the lung due to inhaling asbestos
asthma	AZ-*muh*	chronic lung disease characterized by inflammation and constriction of the airways, with wheezing and excess production of mucus
bronchitis	brong-KEYE-tis	chronic or acute infection or inflammation of the bronchi, with excess production of mucus
chronic obstructive pulmonary disease (COPD)	KRON-ik *uhh*-STRUHKT-iv PUHL-*muh*-ner-ee dih-ZEEZ	a progressive lung condition in which air flow to the lungs is limited by narrowing of the airways due to chronic bronchitis and/or emphysema
emphysema	em-*fuh*-SEE-*muh*, em-*fuh*-ZEE-*muh*	a form of COPD in which the alveoli (air sacs) are destroyed, resulting in abnormally large air spaces in the lungs
dilated cardiomyopathy	deye-LEYT-ed kahr-dee-oh-meye-OP-*uh*-thee	heart disease caused by dilation, or ballooning out, of the heart muscle
restrictive cardiomyopathy	ri-STRIK-tiv kahr-dee-oh-meye-OP-*uh*-thee	heart disease caused by increased stiffness of the heart
coronary artery disease (CAD)	KAWR-*uh*-ner-ee AHR-*tuh*-ree dih-ZEEZ	damage to the heart muscle due to insufficient blood supply in the coronary arteries, caused by atherosclerosis; the leading cause of death in the United States
myocardial infarction (MI)	meye-*uh*-KAHR-dee-*uhl* in-FAHRK-*shuhn*	heart attack
obstructive sleep apnea	*uhh*-STRUHKT-iv SLEEP AP-nee-*uh*	short breathing pauses that happen during sleep due to relaxation of airway tissues causing obstruction in the upper airways

Term	Pronunciation	Meaning
pericarditis	per-i-kahr-DEYE-tis	inflammation or infection of the sac that surrounds the heart
pneumonia	noo-MOHN-*yuh*	inflammation or infection of the lungs
pulmonary fibrosis/interstitial lung disease	PUHL-*muh*-ner-ee feye-BROH-sis/ in-ter-STISH-*uhl* LUHNG dih-ZEEZ	scarring of the lung that can be due to autoimmune disorders, infections, or irritants
tuberculosis (TB)	too-bur-*kyuh*-LOH-sis	infectious disease that primarily attacks the lungs

Gastroenterological Diseases

Digestive diseases can produce many physical symptoms:

- **Dyspepsia** (dis-PEP-see-*uh*) refers to impaired digestion, also called **indigestion** (in-di-JES-*chuhn*).
- **Borborygmi** (bawr-*buh*-RIG-meye) is a rumbling stomach.
- **Nausea** (NAW-zee-*uh*) describes the sensation of needing to vomit.
- **Emesis** (EM-*uh*-sis) is vomiting.
- **Diarrhea** (deye-*uh*-REE-*uh*) refers to loose bowel movements.
- **Constipation** (kon-*stuh*-PEY-*shuhn*) is difficulty evacuating the bowels.

Digestive disorders also can cause a variety of abnormalities. **Achlorhydria** (ey-KLOR-hay-dree-*uh*) is decreased production of stomach acid. Pancreatic problems can cause **steatorrhea** (stee-at-*uh*-ree-*uh*), or fatty, smelly stools. Liver problems can result in **jaundice** (JAWN-dis), also called **icterus** (IK-ter-*uhs*), which is the yellowing of the whites of the eyes and skin.

Bleeding in the digestive tract can result in **hematemesis** (heem-at-*uh*-MEE-*suhs*), or blood in the vomit. **Melena** (*muh*-LEE-nuh, MEL-*uh*-nuh) is bleeding from the upper GI tract that causes dark-colored (tarry) stools. **Hematochezia** (hi-mat-oh-KEE-zee-*uh*) is bleeding in the lower GI tract causing bright red stools. Sometimes **hemorrhoids** (HEM-*uh*-roidz), or dilations of veins around the rectum, can bleed, releasing bright red blood during bowel movements. When veins around the esophagus become dilated, they are called **esophageal varices** (ih-sof-*uh*-JEE-*uhl* VAIR-*uh*-seez).

There are many general terms for digestive disorders. **Gastroparesis** (ga-STROH-*puh*-REE-sis) is delayed stomach emptying. **Bowel obstruction,** also called **ileus** (il-ee-*uhs*), is a blockage of the bowel. **Intussusception** (in-*tuhs*-*suh*-SEP-*shuhn*) happens when part of the intestine collapses into an adjoining part. Chronic constipation can cause **fecal impaction** (im-PAK-*shuhn*), which is when a lump of stool interferes with bowel movements. **Volvulus** (VOL-vy*uh*-*luhs*) is the twisting of a loop of bowel on itself.

Intestinal polyps (POL-ips) are growths that develop over time and can sometimes become cancerous. **Dysbiosis** (dis-bayh-OH-*suhs*, dis-bee-OH-*suhs*) is an imbalance or overgrowth of the commensal bacteria in the gut. **Lactase** (LAK-teys) deficiency, or **lactose** (LAK-tohs) intolerance, is the inability to digest the lactose protein in milk. It is a common problem that is related to genetics and sometimes develops during digestive disorders or the use of antibiotics.

STUDY TIP

Remember to break down the word parts. The ending *-itis* (EYE-tiss) refers to an infection or inflammation and can be applied to many digestive disorders. Examples include appendicitis, colitis, cholecystitis, esophagitis, enteritis, gastritis, gastroenteritis, hepatitis, pancreatitis, and proctitis.

Common Diseases of the Digestive Tract

Term	Pronunciation	Meaning
appendicitis	*uh*-pen-*duh*-SEYE-tis	infection or inflammation of the appendix
celiac disease	SEE-lee-ak dih-ZEEZ	condition caused by an immune reaction to gluten that damages the lining of the small intestine

Term	Pronunciation	Meaning
cirrhosis	si-ROH-sis	scarring of the liver
cholelithiasis	koh-lee-li-THEYE-*uh*-sis	gallstone disease
diverticulitis	Deye-ver-tik-y*uh*-LEYE-tis	condition of having small bulges, or sacs, in the lining of the intestine
diverticulosis	Deye-ver-tik-y*uh*-LOH-sis	infection of diverticula
gastroesophageal reflux disease (GERD)	ga-stroh-ih-sof-*uh*-JEE-*uhl* REE-*fluhks* dih-ZEEZ	condition in which the stomach contents leak into the esophagus
hepatitis	hep-*uh*-TEYE-tis	inflammation or infection of the liver
hernia	HUR-nee-*uh*	protrusion of abdominal contents through a weakened area of tissue; commonly occurs through the diaphragm, inguinal canal, and umbilicus
inflammatory bowel disease (IBD)	in-FLAM-*uh*-tawr-ee BOW-*uhl* dih-ZEEZ	autoimmune disease that causes inflammation in the digestive tract
crohn disease	KROHN dih-ZEEZ	a form of inflammatory bowel disease in which inflammation can occur anywhere in the GI tract, from mouth to anus
ulcerative colitis (UC)	UHL-s*uh*-*ruh*-tiv k*uh*-LEYE-tis	a form of inflammatory bowel disease in which inflammation and ulcers occur primarily in the colon
irritable bowel (IBS) syndrome, spastic colon	IR-i-*tuh*-*buhl* BOW-*uhl* SIN-*druhm*, SPAS-tik KOH-*luhn*	condition characterized by abdominal pain and bloating, alternating bouts of diarrhea and constipation
mallory-Weiss tear	MAL-er-ee-WEYES TAIR	upper GI bleeding caused by forceful, prolonged vomiting or coughing
peptic ulcer disease	PEP-tik UHL-ser dih-ZEEZ	erosion of the mucosa in areas of the stomach or duodenum
toxic megacolon	TOK-sik MEG-uh-*koh*-luhn	sudden distension of the colon, bloating, fever, and pain, caused by inflammatory bowel disease, and infections (*Clostridium difficile*)

> **WORDS OF WARNING**
>
> The standard in medical publishing these days is to omit the 's in the names of diseases, conditions, etc. So although you might see or hear the 's used in instances such as Alzheimer's or Crohn's disease, the more correct practice is to omit the final 's in these terms.

Renal Diseases

Nephropathy (*nuh*-FROP-*uh*-thee) refers to any disorder that damages the kidneys. Many renal diseases cause physiological changes that can damage other organ systems. For example, renal disease can be accompanied by hypertension, which can damage the heart and cause pulmonary or peripheral edema.

Fluid and electrolyte abnormalities also are common in kidney disease. **Uremia** (yoo-REE-mee-*uh*) refers to the buildup in the blood of metabolic waste and other substances normally excreted in the urine. **Azotemia** (az-*uh*-TEE-mee-*uh*, ey-*zuh*-TEE-mee-*uh*) is the buildup of nitrogenous wastes in the blood. **Creatinine** (kree-AT-n-een, kree-AT-n-in), a waste product of muscle metabolism, can build up in the blood and is used as a marker of kidney function.

Renal disease can cause a variety of urinary abnormalities:

- **Hematuria** (hee-*muh*-TOOR-ee-*uh*, hem-*uh*-TOOR-ee-*uh*) is the presence of blood in the urine.
- **Glucosuria** (gloo-kohs-YOOR-ee-*uh*) is excess sugar in the urine.
- **Proteinuria** (proh-tee-NOOR-ee-*uh*) is excess protein in the urine.
- **Pyuria** (peye-YOOR-ee-*uh*) is pus in the urine.
- **Anuria** (an-YOOR-ee-*uh*) is the inability of the kidneys to produce urine.
- **Nocturia** (nok-TUR-ee-*uh*) is excessive production of urine at night.
- **Dysuria** (dis-YOOR-ee-*uh*) refers to difficulty initiating urination or feeling pain on urination.

There are several general terms for kidney disorders. **Nephrolithiasis** (NEF-*ruh*-lith-eye-*uh*-sis) is the condition of having kidney stones, or **calculi** (KAL-*kyuh*-leye). Kidney stones can block urine flow, causing urinary retention and **hydronephrosis** (heye-droh-*nuh*-FROH-sis), or swelling of the kidney.

Nephrosis (*nuh*-FRO-sis) is kidney disease not resulting from an infection or inflammation. **Nephrotic** (*nuh*-FRO-tik) **syndrome** refers generally to a disease process that causes protein to leak into the urine.

In contrast, **nephritis** (*nuh*-FREYE-tis) is kidney disease resulting from infection or inflammation. **Nephritic** (*nuh*-FRI-tik) **syndrome** refers generally to a disease process that primarily affects the glomeruli, or the blood-filtering vessels in the kidney, which allows both blood and protein to leak into the urine. **Glomerulonephritis** (gloh-MER-y*uh*-loh-*nuh*-FREYE-tis) is infection or inflammation of the glomeruli. **Glomerulosclerosis** (gloh-MER-*yuh*-loh-skli-ROH-sis) is scarring of the glomeruli.

Chronic kidney disease (CKD) is the progressive loss of kidney function. **End-stage renal disease** (ESRD) happens when the kidneys no longer function. At this point, **dialysis** (deye-AL-*uh*-sis), or a machine that filters the blood and removes waste, becomes necessary. Kidney problems can be worsened by **nephrotoxins** (NEF-roh-TOK-sinz), like dye used in radiologic studies and nonsteroidal anti-inflammatory (NSAID) drugs.

Common Renal and Urinary Diseases

Term	Pronunciation	Meaning
diabetic nephropathy	deye-*uh*-BET-ik *nuh*-FROP-*uh*-thee	decreased kidney function resulting from damage to the kidneys due to diabetes
hemolytic-uremic syndrome (HUS)	hee-*muh*-LIT-ik yoo-REE-mik SIN-drohm	illness characterized by anemia, sudden kidney failure, and the destruction of platelets; seen mostly in children and associated with recent digestive infection, especially *Escherichia coli* (E. coli)
interstitial cystitis	in-ter-STISH-*uhl* sis-TEYE-tis	bladder condition with unknown cause, characterized by painful, frequent urination or urinary hesitancy
minimal change disease	MIN-*uh*-*muhl* cheynj dih-ZEEZ	disorder in which damage cannot be seen under the microscope, but only at the electron microscopic level; characterized by loss of protein in the urine and edema; most common cause of nephrotic syndrome in children
polycystic kidney disease	POL-ee-SIS-tik	inherited condition in which many cysts form in the kidneys, causing them to become markedly enlarged and lose function
pyelonephritis	peye-el-oh-*nuh*-FREYE-tis	infection of the kidneys, usually caused by a urinary tract infection
urinary tract infection (UTI)	YOOR-*uh*-ner-ee TRAKT	infection of the lower urinary tract (urethra and bladder)

Endocrine Disorders

An endocrine disorder is called an **endocrinopathy** (EN-*duh*-krin-OP-*uh*-thee). Endocrine disorders usually fall into the following broad categories:

- Hormone deficiencies due to endocrine gland **hyposecretion** (heye-poh-si-KREE-*shuhn*) or reduced functioning
- Hormone excess due to endocrine gland **hypersecretion** (heye-per-si-KREE-*shuhn*) or increased functioning
- Endocrine gland tumors

A variety of medical terms are associated with symptoms and abnormalities caused by endocrine disorders.

For example, **Graves disease** is an autoimmune condition caused by too much thyroid hormone. It can cause **goiter** (GOI-ter), which is an enlarged thyroid gland. It also can cause **proptosis** (prop-TOH-sis) or **exophthalmos** (ex-op-THAL-*muhs*), which both describe bulging eyes.

Hyperparathyroidism (HEYE-*per*-par-*uh*-THEYE-roid-iz-*uhm*) is a condition in which the parathyroid glands produce too much parathyroid hormone. It can cause kidney stones and **osteomalacia** (os-tee-oh-*muh*-LEY-*shuh*), which is softening of the bones.

Cushing (KOOSH-ing) **disease** is caused by excess adrenocorticotropic hormone (ACTH), which in turn is due to overgrowth or a tumor of the pituitary gland. Cushing disease causes the adrenal glands to release too much cortisol. **Cushing syndrome** is a more general term that refers to the condition of having too much cortisol. The most common causes of Cushing syndrome are disorders of the adrenal glands or use of steroid medications. Symptoms related to Cushing syndrome include the following:

- **Moon face** describes a round, full face.
- **Striae** (STREYE-ee) are purple stretch marks on the abdomen, hips, or breasts.
- **Buffalo hump** describes a collection of fat around the shoulders and at the base of the neck.

Insulin resistance is the inability of the body's cells to respond to the hormone called insulin. Insulin resistance and inadequate production of insulin by the pancreas causes the chronic disease **diabetes mellitus** (deye-*uh*-BEE-tis MEL-*uh-tuhs*, deye-*uh*-BEE-teez *muh*-LEYE-tis) **type 2**. Diabetes mellitus type 2 was formerly called adult-onset diabetes and non-insulin-dependent diabetes. Type 2 diabetes has strong genetic and lifestyle links. People with obesity are at a much higher risk for developing type 2 diabetes.

WORDS OF WARNING

Type 2 diabetes accounts for most cases of diabetes, but there are other types. Diabetes mellitus type 1 used to be called childhood diabetes and insulin-dependent diabetes (see Chapter 17). Type 1 diabetes is caused by autoimmune destruction of the insulin-producing cells in the pancreas and often occurs after a childhood infection. Other forms of diabetes are **diabetes insipidus** (in-SIP-id-*uhs*), which is due to a problem with the kidneys, and **gestational diabetes**, which occurs during pregnancy.

Even though the underlying dysfunction that causes diabetes may be different for all types of diabetes, they all share common symptoms:

- **Polyuria** (pol-ee-yoor-ee-*uh*) is excess urination.
- **Glucosuria** (gloo-kohs-yoor-ree-*uh*) is excess glucose in the urine.
- **Hyperglycemia** (heye-per-gleye-SEE-mee-*uh*) is a high blood sugar level.
- **Hypoglycemia** (heye-poh-gleye-SEE-mee-*uh*) is a low blood sugar level.
- **Polydipsia** (pol-ee-DIP-see-*uh*) is excess thirst.
- **Polyphagia** (pol-ee-FEY-jee-*uh*) is excess hunger.
- **Acanthosis nigricans** (ey-kan-THOH-*suhs* ni-*gruh*-KANZ) is darkening of the skin around the neck and armpits.

Prolactinoma (proh-LAK-tin-oh-*muh)* is a pituitary tumor that produces too much prolactin, which can cause lactation in men and in women who have not recently given birth. It also causes **amenorrhea** (ey-men-*uh*-REE-*uh*), or the loss of menstrual periods. Amenorrhea can increase the risk for **osteoporosis** (os-tee-oh-*puh*-ROH-sis), or weakened, brittle bones.

Pheochromocytoma (fee-oh-kroh-moh-seye-TOH-m*uh)* is a tumor of the adrenal gland that causes excess adrenal hormones to be produced. It can cause many symptoms of adrenal excess, including high blood pressure and **hyperhidrosis** (heye-per-hi-DROH-sis) or excess sweating.

Common Endocrine Disorders

Term	Pronunciation	Meaning
acromegaly	ak-*ruh*-MEG-*uh*-lee	enlarged head due to excess growth hormone, usually because of a pituitary adenoma (tumor)
Addison disease	AD-*uh-suhn*	adrenal insufficiency, hypocortisolism
carcinoid syndrome	KAHR-*suh*-noid	diarrhea, skin flushing, sometimes heart and lung problems due to a GI tumor that secretes too much serotonin
gigantism	jeye-GAN-tiz-*uhm*	excess stature due to high levels of growth hormone in childhood
Hashimoto thyroiditis	haw-shee-moh-tohz theye-roi-DEYE-tis	autoimmune condition in which bouts of hypothyroidism alternate with hyperthyroidism
metabolic syndrome	met-*uh*-BOL-ik	a constellation of physical symptoms that increases the risk for developing diabetes type 2 and heart disease
polycystic ovary syndrome	pol-ee-SIS-tik	the ovaries develop many cysts and high levels of male sex hormones are present; can result in hirsutism (HUR-soo-tiz-*uhm*), or excess hair growth

DID YOU KNOW?

One of the most famous people to have had an endocrine disorder was John F. Kennedy. He had Addison disease, which is an autoimmune disorder that happens when the adrenal glands cannot produce enough cortisol. Information about JFK's health condition was kept virtually secret throughout his presidency.

The Least You Need to Know

- Conditions of the lungs are often affected by heart conditions, and vice versa.
- Conditions of the heart and blood vessels are the leading killers worldwide.
- Gastrointestinal diseases can be due to infections, autoimmune disorders, lifestyle factors, and diseases in other organ systems.
- Kidney diseases can affect many other organ systems.
- Endocrine disorders often result from hormone hypersecretion, hormone hyposecretion, or tumors of endocrine glands.

Internal Medicine, Part 2

In This Chapter

- Blood diseases
- Diseases of connective tissue
- Diseases of the immune system
- Mental illness
- Diseases of the nervous system

There is a great deal of overlap between the five fields of medicine covered in this chapter. Hematologists treat diseases of the blood and bone marrow and share similar ground with immunologists, who treat diseases of the immune system. Rheumatologists treat rheumatic diseases, many of which have strong autoimmune components and affect blood vessels.

Many medical illnesses produce metabolic and other abnormalities that produce psychiatric symptoms, so there is a lot of overlap between internal medicine, psychiatry, and neurology. Psychiatry is the treatment of mental illness. Neurologists specialize in the pharmacologic treatment of diseases of the nervous system.

Hematologic, Rheumatic, and Immune Diseases

Hematologic, rheumatic, and immune diseases often overlap. For this reason, they are discussed together in this section.

General Terms Related to Hematologic Diseases

There are many general terms associated with hematologic disorders. **Anemia** (*uh-NEE-mee-uh*) is a deficiency of hemoglobin or red blood cells and interferes with the oxygen-carrying capacity of blood. There are several different types of anemia:

- **Aplastic** (ey-PLAS-tik) **anemia** happens when the bone marrow doesn't make enough red blood cells.
- **Hemolytic** (hee-*muh*-LIT-ik) **anemia** happens when red blood cells are destroyed too rapidly.
- **Iron deficiency anemia** happens when there is not enough iron for proper hemoglobin and red blood cell functioning.

STUDY TIP

Word parts can come in handy when learning hematology terms. The ending *-philia* means "an attraction for," so **eosinophilia** (ee-*uh*-sin-*uh*-FIL-ee-*uh*) refers to having increased eosinophils. The ending *-cytosis* means condition or state. So **lymphocytosis** (lim-*fuh*-seye-TOH-sis) refers to the condition of having a lot of lymphocytes. The ending *-penia* means deficiency. So **thrombocytopenia** (throm-boh-seye-*tuh*-PEE-nee-*uh*) refers to a deficiency of blood platelets. The ending *-themia* is a variant of *hemia,* which refers to the blood. So **polycythemia** (POL-ee-seye-thee-mee-*yuh*) refers to a blood condition in which there are too many red blood cells.

Myelo is a word root that means bone marrow and is evident in several terms regarding bone marrow–related conditions:

- **Myelodysplastic** (meye-EL-oh-dis-PLAS-tik) **syndrome** refers to a disorder involving dysfunctional production of white blood cells.
- **Myeloproliferative** (meye-EL-oh-*pruh*-LIF-*uh*-*ruh*-tiv) **disorder** occurs when the bone marrow produces excess blood cells.
- **Myelofibrosis** (meye-EL-oh-feye-BROH-*suhs*) is scarring of the bone marrow.

A **coagulopathy** (koh-AG-*yuh*-lo-*puh*-thee) refers to a condition that interferes with proper blood clotting, also called a **bleeding diathesis** (deye-ATH-*uh*-sis). **Hemorrhage** (HEM-er-ij, HEM-rij) refers to profuse bleeding. **Purpura** (PUR-*pyoor-uh*) are purple discolorations on the skin. A **deep vein thrombosis** (DVT) is a blood clot that can clog blood vessels. It can happen when the blood is **hypercoagulable** (HEYE-per-coh-ag-*yuh-luh-buhl*), or clots too easily.

Common Hematologic Diseases

Term	Pronunciation	Meaning
disseminated intravascular coagulation (DIC)	dih-SEM-*uh*-neyt-ed in-truh-VAS-*kyuh*-ler koh-AG-*yuh*-ley-*shuhn*	condition in which normal coagulation is disrupted, resulting in abnormal clotting within blood vessels and abnormal bleeding
G6PD (glucose-6-phosphate dehydrogenase) deficiency	JEE-SIX-PEE-DEE	genetic disorder of red blood cell metabolism; inherited hemolytic anemia; also called favism
hemophilia	hee-*muh*-FIL-ee-*uh*, hee-*muh*-FEEL-*yuh*	inherited disorder in which there is a deficiency of clotting factors, resulting in an inability to form clots
polycythemia vera	POL-ee-seye-thee-mee-*yuh* VER-*uh*	disorder in which the bone marrow produces too many blood cells
sickle cell disease, sickle cell anemia	SIK-*uhl* SEL	inherited blood disorder in which the red blood cells are sickle-shaped
thalassemia	thal-*uh*-SEE-mee-*uh*	inherited condition in which hemoglobin cannot be properly produced, resulting in anemia
von Willebrand disease	von WIL-*uh*-brand	inherited coagulopathy in which there is a deficient amount of von Willebrand factor, resulting in a tendency to bleed

 WORD ORIGINS

G6PD deficiency is sometimes called favism. People who have this inherited disorder carry a genetic mutation that causes a deficiency in an enzyme needed for the proper manufacture of red blood cells. People with this disorder sometimes develop **hemolysis,** or the breakdown of red blood cells, in reaction to eating Italian fava beans.

General Terms Related to Rheumatic Diseases

There are also many general terms for describing rheumatic disorders and symptoms. **Arthralgia** (ahr-THRAL-*juh*) refers to pain in the joints. **Arthritis** (ahr-THREYE-tis) is inflammation or infection of a joint. When this occurs in one joint, it is called **monoarticular** (MON-oh-ahr-TIK-*yuh*-ler) **arthritis**. Arthritis in multiple joints is **polyarticular** (POL-ee-ahr-TIK-*yuh*-ler) **arthritis**.

A **spondyloarthropathy** (SPAWN-dil-oh-ahr-THROP-*uh*-thee) refers to inflammation of the vertebral column. **Tophi** (TOH-feye) are deposits of uric acid crystals in joints. A **nodule** (NOJ-ool) is the deposition of hard material in tissues, which can affect functioning. **Synovitis** (sin-*uh*-VEYE-tis) is inflammation of the membrane that surrounds joints. A **pannus** (PAN-*uhs*) is a sheath of fibrous tissue that develops in joints of people affected with rheumatoid arthritis. **Fibrosis** (feye-BROH-sis) is scarring of a tissue, which can result from inflammation. **Amyloidosis** (am-*uh*-loi-DOH-sis) is the deposit of amyloid proteins in tissues and organs.

Rheumatic disease often causes inflammation in various tissues. **Uveitis** (yoo-vee-EYE-tis) is inflammation of the uvea of the eye. **Iritis** (eye-REYE-tis) is inflammation of the iris. **Myositis** (meye-*uh*-SEYE-tis) is inflammation of muscles. **Vasculitis** (vas-*kyuh*-LEYE-tis) is inflammation of the lining of blood vessels. **Erythema nodosum** (er-*uh*-THEE-*muh* noh-DOH-*suhm*) are bumpy red skin nodules that result from inflammation of skin, also called **panniculitis** (pan-ik-yoo-LEYE-tis). A **granuloma** (gran-*yuh*-LOH-*muh*) is a type of inflammation that happens when macrophages collect around substances recognized as foreign. **Psoriasis** (*suh*-REYE-*uh*-sis) is a skin condition usually on the elbows, knees, or scalp, in which the skin grows too quickly, becomes itchy, and develops white **plaques** (PLAKS).

Inflammation can cause various physical symptoms. **Keratoconjunctivitis sicca** (ker-*uh*-toh-*kuhn-juhngk-tuh*-VEYE-tis SIK-*uh*) refers to dry eyes. **Xerostomia** (zeer-*uh*-STOH-mee-*uh*) refers to dry mouth. A **malar** (MEY-ler) **rash** is shaped like butterfly whose wings cover the cheeks. **Raynaud** (rey-NOH) **phenomenon** is caused by a spasm of the blood vessels in fingers and toes, resulting in decreased blood flow. It is often triggered by cold and stress.

Many rheumatic disorders overlap with autoimmune disorders. For this reason, rheumatic disorders are often associated with specific antibodies:

Rheumatic (roo-MAT-ik) factor

Antineutrophil (AN-tee-NOO-*truh*-fil)

Cytoplasmic (SEYE-*tuh*-plaz-mik) antibody (ANCA)

Tumor necrosis factor-alpha (TNFα)

Antinuclear (AN-tee-NOO-klee-er) antibody (ANA)

Anticardiolipin (AN-tee-cahr-dee-oh-LEYE-pin) antibody

Rheumatic diseases are also associated with an elevated erythrocyte sedimentation rate (ESR) and high levels of C reactive protein (CRP).

Common Rheumatic Diseases

Term	Pronunciation	Meaning
ankylosing spondylitis	ANG-*kuh*-loh-zing spon-dl-EYE-tis	chronic inflammatory condition primarily affecting joints in the spine
gout	GOUT	sudden inflammatory arthritis of a joint, especially the big toe
Reiter syndrome, reactive arthritis	REYE-ter SIN-*druhm*	inflammatory arthritis that occurs in response to a recent infection
rheumatoid arthritis (RA)	ROO-*muh*-toid	autoimmune disorder with systemic manifestations, especially in synovial joints (especially fingers and toes), lungs, eyes, kidneys, blood vessels, and the pericardium
rheumatic fever	roo-MAT-ik	inflammatory disease of the heart, joints, skin, and brain that develops after infection with Streptococcus pyogenes
sarcoidosis	sahr-koi-DOH-sis	inflammatory condition in which nodules form in various organs, interfering with their functioning

General Terms Related to Immunological Diseases

There is a good deal of overlap between rheumatology and immunology. Many terms that describe rheumatic conditions also apply to immunological disorders. There is also overlap between immune disorders and oncology. Cancers of the immune system are covered in Chapter 22. Immunological conditions usually fall into the following categories.

- **Immune hypersensitivity** (HEYE-per-SEN-si-tiv-*uh*-tee) is an overactivity of the immune system. Asthma and allergies fall into this category.
- **Autoimmune** (aw-toh-i-MYOON) **disease** occurs when the immune system attacks the body's own tissues.
- **Immunodeficiency** (im-*yuh*-noh-di-FISH-*uhn*-see) occurs when parts of the immune system function inadequately and cannot defend against disease.
- **Transplant rejection** occurs when the immune system recognizes a transplanted organ as being foreign and mounts an attack against it.

Common Immune Diseases

Term	Pronunciation	Meaning
acquired immunodeficiency syndrome (AIDS)	EYDZ	immune deficiency disorder caused by the human immunodeficiency virus (HIV)
diabetes mellitus type 1	deye-*uh*-BEE-tis, deye-*uh*-BEE-teez MEL-*uh*-tuhs, *muh*-LEYE-tis	condition resulting from autoimmune destruction of the insulin-producing cells in the pancreas; formerly called childhood diabetes or insulin-dependent diabetes
scleroderma	skleer-*uh*-DUR-*muh*, skler-*uh*-DUR-*muh*	autoimmune disease primarily causing hardening of the skin and vascular abnormalities
Sjögren syndrome	SHOH-grenz	autoimmune disorder in which immune cells attack the glands that produce tears and saliva, resulting in dry eyes and dry mouth
systemic lupus erythematosus (SLE), lupus	si-STEM-ik LOO-*puhs* er-*uh*-THEM-*uh*-TOH-*suhs*	systemic autoimmune disease that often has a characteristic "butterfly" rash on the skin of the cheeks, also affects hearts, joints, blood vessels, liver, kidneys, and nervous system

Psychiatric Disorders

Psychiatric symptoms can be caused by brain abnormalities or by medical and neurological conditions. For this reason, many terms that describe psychiatric symptoms are used in other areas of medicine. **Psychosis** (seye-KOH-sis) is a condition of impaired reality, often accompanied by **delusions**, which are fixed, false beliefs that a person continues to hold even when confronted with proof to the contrary. Someone with psychosis can also experience **hallucinations**, which are sensory experiences that occur without a stimulus and are often auditory. **Paranoia** (par-*uh*-NOI-*uh*) refers to suspiciousness of others.

Depression refers to despondent mood or sadness. **Dysthymia** (dis-THEYE-mee-*uh*) refers to a chronic low mood. A severely depressed mood lasting at least two weeks and interfering with daily functioning is a characteristic of **major depressive disorder**.

Mania (MEY-nee-*uh*) refers to excessively elevated mood—called **euphoria** (yoo-FAWR-ee-*uh*)—and increased energy levels. This mood is sometimes accompanied by sudden anger and impatience. **Bipolar** (beye-POH-ler) **disorder** (BPD), formerly called manic depressive disorder, is a condition characterized by wide mood swings alternating between mania and depression.

Anxiety is excessive, irrational worrying. An irrational, anxious fear of an object, activity, or situation is a **phobia** (FOH-bee-*uh*). A **panic attack** is a period of intense fear and anxiety, often accompanied by difficulty breathing. **Depersonalization** (dee-pur-*suh*-nl-*uh*-ZEY-*shuhn*) describes a feeling of detachments from oneself in response to something that provokes anxiety. **Generalized anxiety disorder** (GAD) is a condition characterized by excessive, irrational worrying and anxiety that occurs for at least 6 months.

An **obsession** is preoccupation with a persistent thought. **Rumination** (ROO-*muh*-ney-*shuhn*) refers to thoughts that repetitively focus on distress. A persistent, repetitive behavior that a person is drawn to perform without any reason or reward is called a **compulsion**. A **ritual** is a set of actions performed compulsively so as to relieve anxiety. A **tic** is the insurmountable urge to perform a repetitive movement or vocalization. **Obsessive-compulsive** (*uhb*-SES-iv *kuhm*-PUHL-siv) **disorder** (OCD) is a disorder characterized by intrusive thoughts and compulsions to engage in ritualized behavior.

Impulsiveness (im-PUHL-siv-nes) is behavior characterized by little forethought regarding the consequences. **Agitation** (aj-i-TEY-*shuhn*) is restlessness. **Insomnia** (in-SOM-nee-*uh*) is the inability to sleep. **Hypersomnia** (hi-pur SOM-nee-*uh*) is excessive sleep.

Substance dependence is physical and mental addiction to a chemical substance, usually mind-altering ones like alcohol or drugs. **Withdrawal** refers to physical and mental symptoms that accompany cessation of an addictive substance like alcohol or heroin.

Common Psychiatric Disorders

Term	Pronunciation	Meaning
anorexia nervosa	an-*uh*-REK-see-*uh* nurv-OH-*suh*	eating disorder characterized by restricted food intake and irrational fear of gaining weight
attention deficit hyperactivity disorder (ADHD)	*uh*-TEN-*shuhn* DEF-*uh*-sit heye-per-ak-TIV-i-tee	a disorder characterized by inattention and difficulty controlling impulses; may have a hyperactivity component; usually starts in childhood and often continues into adulthood
autism	AW-tiz-*uhm*	childhood disorder involving impaired social interaction, limited speech, repetitive behaviors, and sometimes seizures
bulimia nervosa	*buh*-LEE-mee-*uh* nurv-OH-*suh*	eating disorder characterized by binge eating and purging, often by vomiting
hypochondria	heye-*puh*-KON-dree-*uh*	excessive worry and preoccupation about one's health
personality disorder		disorder that causes a person to behave outside society's norms and causes significant distress or disruption in social functioning
posttraumatic stress disorder (PTSD)	POHST-*truh*-MAT-ik STRES	disorder characterized by severe anxiety that develops after experiencing psychological trauma
seasonal affective disorder (SAD)	SEE-*zuh*-nl AF-ek-tiv	depressed mood that occurs only during certain seasons
schizophrenia (SCZ)	skit-*suh*-FREN-ee-*uh*, skit-*suh*-FREEN-ee-*uh*	disorder characterized by disorganized thinking, speech, and behavior; hallucinations; delusions; and impaired cognition
Tourette syndrome	TAWR-et	disorder characterized by tics

WORDS OF WARNING

Schizophrenia comes from the word roots *schizo*, which means split, and *phrenia*, which means brain. Sometimes people think that those who have schizophrenia have a split personality, but this is not entirely accurate. People with schizophrenia have a breakdown, or splitting, of mental functioning but not necessarily multiple personalities. The terms **multiple personality disorder** and **dissociative personality disorder** refer to a person who has split personalities.

Neurological Disorders

Neurological disorders can result from trauma, sudden events like stroke that interfere with blood flow to the brain, and chronic disease processes that damage the nerves or the brain. Many general terms describe neurological disorders and symptoms. **Neuropathy** (noo-ROP-*uh*-thee) refers to any condition that causes the nervous system to become diseased and is commonly used to refer to diseases of the peripheral nervous system.

Cognition (kog-NISH-uhn) refers to thinking and reasoning abilities. **Dementia** (dih-MEN-*shuh*) refers to a decline in cognitive abilities due to normal aging or disease. The worsening of dementia symptoms in the evening is called **sundowning** (SUHN-down-ing). **Delirium** (dih-LEER-ee-*uhm*) refers to sudden altered mental functioning due to medical illness.

Several medical terms describe symptoms of disordered cognition. **Aphasia** (*uh*-FEY-*zhuh*) is difficulty forming and understanding speech. **Dysarthria** (dis-AHR-three-*uh*) is difficulty pronouncing words. **Apraxia** (ey-PRAK-see-*uh*) refers to problems organizing the patterns and sequence of movements. **Agnosia** (ag-NOH-*zhuh*) is difficulty identifying people or things. **Amnesia** (am-nee-*zhuh*) is the loss of memory.

Other terms describe changes in consciousness. **Syncope** (SING-*kuh*-pee) is fainting. **Coma** (KOH-*muh*) is a period of unconsciousness from which a person cannot be stimulated to retain consciousness.

Seizure is abnormal brain electrical activity caused by excessive firing of neurons in the brain. **Ictal** (IK-*tuhl*) is a term that refers to events associated with seizures, such as an ictal headache. An **aura** is a perceptual disturbance that precedes a seizure or migraine. A **migraine** (MEYE-greyn) is a headache that usually appears on one side. In addition to an aura, other symptoms of a migraine can include nausea, vomiting, photophobia, and phonophobia. **Photophobia** (foh-*tuh*-FOH-bee-*uh*) is sensitivity to light. **Phonophobia** (fohn-oh-FOH-bee-*uh*) is sensitivity to sound.

Several medical terms describe sensory disturbances. **Hyperacusis** (HEYE-per-*uh*-kyoo-*suhs*) is heightened sensitivity to certain sound frequencies. **Tinnitus** (ti-NEYE-*tuhs*, TIN-i-*tuhs*) is ringing in the ears. **Vertigo** (VUR-ti-goh) is a sensation of feeling like one's body is spinning or whirling around. **Paresthesia** (par-*uhs*-THEE-*zhuh*) refers to a burning or tingling sensation of the skin.

Paralysis is the inability to move a body part. **Paraplegia** (par-*uh*-PLEE-*juh*) is paralysis of both lower limbs. **Quadriplegia** (kwod-*ruh*-PLEE-*juh*) is paralysis of all four limbs. **Hemiplegia** (hem-i-PLEE-*juh*) is paralysis of one side of the body.

Paralysis can cause abnormal physical symptoms, for which there are many medical terms. **Hyperreflexia** (HEYE-per-ri-FLEKS-ee-*yuh*) refers to overactive reflexes. **Flaccidity** (*fluh*-SID-*uh*-tee) describes muscles with decreased tone. **Spasticity** (spas-TI-*suh*-tee) and **hypertonicity** (HEYE-per-taw-NI-*suh*-tee) both describe muscles with increased tone. **Atrophy** (A-*truh*-fee, EY-*truh*-fee) is wasting away of a muscle. **Fasciculation** (*fuh*-sik-yuh-LEY-*shuhn*) is a small muscle twitch. **Myoclonus** (meye-*uh*-KLOH-*nuhs*) is a brief twitch of a muscle group. **Nystagmus** (ni-STAG-*muhs*) is a rapid involuntary movement of the eyeball from side to side. **Ptosis** (TOH-*suhs*) is drooping of the eyelids. **Chorea** (kaw-REE-*uh*) refers to uncontrollable dancelike movements.

DID YOU KNOW?

Chorea used to be called St. Vitus's dance when it was used to describe the jerky movements of children with rheumatic fever. St. Vitus is the patron saint of dancers. His name was applied to this disorder possibly because of the wild dances that occurred during the feast of St. Vitus in places like Bohemia and Germany. Another name for chorea found in children is Sydenham chorea.

Infections of the nervous system have their own associated terms. **Meningitis** (men-in-JEYE-tis) is infection or inflammation of the meninges. **Encephalitis** (en-sef-*uh*-LEYE-tis) is an infection or inflammation of the brain. **Hydrocephalus** (heye-*druh*-SEF-*uh*-luhs) is increased cerebrospinal fluid (CSF) in the ventricles of the brain and can result from brain infections, tumors, hemorrhages, or congenital disorders.

Common Neurological Disorders

Term	Pronunciation	Meaning
Alzheimer disease	ALZ-heye-merz	dementia characterized by memory loss that cannot be attributable to normal aging; often includes confusion, speech difficulties, and mood swings
amyotrophic lateral sclerosis, Lou Gehrig disease	am-ee-oh-TROH-fik LAT-er-*uhl* skli-ROH-sis, LOO GAIR-ig	motor neuron disease characterized by rapid, progressive weakness, paralysis, and then death
Bell palsy	BEL PAWL-zee	paralysis of the muscles, usually only on one side of the face
carpal tunnel syndrome	KAHR-*puhl* TUHN-l	entrapment of the nerves that go from the wrist to the hand, causing weakness and numbness in the muscles in the hand
cervical spinal stenosis	SUR-vi-*kuhl* SPEYEN-l sti-NOH-sis	abnormal narrowing of the spinal vertebrae, which constricts the spinal cord and causes neurological symptoms
diabetic neuropathy	deye-*uh*-BET-ik noo-ROP-*uh*-thee	condition characterized by nerve damage caused by diabetes
epilepsy	EP-*uh*-lep-see	group of neurological disorders characterized by the presence of seizures
Erb palsy	ERB PAWL-zee	paralysis of the arm due to injury of nerves in the shoulder
fibromyalgia	feye-broh-meye-AL-*juh*	disorder characterized by pain or tingling in at least nine separate points on the body, sometimes with fatigue and joint stiffness
Guillain-Barré syndrome	GEE-yawn *buh*-rey	a neuropathy that can cause ascending paralysis; often occurs after an infection
Huntington disease	HUHN-ting-*tuhn*	an inherited disorder that causes cognitive degeneration, poor muscle coordination, and psychiatric symptoms

continues

Common Neurological Disorders   (continued)

Term	Pronunciation	Meaning
Ménière disease	*muhn*-YAIRZ	inner ear disorder causing vertigo, tinnitus, and hearing loss
multiple sclerosis	MUHL-*tuh-puhl* skli-ROH-sis	inflammatory disease that destroys the myelin sheaths of nerves in the brain and spinal cord, interfering with nerve transmission and causing muscle weakness and cognitive decline
muscular dystrophy	MUHS-*kyuh*-ler DIS-*truh*-fee	a group of muscle disorders causing muscle weakness and wasting
myasthenia gravis	meye-*uhs*-THEE-nee-*uh* GRAV-*uhs*	autoimmune disorder in which the nerve transmission to muscles is destroyed, causing muscle weakness
neurofibromatosis	noor-oh-feye-broh-meye-TOH-*suhs*	inherited disorder in which nerve tissues grow tumors, interfering with function
optic neuritis	op-TIK noo-REYE-tis	inflammation of the optic nerve, can cause partial or complete vision loss
Parkinson disease	PAHR-kin-*suhn*	degenerative condition caused by death of certain brain cells; characterized by tremor, a shuffling walk, rigidity, and psychiatric symptoms
restless legs syndrome		condition characterized by uncomfortable sensations in the legs and the overwhelming urge to move them
stroke, cerebrovascular accident (CVA)	STROHK, se-ree-broh-VAS-*kyuh*-ler AK-si-*duhnt*	loss of blood supply to part of the brain, causing sudden loss of function and sometimes death of that brain region
transient ischemic attack	TRAN-*shuhnt* ih-SKEE-mik *uh*-TAK	short period of neurological dysfunction caused by decreased oxygen supply to an area of the brain
traumatic brain injury (TBI)	*truh*-MAT-ik BREYN IN-*juh*-ree	death of part of the brain as the result of trauma and injury

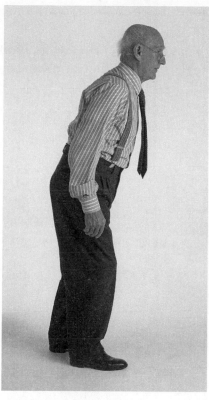

This man has the characteristic shuffling gait and stance of Parkinson disease. The parkinsonian gait is described in Chapter 11.
© Dorling Kindersley

The Least You Need to Know

- Hematological disorders can result from processes that interfere with the abnormal production, formation, or destruction of red blood cells, white blood cells, and platelets.
- Rheumatic disorders affect a wide variety of tissues and organ systems and often have an autoimmune component.
- Immunological disorders are usually caused by autoimmune problems, immune deficiencies, or transplant rejection.

- Psychiatric symptoms can be caused by brain abnormalities or by medical and neurological conditions.
- Neurological disorders can result from trauma, sudden events that interfere with blood flow to the brain, and chronic disease processes that damage the nerves or the brain.

Chapter

Pediatrics

18

In This Chapter

- Medical problems in newborns
- Organ and tissue abnormalities in newborns
- Childhood illnesses
- Growth and sexual development disorders
- Cancer in children

Pediatricians treat medical diseases of infants, children, and adolescents. Due to their growing bodies and other issues related development, children are susceptible to different diseases than adults. They also respond differently to medications and treatments. These differences necessitate a branch of medicine, even entire hospitals, dedicated just to children.

Some of the medical terms used to describe childhood illnesses overlap with terms used to describe adult illnesses. Other terms are specific to pediatrics. Knowing some of the specific terms will expand your knowledge of medical terminology. While reading this chapter, see whether you can pick out the terms that overlap with adult medicine and the ones that are more specific to pediatrics.

Neonatology

Neonatology (nee-oh-ney-TOL-*uh*-jee) deals with the treatment of newborn infants, especially seriously ill infants who need to be cared for in neonatal intensive care units, or NICUs. Such infants usually have medical problems resulting from one or more of the following conditions: premature or preterm birth, **intrauterine growth retardation** (low birth weight), **congenital malformations** (birth defects), medical conditions, and birth complications.

> **DID YOU KNOW?**
>
> Alcohol use by the mother during pregnancy can cause growth delay, low birth weight, and birth defects in the fetus. Alcohol is a **teratogen** (*tuh*-RAT-*uh-juhn*), or a substance that causes birth defects. The constellation of disorders caused by maternal alcohol consumption is called **fetal alcohol syndrome** (FAS) and includes abnormal facial features, neuronal and brain damage, heart defects, joint abnormalities, kidney malformations, and many other types of abnormalities. Long-term effects can include growth delays and psychiatric problems. Fetal alcohol syndrome is one of the leading causes of mental retardation in the United States.

Complications of Preterm Birth

Preterm birth is defined as birth before 37 weeks of gestational age. An infant who is born before this age is considered to be premature. **Viability** (veye-*uh*-BIL-i-tee) refers to the gestational age at which a premature infant is able to survive outside the uterus. Due to advances in modern medical technology, this age has decreased over the past decades. Currently, birth before 24 weeks of gestational age is generally considered to be the limit of viability, or the point at which there is a 50 percent chance of survival outside the uterus. Because severely preterm birth can result in brain damage and lifelong disability, there are ethical considerations surrounding the use of medical technology to decrease the limit of viability.

Premature infants are born before many organ systems are fully developed and therefore have problems related to inadequately developed organ systems. Due to low fat stores and an immature nervous system, premature infants can have difficulties regulating body temperature and other homeostatic processes. These difficulties can cause a number of related abnormalities:

- **Hypoglycemia** (heye-poh-gleye-SEE-mee-*uh*): low blood sugar levels
- **Hypocalcemia** (heye-poh-kal-SEE-mee-*uh*): low levels of calcium in the blood
- **Thrombocytopenia** (throm-boh-seye-*tuh*-PEE-nee-*uh*): low levels of blood platelets
- **Anemia** (*uh*-NEE-mee-*uh*): low levels of hemoglobin and red blood cells

Because the lungs are among the last organs to develop, most premature infants have respiratory problems and require the assistance of a **ventilator** (ven-tl-ey-ter), a mechanical device that helps infants breathe. Premature infants might have short periods of rapid breathing, which is called **transient tachypnea** (TRAN-*shuhnt* tak-IP-NEE-*uh*). Or they might have periods when they stop breathing entirely, which is called **apnea** (AP-nee-*uh*). Premature infants may also have low heart rates, or **bradycardia** (brad-i-kahr-dee-*uh*); and low blood pressure, or **hypotension** (heye-*puh*-ten-*shuhn*).

Premature infants are at risk of developing **sepsis** (SEP-sis), which is a blood infection, and/or other infections. They are also at risk of developing **pneumonia** (noo-MOHN-yuh), which is an infection or inflammation of the lungs. Long-term complications of preterm birth include growth delay, learning disabilities, mental retardation, chronic lung problems, hearing and vision loss, and other physical and mental disabilities.

Conditions Resulting from Preterm Birth

Term	Pronunciation	Meaning
anemia of prematurity	*uh*-NEE-mee-*uh uhv* pree-*muh*-CHOOR-*uh*-tee	condition in which the blood system is not developed enough to make adequate red blood cells
cerebral palsy	*suh*-REE-*bruhl* PAWL-zee	long-term nervous system disability that can result from preterm birth
hyperbilirubinemia of prematurity and jaundice	HEYE-per-bil-ee-roo-bin-EE-mee-*yuh*, JAWN-dis	condition in which the infant's liver is not developed enough to properly break down heme, resulting in high blood levels of bilirubin—the normal break-down product of heme—and causing a yellowing of the skin and white parts of the eyes
intraventricular hemorrhage	in-*truh*-ven-TRIK-*yuh*-ler HEM-er-ij, HEM-rij	bleeding in the brain that results from immature blood vessels not being able to handle increased blood pressures after birth
kernicterus	kur-NIK-tur-*uhs*	brain dysfunction or damage due to hyperbilirubinemia

continues

Conditions Resulting from Preterm Birth   (continued)

Term	Pronunciation	Meaning
necrotizing enterocolitis	NEK-*ruh*-teyez-ing en-*tuh*-roh-*kuh*-LEYE-tis	condition in which parts of the bowel die
patent ductus arteriosus (PDA)	PAT-nt DUHKT-*uhs* ahr-teer-ee-OH-*suhs*	failure of a blood vessel connecting the pulmonary artery to the aorta to close, resulting in breathing difficulties and long-term heart problems
respiratory distress syndrome	RES-per-*uh*-tawr-ee dih-STRES SIN-*druhm*	condition in which the lungs are not developed enough to breathe properly
retinopathy of prematurity	ret-n-OP-*uh*-thee *uhv* pree-*muh*-CHOOR-*uh*-tee	eye condition that can result in blindness
sudden infant death syndrome (SIDS)	SUHD-n IN-*fuhnt* DETH SIN-*druhm*	sudden death without warnings or symptoms of an infant under age one

Complications of Term Birth

Complications can also occur in term births, which are those that occur after 37 weeks of gestation. Problems can result from obstetrical difficulties (see Chapter 19), medical illness in the mother, or problems with the fetus. **Respiratory depression** can sometimes happen during delivery, but it may not cause problems if it occurs for a short time. **Intrapartum asphyxiation** (in-*truh*-PAHR-*tuhm* as-FIK-see-ey-*shuhn*), or decreased oxygen supply during the birth process, is more serious and can result in **hypoxic ischemic encephalopathy** (heye-POK-sik ih-SKEE-mik en-sef-*uh*-LOP-*uh*-thee), or brain damage that can cause long-term disabilities like cerebral palsy.

Damage also can occur to the peripheral nerves during birth. **Brachial** (BREY-kee-*uhl*) **nerve damage** refers to injury to the nerves that course through the shoulder to innervate the arm and hand. It can occur as a consequence of shoulder **dystocia** (dis-TOH-*shuh*), when the shoulder has trouble clearing the birth canal. Long-term complications of this injury include **Erb palsy** (ERB PAWL-zee) and **Klumpke paralysis** (KLUMPK *puh*-RAL-*uh*-sis), or paralysis of the muscles in the arm, wrist, or hand. **Fetal macrosomia** (MAK-*ruh*-SOH-mee-*yuh*), or a large birth weight, is a risk factor for this kind of complication.

Perinatal infections can also be acquired through vertical transmission, or mother-to-child transfer. **Neonatal sepsis** typically results from a type of bacteria called **group B** *Streptococcus* (strep-*tuh*-KOK-*uhs*). Several other types of bacteria also can cause infections in newborns. One of the most serious complications of neonatal infection is **herpes encephalitis** (HUR-peez en-sef-*uh*-LEYE-tis), which is a brain infection caused by the herpes virus.

Like preterm infants, full-term infants also can develop hyperbilirubinemia and jaundice, which are often easily treatable without long-term consequences. **Rh disease** of the newborn happens when the mother has a different blood type than the fetus. In such scenarios, the mother makes antibodies against the fetus, which can cause benign disease; severe anemia in the newborn; and sometimes **hydrops fetalis** (HEYE-drops fee-TAL-*uhs*), or stillbirth.

STUDY TIP

A group of infections that most commonly occurs in newborns is called the TORCH complex. Each letter in the acronym stands for an infection. *T* stands for **toxoplasmosis** (tok-soh-plaz-MOH-sis). *O* stands for other infections. These infections are **Coxsackie** (COX-sak-ee) **virus**, **syphilis** (SIF-*uh*-lis), **varicella-zoster** (var-*uh*-SEL-*uh* zos-ter) **virus**, HIV, and **parvovirus** (PAHR-voh-veye-*ruhs*). R stands for **rubella** (roo-BEL-*uh*). *C* stands for **cytomegalovirus** (seye-toh-meg-*uh*-loh-VEYE-*ruhs*). *H* stands for **histoplasmosis** (his-toh-plaz-MOH-sis).

Birth Defects

Birth defects are also called **congenital** (*kuhn*-JEN-i-tl) **defects**. Structural abnormalities of body parts or organs are called **congenital anomalies** (*uh*-NOM-*uh*-leez) and can be due to abnormalities that occur during embryonic and fetal development. **Malformation** (mal-fawr-MEY-*shuhn*) refers to abnormalities in tissue development. **Dysplasia** (dis-PLEY-*zhuh*) refers to abnormalities in organ development. **Deformation** (dee-fawr-MEY-*shuhn*) refers to a body structure whose tissues develop normally but whose physical appearance is abnormal due to factors like external pressure or constriction in the uterus.

Common types of birth defects include **neural** (NOOR-*uhl*) **tube defects**, which are abnormalities in the formation of the spinal cord. Neural tube defects include the following.

- **Spina bifida** (SPEYE-*nuh* BIF-i-*duh*) is unfused vertebrae over the spinal cord, which sometimes allow the spinal cord to protrude.
- **Meningomyelocele** (mi-NINJ-oh-meye-EL-*uh*-seel) is the most serious form of spina bifida, in which a portion of the spinal cord protrudes in a fluid-filled sac. It often results in paralysis.
- **Anencephaly** (an-en-SEF-*uh*-lee) is lacking parts of the brain, skull, and scalp.
- **Arnold-Chiari malformation** (AHR-nld kee-AWR-ee mal-fawr-MEY-*shuhn*) is a brain deformation that can cause hydrocephalus.

Limb abnormalities are called **dysmelias** (dis-MEE-lee-*uhz*). Sometimes, more than five fingers can form, which is called **polydactyly** (pol-ee-DAK-*tuh*-lee). **Amelia** (*uh*-MEL-ee-*uh*, ey-MEE-lee-*uh*) refers to an arm or leg that fails to form. **Amniotic** (am-nee-OT-ik) **band syndrome** occurs when fibrous bands break loose from the amnion and wrap around a developing limb or digit, interfering with its development. **Congenital talipes equinovarus** (TAL-*uh*-peez e-KWEYN-oh VAIR-*uhs*), or clubfoot, refers to one or both feet turning inward at the ankle.

Other physical birth defects include cleft lip, or **cheiloschisis** (keyel-*uh*-SKI-*suhs*), and cleft palate, or **palatoschisis** (*puh*-LAT-*uh*-ski-*suhs*). These defects cause facial deformities when the tissues that form the lips and palate fail to fuse. **Congenital dysplasia** (dis-PLEY-*zhuh*) **of the hip** refers to a condition in which the hip socket forms improperly, which can cause hip dislocation.

Organs also can fail to undergo proper **morphogenesis** (mawr-*fuh*-JEN-*uh*-sis), or development. **Gastrointestinal atresia** (*uh*-TREE-*zhuh*) refers to the narrowing of part of the intestine. **Pyloric stenosis** (peye-LOR-ik stuh-NOH-sis) refers to the narrowing of the opening from the stomach to the duodenum, which can cause severe projectile vomiting. **Meckel diverticulum** (MEK-*uhl* deye-ver-TIK-*yuh-luhm*) is a small pocket that develops in the small intestine. It is asymptomatic in most people, but it can sometimes cause pain, blood in the stool, and intestinal obstruction. Sometimes the lungs do not form properly, which is called **lung aplasia** (*uh*-PLEY-*zhuh*). Failure of the kidneys to form is called **renal agenesis** (ey-JEN-*uh*-sis). A **septal** (SEP-tl) **defect** is a hole in the septum between the atria or ventricles that allows blood to flow between the left and right sides of the heart.

Genetic disorders can also cause birth defects. **Achondroplasia** (ey-kon-*druh*-PLEY-*zhuh*) is due to an inherited genetic mutation and refers to short stature, abnormalities in body proportions, and other physical deformities. Down syndrome, also called **trisomy** (TREYE-soh-mee) **21** is very common and causes mental retardation, facial and other physical abnormalities, and several medical complications. Other genetic mutations can result in metabolic problems and are called inborn errors of metabolism. Genetic disorders are more fully covered in Chapter 21.

Diseases of Childhood and Adolescence

Children's developing bodies are physiologically different from adult's bodies. Children's growing bodies have different nutritional and other requirements and are susceptible to different diseases than adults. Children's special needs also make them more vulnerable to the effects of some medications and treatments.

The immune system is still developing throughout much of childhood. This fact, combined with greater exposure to microbes at school, makes infectious disease an important category of childhood illnesses. Vaccinations are provided to children during childhood to help their developing immune systems fight infections, many of which were deadly before the widespread use of vaccines.

STUDY TIP

Certain inoculations combine vaccines for several viruses all into one shot. In such cases, the name for the shot is an abbreviation of the first letters of the names of the viruses. For example, the shot that vaccinates against diphtheria, tetanus, and pertussis is called DTaP. And the shot that vaccinates against measles, mumps, and rubella is called MMR.

The increased metabolic requirements needed during rapid childhood growth also put certain children in resource-poor environments at risk for nutritional deficiencies. Growth is also a hormonal phenomenon, and children are susceptible to particular endocrine disorders during this period of life. Genetic disorders also play a big role in childhood illnesses and are covered more fully in Chapter 21.

Common Childhood Diseases and Illness Symptoms

Term	Pronunciation	Meaning
asthma	AZ-*muh*	chronic lung disease characterized by inflammation and constriction of the airways, with wheezing and excess mucus production
congenital diaphragmatic hernia	deye-*uh*-frag-MAT-ik HUR-nee-*uh*	protrusion of part of the abdominal contents into the chest cavity through a weakened part of the diaphragm; can interfere with lung development
croup	KROOP	swelling around the vocal cords, causing breathing difficulties
cryptorchidism	krip-TAWR-ki-diz-*uhm*	undescended testicle
cystic fibrosis	SIS-tik feye-BROH-sis	inherited disorder characterized by thick mucus that causes breathing and digestive problems
diphtheria	dip-THEER-ee-*yuh*	bacteria that causes serious respiratory illness and can result in heart problems; common childhood vaccine
encopresis	en-*kuh*-PREE-sis	soiling the pants with stool after having been potty trained; due to constipation or medical or psychiatric conditions
fifth disease, erythema infectiosum	er-*uh*-THEE-*muh* in-*fek*-shee-OH-sum	infection with parvovirus B19 that causes a characteristic red rash on both cheeks; formerly called "slapped cheek syndrome"
haemophilus influenzae type b (Hib)	heem-AW-*fuh-luhs* in-floo-EN-*zuh*	bacteria that that causes serious flulike symptoms and was the leading cause of meningitis and pneumonia before the Hib vaccine; in the past, H. flu was incorrectly thought to be the cause of the flu illness, which instead is caused by a virus
hand-foot-and-mouth disease		common viral illness that causes a characteristic rash on the mouth, palms, and bottoms of the feet

Term	Pronunciation	Meaning
Hirschsprung disease	HURSH-*sprung*	congenital condition in which the intestinal nerves do not develop, impairing bowel movements and causing blockage
infant colic	KOL-ik	irritability and crying in a baby, often due to intestinal discomfort
Kawasaki syndrome	KAH-wah-SAH-kee	autoimmune disease that causes high fever, rash, "strawberry" tongue, and vasculitis; can result in heart problems
kwashiorkor	kwah-shee-AWR-kawr	protein malnutrition
Marfan syndrome	MAHR-*fuhn*	genetic connective tissue disorder characterized by unusual tallness and heart problems
meningococcal meningitis	*muh*-ning-goh-KOK-*uhl* men-in-JEYE-tis	bacteria that causes inflammation of the covering of the brain and spinal cord; common vaccine for children and adolescents
mononucleosis	MAW-noh-noo-klee-OH-*suhs*	infectious disease that causes fever, sore throat, and marked tiredness, as well as hepatitis, enlarged liver, and jaundice in adolescents
mumps		virus that causes painful swelling of salivary glands; common childhood vaccine
nocturnal enuresis	nok-TUR-nl en-*yuh*-REE-sis	bedwetting, urination at night
otitis externa	oh-TEYE-tis ex-STUR-*nuh*	outer ear infection
otitis media	oh-TEYE-tis MEE-dee-*uh*	middle ear infection
pertussis, whooping cough	per-TUHS-is	bacteria that causes severe coughing; common childhood vaccine
polio myelitis	POH-lee-oh meye-*uh*-LEYE-tis	virus that can cause neurological damage and paralysis; common childhood vaccine
pneumococcal disease	noo-*muh*-KOK-*uhl*	bacteria that can cause pneumonia; common childhood vaccine

continues

Common Childhood Diseases and Illness Symptoms   (continued)

Term	Pronunciation	Meaning
respiratory syncytial virus (RSV)	RES-per-*uh*-tawr-ee sin-SISH-*uhl*	virus that can cause pneumonia and bronchiolitis
rhinitis	reye-NEYE-tis	infection or inflammation of the tissues lining the nasal passages; runny nose
rickets	RIK-*uhts*	softening of the bones (osteomalacia) due to vitamin D deficiency
ringworm	RING-*wurm*	parasite that causes a circular skin rash
rotavirus infection	ROH-*tuh*-VEYE-*ruhs*	most common cause of diarrhea in infants and children; common childhood vaccine
rubella, German measles	roo-BEL-*uh*	virus that causes flulike illness and a characteristic rash; common childhood vaccine
rubeola, measles	roo-bee-OH-*luh*	virus that causes a respiratory illness; common childhood vaccine
scabies	SKEY-beez	itchy skin rash caused by a mite
scoliosis	skoh-lee-OH-sis	abnormally curved spine
streptococcal pharyngitis	strep-*tuh*-KOK-*uhl* far-in-JEYE-tis	an infection of the throat caused by group A *Streptococcus*; strep throat
tetanus, lockjaw	TET-n-*uhs*	bacteria that infects the nervous system and can cause jaw and whole-body spasms; childhood vaccine
torticollis	tawrt-i-KUHL-is	twisted neck that can be caused by tight positioning in the uterus, congenital defects, infection, trauma, or reaction to medications
urticaria	ur-ti-KAIR-ee-*uh*	hives
varicella-zoster virus	var-*uh*-SEL-*uh* ZOS-ter	chickenpox; common childhood vaccine

Abnormal Growth and Disorders of Puberty

Medical disease and malnutrition affect growth and sexual development. Inadequate weight gain and growth is called **failure to thrive** and has a number of medical and psychological causes. Short stature can also be caused by growth hormone deficiency, which can be due to a number of genetic and congenital causes.

Sexual development and puberty can be delayed if sex hormones are produced in inadequate amounts or the body is unable to respond to these hormones. **Congenital adrenal hyperplasia** (heye-per-PLEY-*zhuh*) is a genetic disorder that can cause inadequate cortisol and too much **androgens** (AN-druh-*juhnz*), or sex hormones. This condition can cause **precocious** (pri-KOH-*shuhs*), or early, puberty. Paradoxically, it can also delay puberty and interfere with the development of external sex organs.

> **DID YOU KNOW?**
>
> Puberty has different stages, and each has its own name. **Pubarche** (PYOO-bahr-kee) refers to the development of pubic hair. **Thelarche** (thee-LAHR-kee) refers to breast development in young women. **Menarche** (MEN-ahr-kee) refers to the beginning of menstrual periods. **Gonadarche** (GOH-nad-ahr-kee) refers to the onset of testicular growth in young men.

Gonadal development can be affected by genetic diseases and can result in **hypogonadism** (heye-*puh*-GOH-na-diz-*uhm*), or small or inadequately developed gonads. **Kallman syndrome** is a genetic disorder that results in low levels of circulating sex hormones and small gonads. This delays puberty or blocks it from occurring. **Klinefelter** (KLEYEN-felt-er) **syndrome** is a genetic disorder that affects males and causes impaired fertility and hypogonadism. A similar genetic disorder affects women and is called **Turner** (TURN-er) **syndrome**. It causes **amenorrhea** (ey-men-*uh*-REE-*uh*), or lack of menstrual periods. It also causes minimally developed ovaries, short stature, poorly developed breasts, and a number of medical problems.

Pediatric Oncology

Brain tumors are a common type of pediatric cancer. Brain tumors are named after the type of nerve cell that becomes cancerous. The most common types of brain tumors in children are **medulloblastomas** (*muh*-DUHL-*uh*-bla-STOH-*muhz*), **ependymomas** (*uh*-pen-dim-OHM-*uhz*), and **gliomas** (gleye-OH-*muhz*).

Other common types of pediatric cancer are **leukemia** (loo-KEE-mee-*uh*), which is cancer of the blood; and **lymphoma** (lim-FOH-*muh*), which is cancer of white blood cells that occurs in the lymph nodes, spleen, and bone marrow. By far the most common type of childhood leukemia is **acute lymphocytic leukemia** (*uh*-KYOOT lim-*fuh*-SIT-ik loo-KEE-mee-*uh*), also called **acute lymphoblastic** (lim-*fuh*-BLAST-ik) **leukemia**, which is cancer of white blood cells. The most common type of pediatric lymphoma is **non-Hodgkin lymphoma** (lim-FOH-*muh*), which is a group of cancers of white blood cells that can range from slow-growing to aggressive.

Other cancers that primarily affect children include the following:

- **Neuroblastoma** (noor-oh-bla-STOH-*muh*): a **neuroendocrine** (noor-oh-EN-*duh*-krin)—meaning arising from neural and endocrine cells—tumor that primarily affects the adrenal glands
- **Wilms tumor** (WILMZ TOO-mer): cancer of the kidneys
- **Rhabdomyosarcoma** (RAB-doh-MEYE-oh-sawr-KOH-*muh*): cancer of connective tissues
- **Retinoblastoma** (ret-noh-bla-STOH-*muh*): cancer of retinal cells
- **Osteosarcoma** (os-tee-oh-sahr-KOH-*muh*): bone cancer
- **Ewing sarcoma** (YOO-ing sahr-KOH-*muh*): cancer that forms in bones or soft tissues, especially in the pelvis, femur, humerus, ribs, or clavicle

The Least You Need to Know

- Neonatologists care for premature and medically ill infants needing care in a neonatal intensive care unit.
- Congenital defects can result from genetic disorders, problems with morphogenesis, medical issues in the mother, and alcohol or use of illicit substances by the mother.
- Pediatric illnesses can result from infectious diseases; nutritional deficiencies; and autoimmune, endocrine, and genetic disorders.
- Abnormal growth and disorders of puberty can be due to nutritional, medical, genetic, and endocrine causes.
- Leukemia, lymphoma, and some types of brain tumors are the most common types of cancers in children.

Surgery and Related Disciplines

In This Chapter

- Terms and word endings used by most surgeons
- Orthopedic, heart surgery, and urology procedures
- OB-GYN and brain surgery operations
- Anesthesia and x-rays
- Skin, eye, ear, nose, and throat specialists

Surgery is the use of manual and instrumental techniques to treat human disease. General surgeons operate on abdominal organs. Diseases in the other areas of the body are treated by a surgeon who specializes in one of the surgical subfields.

In many surgical terms, the word root tells you what part of the body is being operated on. The word ending tells you what kind of operation it is. Knowing some of the word roots and surgical word endings will help you figure out many surgical terms in the various surgical subfields.

Surgical Suffixes and Common Terms

All the surgical fields share similar terms for surgical procedures. The end of a surgical term provides a clue about the kind of procedure it is.

Becoming familiar with surgical word endings is one of the keys to learning surgical terms. These endings include the following:

- **–centesis:** Surgical puncture. In **arthrocentesis** (ahr-throh-cen-TEE-*suhs*), for example, a surgeon makes a puncture and drains a joint of excess fluid.
- **–desis:** To fuse in order to provide stabilization. For example, **arthrodesis** (ahr-throh-DEE-sis) is the surgical fusion of a joint.

- **-ectomy:** A procedure that **excises** (ik-SAHZ-ez), or cuts out, a body part. For example, an **appendectomy** (ap-*uhn*-DEK-*tuh*-mee) cuts out the appendix.

- **–opsy:** Inspection. For example, an **autopsy** (AW-top-see) is the inspection of a dead body.

- **–otomy:** To cut into. For example, a **lobotomy** (*luh*-BOT-*uh*-mee) cuts into a lobe of the brain, usually in order to remove it.

- **–ostomy:** Creation of a **stoma** (STOH-*muh*), or opening. An **ileostomy** (il-ee-OS-*tuh*-mee), for example, is an opening from the ileum through the abdominal wall.

- **–plasty:** Reconstruction of a body part. **Rhinoplasty** (REYE-*nuh*-plas-tee) is reconstruction of the nose, for example.

- **–rrhaphy:** Repairing a damaged area. For example, **herniorrhaphy** (hur-nee-AWR-*uh*-fee) repairs a hernia.

- **–pexy:** To create an attachment. **Gastropexy** (gas-troh-PEX-ee) attaches the stomach to the abdominal wall, for example.

- **–scopy:** To view. **Endoscopy** (en-DOS-*kuh*-pee), for example, uses an instrument to view inside the body.

 WORD ORIGINS

The term *surgery* comes from the Latin term *chirurgiae*, which means handwork. That's what surgeons do. They use their hands and surgical instruments to diagnose and treat diseases. Surgery is an ancient medical specialty and may date as far back as the Neolithic period. The oldest known surgical texts come from ancient Egyptian papyri.

Common Surgical Terms

Term	Pronunciation	Meaning
amputation	am-pyoo-TEY-*shuhn*	cutting off a body part
anastomosis	*uh*-nas-*tuh*-MOH-sis	joining or connecting two organs that were not previously connected
aseptic	ey-SEP-tik	technique used in the operating room to keep it free of microbes

Term	Pronunciation	Meaning
debridement	dih-BREED-*muhnt*	cleaning a wound by surgically removing dead tissue and debris
excision	ek-SIZH-*uhn*	cutting out an organ or tissue
graft		attaching tissue from one area of the body to a different area
incision	in-SIZH-*uhn*	cutting into
ligation	leye-GEY-*shuhn*	tying off, especially a bleeding vessel
prosthesis	pros-THEE-sis	an artificial object that substitutes for a missing or damaged body part or structure
reduction	ri-DUHK-*shuhn*	realigning a body part to its normal position
replantation	ree-plan-TEY-*shuhn*	reattaching a body part
resection	ri-SEK-*shuhn*	cutting out part of an organ or tissue
suture	SOO-cher	stitching a wound together
transplant	trans-PLANT	replacing a damaged body part with a foreign one

Orthopedic Surgery

Orthopedic (awr-*thuh*-PEE-dik) surgeons treat conditions of the musculoskeletal system. Orthopedics grew largely out of experiences treating battle injuries, and orthopedists continue to treat injuries due to **trauma** (TRAW-*muh*), including amputations and broken bones (see Chapter 20). Amputations can also become necessary due to medical diseases, like diabetes. Orthopedists also treat bone deformations resulting from cancer and genetic and degenerative disorders. They treat sports injuries, which include joint, ligament, and tendon problems (see Chapter 20).

Orthopedists use many general terms to refer to musculoskeletal deformities and treatments, such as the following:

- A **bunion** (BUHN-*yuhn*) is a deformation of the head of the first toe joint.
- **Planus** (PLEY-*nuhs*, PLAN-*uhs*) refers to a flat foot.
- **Kyphosis** (keye-FOH-*suhs*) is a rounded curvature of the spine, or hunchback.

- **Lordosis** (lawr-DOH-sis) is forward curvature of the spine, or swayback.
- An **exostosis** (ek-so-STOH-sis) is a bony overgrowth.
- **Bursitis** (ber-SEYE-tis) refers to inflammation of the sac around a joint.
- **Chondromalacia** (kon-droh-*muh*-LEY-*shuh*) is softening of joint surfaces due wear and tear.
- **Crepitus** (KREP-*uh*-*tuhs*) is a grinding sound that occurs between two joints when they have lost their fibrous cushioning.

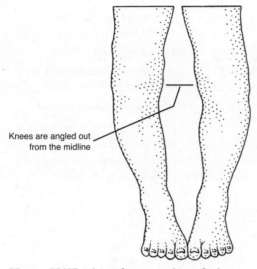

Varus (VAIR-uhs) refers to angling of a bone away from the midline, such as in **genu varum** *(JEN-oo VAIR-uhm), or bowleggedness.*
Halli Verinder © Dorling Kindersley

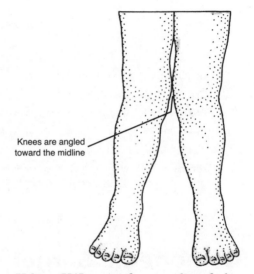

Valgus (VAL-gus) refers to angling of a bone toward the midline, such as in **genu valgum** *(JEN-oo VAL-guhm), or knock-knees.*
Halli Verinder © Dorling Kindersley

Some general terms refer to orthopedic conditions. **Compartment syndrome** is increased pressure in a compartment of the body—an enclosed space that is bounded by fascia, like areas of the arms and lower limbs—causing pain, loss of sensation, and paralysis. Compartment syndrome is an emergency that can cause loss of the body part in which it occurs if left untreated. **Impingement** (im-PINJ-*muhnt*) **syndrome** is shoulder pain due to inflammation in the rotator cuff area. **Subluxation** (suhb-luhk-SEY-*shuhn*) is partial dislocation of a joint. **Diastasis** (deye-AS-*tuh*-sis) is separation of the distal tibia from the fibula. A **dislocation** is complete separation of a joint.

Orthopedists sometimes **aspirate** (AS-*puh*-reyt) or remove fluids from a joint using a needle. They use **fixation** (fik-SEY-*shuhn*) to stabilize broken bones, and sometimes use **traction** (TRAK-*shuhn*) to pull on broken bones and correctly align them.

Cardiothoracic Surgery

Cardiothoracic (KAHR-dee-oh-thaw-RAS-ik) surgery treats conditions of the heart, great vessels, and lungs. Cardiothoracic surgery is further subdivided into **cardiac** (KAHR-dee-ak), or heart, and **thoracic** (thaw-RAS-ik), or lung and chest, surgery.

Cardiac surgeons perform open-heart surgery. During this operation, the heart is stopped and a **cardiopulmonary bypass** (KAHR-dee-oh-PUHL-*muh*-ner-ee BEYE-pas) machine takes over pumping and oxygenating the blood. Cardiac surgeons repair damaged heart valves, which is called **valvuloplasty** (valv-yoo-loh-PLAS-tee). They also repair congenital defects, such as a **patent ductus arteriosus** (PDA) or **coarctation** (koh-ahrk-TEY-*shuhn*), narrowing, of the aorta. Cardiac surgeons also repair **aneurisms** (AN-*yuh*-riz-*uhmz*). Aneurisms are bulging, weakened areas of blood vessels that can sometimes burst. Sometimes these vessels can be treated through **percutaneous** (pur-kyoo-TEY-nee-*uhs*) procedures, in which small instruments for repairing the aneurysm are inserted through blood vessels in the groin area.

WORDS OF WARNING

Another spelling for the word *aneurism* is *aneurysm*. Both spellings are correct, and both are commonly used. The different spellings may be due to different translations of the Greek word from which the term originates, *aneurysma*, which means dilation. For the sake of consistency, this book uses the spelling *aneurism*.

If the pacemaker of the heart is damaged, cardiac surgeons can install artificial cardiac pacemakers. Some types of cardiac **arrhythmias** (*uh*-RITH-mee-*uhz*, ey-RITH-mee-*uhz*), or irregular heart rhythms, are treated with cardiac **ablation** (a-BLEY-*shuhn*), which destroys the damaged area of the heart where irregular electrical signals are originating.

One of the major operations that cardiac surgeons perform is **coronary artery bypass grafting**, or **CABG** (KAB-ij), in which a blocked and diseased coronary artery is replaced with a **graft** of a vessel from another part of the body. Sometimes, cardiac surgeons can use **balloon angioplasty** (AN-jee-*uh*-plas-tee) to widen diseased coronary arteries. They also place **stents** (STENTS) in arteries to keep them open.

Cardiac surgeons also perform cardiac **transplants** (TRANS-plants), which is the replacement of a diseased heart with a donor heart.

Thoracic surgeons perform **lobectomies** (loh-BEK-*tuh*-meez), which is the removal of part of the lung that is dead or diseased due to infection, cancer, or other disease processes. This operation can sometimes be done via **video-assisted thorascopic surgery** (VATS). In this minimally invasive technique, a surgeon cuts a small hole into the chest wall and inserts a small camera into the chest cavity. The surgeon does the lung surgery with the assistance of the video camera. Thoracic surgeons also perform lung transplants, which require a **pneumonectomy** (noo-*muh*-NEK-*tuh*-mee), or removal of the diseased lung.

Thoracic surgeons also operate on the esophagus. Sometimes treatment for esophageal cancer requires an **esophagogastrectomy** (ih-SOF-*uh*-goh-ga-STRECT-*uh*-mee), which is removal of the cancerous part of the esophagus and reconstruction of the digestive tract. Esophageal tissue damaged by **gastroesophageal reflux disease** (GERD) and **hiatal** (heye-EY-*tuhl*) **hernias**, or protrusion of the stomach into the chest cavity, are treated by **Nissen fundoplication** (fuhnd-oh-pleye-KEY-*shuhn*). In this technique, the upper part of the stomach is stitched around the lower part of the esophagus. **Achalasia** (ak-*uh*-LEY-*zhuh*), in which the lower esophageal sphincter fails to relax to allow food to pass into the stomach, can be treated with a **myotomy** (meye-OT-*uh*-mee), or cutting the muscles in the lower esophageal sphincter.

In **bronchoscopies** (brong-KOS-*kuh*-peez), thoracic surgeons insert an instrument through the mouth to look at the inside of the airways. **Biopsies** (BEYE-op-seez), or samples of tissue, are sometimes collected for further analysis during bronchoscopies. Another procedure that thoracic surgeons often perform is a **thoracentesis** (thawr-*uh*-sen-TEE-sis), which involves using a needle to drain fluid from the chest.

Urological Surgery

Urologists use surgical techniques and medical management to treat diseases of the urinary and male reproductive tract. Surgical techniques that urologists perform include **nephrectomies** (*nuh*-FREK-*tuh*-meez), or removal of a kidney to treat cancer or other diseases. They also perform **nephrolithotomies** (nef-*ruh-li*-THOT-*uh-meez*) to remove **renal calculi** (KAL-*kyuh*-leye), which are kidney stones. This process sometimes entails the placement of ureteral stents to prevent future obstructions. Urologists can treat bladder cancer with **transurethral** (tranz-yoo-REE-*thruhl*) **resections** and **cystectomies** (si-STEK-*tuh*-meez).

Urogynecologists (yoor-oh-geye-ni-KOL-*uh*-jists) specialize in the treatment of female urinary conditions. Many of these conditions develop as a result of childbirth. When a woman's pelvic floor becomes weakened, **pelvic organ prolapse** can result. **Cystocele** (sis-*tuh*-seel) is protrusion of the bladder into the vagina, and **rectocele** (rek-*tuh*-seel) is protrusion of the rectum into the vagina. **Pelvic floor reconstruction** can improve these conditions.

For example, when a woman's bladder drops down from its normal position, urinary **incontinence** (in-KON-tn-*uhn-nuhns*) can result. It can be treated through the following procedures:

- **Bladder repositioning** (ree-*puh*-ZISH-*uhn*-ing) lifts the bladder and urethra.
- **Retropubic suspension** (RE-troh-PYOO-bik *suh*-SPEN-*shuhn*) secures the urethra and neck of the bladder.
- **Urethral slings** (yoo-REE-*thruhl* SLINGZ) lift the urethra to its normal position.

Urologists also treat neurological conditions that can result in urinary incontinence, such as **spastic** (SPAS-tik) **bladder**. This condition results from a lesion in the spinal cord.

Urologists perform surgeries on the male reproductive tract as well. They treat **testicular torsion** (TAWR-*shuhn*), or twisting of the testicle in its sac, which cuts off its blood supply and can result in death of the testicle. **Orchiopexy** (awr-kee-oh-PEX-ee) is used to move an undescended testicle into the scrotum. If left untreated, an undescended testicle can be a risk factor for testicular cancer.

Treatment for testicular cancer can necessitate an **orchiectomy** (awr-kee-EK-*tuh*-mee), or removal of a testicle. Urologists also perform **prostatectomies** (pros-*tuh*-TEK-*tuh*-mee), or removal of the prostate when it is cancerous. Sometimes the prostate can require removal due to **benign prostatic hypertrophy** (bih-NEYEN pro-STAT-ik heye-PER-truh-fee), or BPH, which is enlargement of the prostate that can obstruct urinary flow. Note that the H in BPH also can stand for **hyperplasia** (heye-per-PLEY-*zhuh*).

Urologists also operate on the penis. They can treat **erectile** (ih-REK-tl, ih-REK-teyel) **dysfunction**, or the inability to attain an erection, with medication or penile implants. Urologists can also correct congenital malformations of the male reproductive tract, such as **hypospadias** (HEYE-poh-SPEY-dee-*uhs*), which is when the urethral opening occurs in an abnormal position on the penis.

Obstetrics and Gynecology

An obstetrician-gynecologist (OB-GYN) uses both surgery and medical management to treat gynecologic conditions, obstetrical emergencies, medical complications of pregnancy and childbirth, and gynecological cancers.

OB-GYNs treat conditions like **endometriosis** (en-doh-mee-tree-OH-sis) and **fibroids** (FEYE-broidz), which are also called **leiomyomas** (leye-oh-meye-OH-*muhz*) and are benign fibrous tumors of the uterus. These conditions can cause **dysmenor-rhea** (dis-men-*uh*-REE-*uh*), which is painful menstruation, and **menorrhagia** (men-*uh*-REY-*juh*), which is heavy bleeding during menstruation. **Amenorrhea** (ey-men-*uh*-REE-*uh*) is the absence of menstrual periods and can be due to a number of causes. A **myomectomy** (meye-*uh*-MEK-*tuh*-mee) can be used to cut out fibroids. **Dilation** (deye-LEY-*shuhn*) **and curettage** (kyoor-i-TAHZH), or D&C, which is dilating the uterus and scraping its contents, is used to diagnose many gynecological conditions.

OB-GYNs also treat obstetrical emergencies that develop during labor and childbirth. Birth can be complicated by medical problems in the mother, such as **preeclampsia** (pree-i-KLAMP-see-*uh*), which is high blood pressure accompanied by protein in the urine. Preeclampsia can progress to life-threatening **eclampsia** (i-KLAMP-see-*uh*), or seizures in the mother.

Dystocia (dis-TOH-*shuh*) refers to prolonged or difficult birth. Birth complications can include **umbilical cord prolapse** (PROH-laps), which is an emergency because it cuts off oxygen supply to the fetus.

DID YOU KNOW?

The placenta can form abnormally, causing profuse bleeding at delivery. A **placenta accreta** (*uh*-KREET-*uh*) grows into the uterine lining, but does not reach the muscle. A **placenta increta** (IN-KREET-*uh*) grows into the uterine muscle. A **placenta percreta** (PER-KREET-*uh*) grows through the full thickness of the uterus, and sometimes attaches to pelvic organs. Development of one of these conditions, especially placenta percreta, can require removal of the uterus.

A serious complication of labor is **uterine rupture**, in which the wall of the uterus bursts and necessitates hysterectomy. A **hysterectomy** (his-*tuh*-REK-*tuh*-mee) is the removal of the uterus.

Labor and delivery complications often lead to **cesarean** (si-ZAIR-ee-*uhn*) **section**, in which the abdominal and uterine walls are cut in order to extract the fetus. At this time, **tubal ligation** (TOO-*buhl* leye-GEY-*shuhn*), or tying the tubes, is sometimes done to induce infertility in women not desiring subsequent pregnancies.

Cancers of the female reproductive tract include uterine, ovarian, cervical, and vulvar cancer. Surgical techniques in the treatment of these cancers include hysterectomy; **vulvectomy** (vuhl-VEK-*tuh*-mee), which is removal of the cancerous parts of the vulva; and **oophorectomy** (oh-*uh-fuh*-REK-*tuh*-mee), or removal of the ovaries. Cervical cancer is sometimes treated with a **loop electrocautery excision procedure** or **cone biopsy** (KOHN BEYE-op-see), both of which excise the cancerous cells. Some gynecological cancers also are treated with concurrent **chemotherapy** (kee-moh-THERE-*uh*-pee), which is cancer medication, and **radiation** (rey-dee-EY-*shuhn*) **therapy**.

OB-GYNs also treat **infertility** (in-fur-TIL-*uh*-tee), or the inability to conceive, through hormonal means and **artificial insemination** (in-SEM-*uh*-ney-*shuhn*). In this procedure, sperm is artificially introduced into the female reproductive tract near the time of ovulation.

Neurosurgery

Neurosurgeons (noor-oh-SUR-*juhnz*) treat diseases and disorders of the nervous system. Such diseases include cancer and tumors of the brain, spinal cord, and peripheral nerves; stroke and other conditions that can cause bleeding or blood clots in the brain; disorders of the spinal cord and vertebrae; and other disorders of the nervous system caused by medical or neurological illnesses.

DID YOU KNOW?

Neurosurgeons can treat movement disorders caused by Parkinson disease with deep brain stimulation. They implant a device called a brain pacemaker into the brain. This device sends electrical signals to different parts of the brain to affect brain activity. These effects are reversible. The pacemaker sometimes needs to be recalibrated by a physician or nurse. Deep brain stimulation has also been used to treat chronic pain, essential tremor, dystonia, and major depression.

Brain Tumors

Neurosurgeons treat brain tumors with surgical resection and/or chemotherapy and radiation treatment. Primary tumors of the nervous system are tumors that begin in the nervous system and aren't the result of spreading from other parts of the body to the nervous system. Primary tumors of the nervous system are named according the type of cell that becomes cancerous. For example, **meningiomas** (*muh*-nin-jee-OH-*muhz*) are a group of mostly benign tumors that arise from the meninges. **Oligodendrogliomas** (OL-*uh*-goh-den-DROH-glee-OH-*muhz*) are slowly growing, malignant tumors that arise from oligodendrocytes. **Oligodendrocytes** (OL-*uh*-goh-DEN-*druh*-seyets) are cells that support nerve axons.

Other examples include **pituitary adenomas** (ad-n-OH-*muhz*). These benign pituitary tumors can cause excess pituitary hormones, endocrine abnormalities, visual defects, and psychiatric symptoms. Nerve sheath tumors are primary tumors that arise from **myelin** (MEYE-*uh*-lin), the substance that surrounds nerves.

Astrocytomas (AS-*truh*-seyet-OH-*muhz*) are a group of benign and malignant primary tumors that arise from astrocytes. **Astrocytes** (AS-*truh*-seyets) are cells that provide support for the brain. A subgroup of astrocytomas, **glioblastomas** (glee-oh-blast-OH-*muhz*) are a group of malignant tumors. The most deadly type of primary brain tumor is a **glioblastoma multiforme** (glee-oh-blast-OH-*muh* muhl-*tuh*-form), which usually causes death within about 1 year of diagnosis.

Secondary or metastatic tumors are the most common type of tumor found in the brain. These tumors are spread most commonly from cancer of the lung, breast, skin, kidney, and colon (see Chapter 22).

Some brain tumors take up space in the skull and cause **mass effect**, which compresses the brain and increases intracranial pressure. Mass effect can also cause a **midline shift** in which the central axis of the brain moves past its normal position. This can cause physical symptoms like behavioral changes, vomiting, headaches, movement problems, and seizures. **Brain herniation** (hur-nee-EY-*shuhn*), in which parts of the brain shift past cranial structures, can occur. Brain herniation that causes the brain stem to protrude into the **foramen magnum** (*fuh*-REY-*muhn* MAG-*nuhm*), or opening at the base of the skull, can be deadly. Bleeding also can cause mass effect.

Bleeding in the Brain

Intracranial hemorrhages (in-*truh*-KREY-nee-*uhl* HEM-er-ij-ez), or bleeding inside the skull, can result from hemorrhagic stroke or traumatic brain injury.

When the bleeding collects and clots in a certain location, it is called a **hematoma** (hee-ma-TOH-*muh*).

Intracranial hemorrhages and hematomas are named based on their location:

- An **epidural** (ep-i-DOOR-*uhl*) **hematoma** is found between the skull and the dura mater, the tough outer covering of the brain.
- A **subdural** (suhb-DOOR-*uhl*) **hematoma** is found between the dura mater and the arachnoid mater, which is the middle, spider weblike layer of the covering of the brain.
- A **subarachnoid** (*suhb-uh*-RAK-noid) **hemorrhage** is found between the arachnoid mater and the pia mater, the delicate inner layer of the covering of the brain.
- An **intraparenchymal** (in-*truh-puh*-RENG-*kuh-muhl*) **hemorrhage** is bleeding into the tissue of the brain.
- An **intraventricular** (in-*truh*-ven-TRIK-*yuh*-ler) **hemorrhage** is bleeding into the ventricles of the brain, where cerebrospinal fluid (CSF) circulates.

Neurosurgeons also treat vascular malformations that can cause bleeding into the brain if they rupture. **Cerebral arteriovenous** (ahr-teer-ee-oh-VEE-*nuhs*) **malformations** are abnormal connections between arteries and veins that are often present at birth. Other blood vessel malformations include **hemangiomas** (hi-man-jee-OH-*muhz*), which are benign tumors of blood vessel walls, and **capillary telangiestasias** (*tuh*-lan-jee-ek-TEY-*shuhz*), which are dilated blood vessels in the brain.

Sometimes neurosurgeons are needed to treat complications that arise from **cerebral venous sinus thrombosis** (throm-BOH-sis), a clot that forms in the venous sinuses of the brain. This condition is often treated nonsurgically with anticoagulant medication. Blood clots can raise intracranial pressure, contributing to the buildup of CSF and hydrocephalus. Neurosurgeons can treat this condition by inserting a cerebral shunt, which drains off excess CSF.

Spinal Cord Disorders

Neurosurgeons also treat disorders of the spinal cord and vertebrae, such as spinal tumors and spinal cord trauma (see Chapter 20). **Spinal stenosis** (sti-NOH-sis) is the narrowing of the vertebral column. It constricts the spinal cord and can cause symptoms like discomfort while standing, numbness, and weakness. It can also cause a **radiculopathy** (*ruh*-dik-yoo-LAWP-*uh*-thee), which is dysfunction of the spinal nerve roots, and cauda equina syndrome.

> **WORD ORIGINS**
>
> The term *cauda equina* comes from Latin and means "horse's tail." The **cauda equina** is a loose bundle of nerves that look like a horse's tail and lie at the bottom of the spinal cord. **Cauda equina** (KAW-*duh* ik-WEYEN-*uh*) **syndrome** is an emergency and refers to sudden loss of function, including lower limb paralysis, urinary and bowel incontinence, pain, and loss of sensation. Cauda equine syndrome can be caused by tumors, injury, inflammation, infection, spinal stenosis, and disc herniation.

Spinal disc herniation (hur-nee-AY-shuhn) is a condition in which the soft portion of an intervertebral disc called the **nucleus pulposus** (NOO-klee-*uhs* puhlp-OH-*suhs*) bulges outward. This condition can result in numbness, muscle weakness, erectile dysfunction, urinary incontinence, and sciatica. **Sciatica** (seye-AT-i-*kuh*) is lower-back pain that runs down the side of the leg. Neurosurgeons can treat severe cases of disc herniation with several types of operations, including discectomy, laminectomy, and disc replacement. **Discectomy** (disk-EK-*tuh*-mee) is the partial or full removal of an intervertebral disc; **laminectomy** (lam-*uh*-NEK-*tuh*-mee) is the removal of part of the arch of a vertebra.

Anesthesiology

Anesthesiologists deal with pain management during surgical procedure and chronic pain control. The sensation of pain is called **nociception** (noh-see-CEP-*shuhn*). **Analgesia** (an-l-JEE-zee-*uh*) refers to the condition of not feeling pain. During surgery, anesthesiologists monitor the patient for many abnormalities, including changes in blood pressure, heart rate, blood composition, and oxygen saturation of the blood, which is also called **pulse oximetry** (ok-SIM-i-tree). When necessary, anesthesiologists administer medication to keep the patient alive during surgery. They also monitor the levels of anesthetic agent in the patient's blood.

There are several types of anesthesia. **General anesthesia** blocks pain at the level of the brain, resulting in unconsciousness and loss of memory of the procedure. During general anesthesia, certain breathing reflexes are lost. Anesthesiologists **intubate** (IN-too-beyt), or place a breathing tube down the throat, and provide airway management to ensure that the patient breathes properly.

Regional anesthesia provides pain control of a body region. In **epidural** (ep-i-DOOR-*uhl*) **anesthesia**, the anesthetic agent is injected into the epidural space outside the sac containing the spinal cord and normally requires placement of a **catheter** (KATH-i-ter), or tube through which more medication can be administered. Epidural anesthesia is frequently used during childbirth. During administration of **spinal anesthesia,** the anesthetic agent is injected into the spinal fluid and does not involve placement of a catheter. Epidural and spinal anesthesia are usually injected into the lower back and provide pain control to the lower body. A **saddle block,** or caudal anesthesia, produces numbness in the buttocks, inner thighs, and **perineum** (per-*uh*-NEE-*uhm*), or area containing the external genitalia. A **plexus block** is anesthesia provided to a particular nerve **plexus** (PLEK-*suhs*), or group of nerves that innervates a body area. For example, the **brachial plexus** innervates much of the shoulder, arm, and hand.

Local anesthesia provides pain control of a particular body area or part. **Topical** (TOP-i-*kuhl*) anesthetics are applied to the surface of a tissue and to numb the top layers of it.

Ophthalmology

Ophthalmologists (off-*thuhl*-MOL-*uh*-jists) use various surgical techniques to treat diseases of the eye, including laser surgery, cauterization, and cryotherapy. **Cauterization** (KAW-*tuh*-ruh-ZEY-*shuhn*) is the use of extreme heat to burn abnormal tissue, and **cryotherapy** (kreye-oh-THER-*uh*-pee) is the use of extreme cold to freeze abnormal tissue.

Surgery can be used to treat cataracts and glaucoma. **Cataracts** (KAT-*uh*-rakts) are **opacifications** (oh-pas-*uh*-*fuh*-KEY-*shuhnz*), or cloudiness, of the lens of the eye that can cause vision loss. **Glaucoma** (glaw-KOH-*muh*) is a disease of the optic nerve that causes pressure to build inside the eye and can cause blindness.

Ophthalmologists also use various techniques to perform **refractive** (ri-FRAK-tiv) surgery, which are operations on the cornea that improve refractive errors in vision, often making glasses unnecessary. Ophthalmologists also perform **retinopexies** (ret-noh-PEX-eez), in which they reattach detached retinas.

Ophthalmologists also can perform laser surgery to slow down vision loss in people with some types of **macular** (MAK-*yuh*-ler) degeneration, which is a process of deterioration often associated with age that results in loss of the central field of vision. Ophthalmologists also perform surgery on the ocular muscles to correct strabismus (struh-BIZ-*muhs*), or misaligned eyes, in children. Another procedure that ophthalmologists perform is called **blepharoplasty** (BLEF-er-*uh*-PLAS-tee), which is surgery on the eyelids to remove excess tissue. Sometimes trauma and other processes require removal of the entire eye, which is called **enucleation** (ih-noo-klee-EY-*shuhn*).

Ear, Nose, and Throat (ENT)

Surgeons who treat conditions of the head and neck are called ear, nose, and throat surgeons, or ENTs. Another name for this surgical subspecialty is **otolaryngology** (oh-toh-lar-ing-GOL-*uh*-jee). ENTs treat many types of disorders. Hearing loss in children is sometimes treated by inserting **cochlear** (KOK-lee-er) implants. Complications from multiple middle ear infections can be treated with a **myrin-gotomy** (mir-in-GOT-*uh*-mee), or an incision in the eardrum, and placement of **tympanostomy** (tim-pan-OST-*uh*-mee) tubes to prevent buildup of fluid and pus. ENTs also excise vocal cord **nodules** (NOJ-oolz) and **polyps** (POL-ips), which are small growths on the vocal cords that can cause hoarseness. ENTs sometimes treat sinus disorders with **endoscopic** (*en*-duh-SKAWP-ik) surgery, in which surgery is conducted via a small tube that has been inserted through the nostrils.

WORD ORIGINS

Some people who have trouble getting words out of their mouths are literally tongue-tied in a medical sense. **Tongue-tie**, or **ankyloglossia** (ang-*kuh*-loh-GLAW-see-*uh*), is a congenital malformation in which a membrane called the **lingual frenulum** (LING-*gwuhl* FREN-*yuh-luhm*) attaches the bottom of the tongue to the floor of the mouth. ENTs or dentists sometimes perform **frenectomies** (fren-EK-*tuh*-mee) to remove the frenulum and improve tongue movement.

ENTs also treat cancer and other growths in the head and neck. Thyroid growths are treated with a **thyroidectomy** (theye-roi-DEK-*tuh*-mee), which is a complete removal of the thyroid, or a **lobectomy** (loh-BEK-*tuh*-mee), which is a removal of one of the lobes, and often removal of the surrounding lymph nodes.

ENTs treat obstructive sleep apnea with various types of surgeries:

- **Septoplasty** (sep-toh-PLAS-tee) straightens a deviated, or crooked, nasal septum.
- **Tonsillectomy** (ton-*suh*-LEK-*tuh*-mee) is removal of the tonsils.

- **Uvulopalatopharyngoplasty** (YOO-vyuh-loh-PAL-it-oh-far-IN-joh-PLAS-tee) is removal of parts of the uvula, soft palate, and adenoids, and reconstruction of the pharynx.

ENTs also do some forms of plastic and reconstructive surgery, including **maxillofacial** (mak-SIL-oh-FEY-*shuhl*) surgery, or reconstruction of the bones in the jaw and face. Reconstructive surgery is also used to repair a cleft lip and palate, a congenital facial malformation that results when the palates fail to fuse during development.

Dermatology

Dermatology is the pharmacologic and surgical treatment of skin disorders. Some types of skin problems that dermatologists treat are infections, autoimmune conditions, cancer, and skin conditions that result from aging and excess sun exposure. The latter sometimes includes cosmetic dermatology or the treatment of skin conditions to improve appearance. General terms that dermatologists use include the following:

Bulla (BUHL-*uh*): blister

Cicatrix (SIK-*uh*-triks): scar

Comedo (KOM-i-doh): blackhead

Ichthyosis (ik-thee-OH-sis): fishlike scales

Keloid (KEE-loid): abnormally thick scar

Nevus (NEE-*vuhs*): mole

Papule (PAP-yool): nonpustulous skin elevation

Pruritus (proo-REYE-*tuhs*): itchiness

Pustule (PUS-tyool): pimple

Urticaria (ur-ti-KAIR-ee-*uh*): hives

Verruca (*vuh*-ROO-*kuh*): wart

Acne vulgaris (AK-nee vuhl-GEYR-*uhs*), or cystic acne, is a common condition that dermatologists treat and is characterized by scaly, red skin; pimples; and often scarring. **Rosacea** (roh-ZEY-*shuh*) is a skin disorder that causes facial **erythema** (er-*uh*-THEE-*muh*), or redness, and may resemble acne but is not a form of it.

Vitiligo (vit-l-EYE-goh) is a condition that causes skin depigmentation. **Eczema** (EK-*zuh-muh*), or atopic dermatitis, is a red, itchy, scaly rash associated with allergies. **Psoriasis** (*suh*-REYE-*uh*-sis) is a red, itchy, silver-white scaly rash. **Impetigo** (im-pi-TEYE-goh) is the most common skin infection in children and is characterized by blisters that ooze and crust over. **Seborrheic dermatitis** (seb-*uh*-REE-ik dur-*muh*-TEYE-tis) is a common patchy, red, scaly rash that usually is found on the face, trunk, or scalp.

Types of cancers that dermatologists treat include the following:

- **Basal** (BEY-*suhl*) **cell carcinoma** is the most common, least lethal skin cancer. It originates from the bottom layer of the epidermis and is translucent.
- **Squamous** (SKWEY-*muhs*) **cell carcinoma** originates from the middle layer of epidermis and is likely to spread.
- **Melanoma** (mel-*uh*-NOH-*muh*) originates from **melanocytes** (*muh*-LAN-*uh*-seyets), which make skin pigment, and is the most likely to spread and the most lethal.

Dermatologists also treat conditions that affect the nails. **Paronychia** (par-*uh*-NIK-ee-*uh*) is a skin infection around the nail bed. **Onychomycosis** (ong-koh-meye-KOH-*suhs*) is nail fungus; **onychocryptosis** (ong-koh-krip-TOH-*suhs*) is an ingrown nail. Dermatologists treat conditions that affect the hair as well, including **alopecia** (al-*uh*-PEE-*shuh*), which is hair loss.

The Least You Need to Know

- Surgical suffixes help you decipher the type of surgical procedure a word is describing.
- Surgical subfields include orthopedics, cardiology, urology, neurosurgery, and ophthalmology. Each of these is dedicated to a different body system.
- Surgeons use their hands and instruments to perform procedures to treat disorders, correct deformities, remove cancerous tumors, and repair injuries.
- Anesthesiologists manage a patient's pain during and after surgical procedures.

Emergency Medicine and Acute Illnesses

Chapter 20

In This Chapter

- Trauma, broken bones, and bleeding
- Heart attacks and breathing difficulties
- Shock, infections, and poisoning
- Strokes, seizures, and head and spine injuries
- Psychosis and recurrent suicidal or homicidal thoughts

Emergency medicine is a medical specialty in which physicians care for acute illnesses and emergencies in the setting of the emergency department (ED) or emergency room (ER). These physicians treat and attempt to stabilize critically ill patients for admission to the hospital or release home. Emergency medicine physicians call on the services of many other types of medical specialists, such as surgeons, neurologists, and psychiatrists.

Emergency medicine physicians also work in urgent care facilities that provide **ambulatory** (AM-*byuh-luh*-tawr-ee), or outpatient, care for some types of acute illnesses and injuries. These facilities are not located adjacent to an emergency room or hospital, so the types of problems they can treat are limited.

Some emergencies occur within hospitals, especially in critical care, or intensive care, units. In such cases, intensive care and other medical specialists are called upon.

Orthopedic and Vascular Emergencies

Orthopedic and vascular emergencies are normally treated in the ED and operating room by emergency medicine physicians and surgeons.

Trauma

Trauma (TRAW-*muh*) refers to physical and psychological injury resulting from sudden events like accidents and violence. Several categories describe these types of injuries.

Blunt-force trauma is also called **nonpenetrating trauma** and happens when soft-tissue injury occurs as a result of physical impact or attack. Blunt-force trauma can result in one or more of the following:

- **Ecchymosis** (ek-*uh*-MOH-sis): a skin bruise
- **Contusion** (*kuhn*-TOO-*zhuhn*): a bruise anywhere in the body, including the internal organs
- **Abrasion** (*uh*-BREY-*zhuhn*): a scrape in tissue like the skin that results from rubbing it against a surface
- **Laceration** (las-*uh*-REY-*shuhn*): a tear in a tissue
- **Fracture** (FRAK-cher): a broken bone (see table in this chapter for names of common fractures)

Blunt-force trauma to the abdomen can damage internal organs, such as the kidneys and spleen, and cause internal bleeding. Diagnostic techniques such as bedside ultrasound, **diagnostic peritoneal lavage** (*luh*-VAHZH), and surgical laparotomy are sometimes used to diagnose abdominal injuries.

Penetrating trauma occurs when the skin is pierced, as in a stab wound. Penetrating wounds to the chest and broken ribs can cause **pneumothorax** (noo-*muh*-THAWR-aks), or air in the chest cavity, which can cause a lung to deflate. A **tension** (TEN-*shuhn*) **pneumothorax** causes significant respiratory distress, including **tachycardia** (tak-i-KAHR-dee-*uh*), or fast heart rate, and **tachypnea** (tak-ip-NEE-*uh*), or fast breathing. **Flail** (FLEYL) **chest** is a serious condition that can sometimes result when multiple ribs are broken, allowing the section with the broken ribs to detach from the chest wall and move in the opposite direction from the chest wall during breathing movements.

Ballistic (*buh*-LIS-tik) **trauma** refers to gunshot wounds. These wounds can cause profuse bleeding and **hypovolemic** (heye-*puh*-*vuh*-LEE-*muhk*) shock, which occurs when there is not enough blood to supply critical organs with oxygen. Death can occur as a consequence of the bullet hitting a critical organ, such as the heart or brain, and by **exsanguination** (eks-sang-*gwuh*-NEY-*shuhn*), or bleeding out.

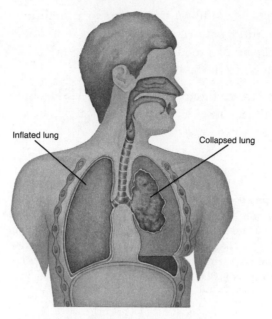

A pneumothorax is a collapsed lung.
© Dorling Kindersley

Burns can cause trauma to the skin and other organs. Fires, chemicals, sunlight, radiation, and electricity can cause burns (see Chapter 5 for information on types of burns). Electrical shocks also can injure other areas of the body, like the heart and nervous system. Death by electric shock is called **electrocution** (ih-LEK-*truh*-kyoo-*shuhn*).

Emergency medicine physicians are often required to remove **foreign bodies**, such as a needle that gets stuck in a foot. Depending on the body part, surgical specialists may be called upon. **Foreign-body aspiration** (as-*puh*-REY-*shuhn*), in which objects are breathed into the lungs, is often treated by thoracic surgeons.

The trauma resulting from sexual assault and/or rape is also treated by emergency medicine physicians, gynecologists, and psychiatrists. Physicians follow specific legal and medical protocols, or guidelines, for treating victims of sexual assault.

Sports Injuries

Sports injuries include bone and soft-tissue problems as well as some neurological injuries. A **sprain** involves ligaments and happens when a joint is overextended, which causes the ligament to tear or stretch too far. A **strain**, or a pulled muscle, involves muscles and tendons and happens when they are overstressed or pulled too far.

Tendinopathy (ten-duhn-OP-*uh*-thee) refers to a condition in which a tendon has been torn or is painful from overuse. **Tendonitis** (ten-*duh*-NEYE-tis) is inflammation, swelling, and pain of a tendon. A **ruptured tendon** happens when the tendon pulls completely away from the bone.

Sports doctors also treat **concussions** (*kuhn*-KUHSH-uhnz), which can result from a blow to the head that causes a brief neurological deficit. Head trauma is discussed later in this chapter.

STUDY TIP

The **unhappy triad** refers to a knee injury that commonly occurs among football, soccer, and basketball players. This term refers to three structures in the knee that are often torn together: the anterior cruciate ligament (ACL), the medial collateral ligament (MCL), and the medial meniscus. Sometimes the lateral meniscus is also injured. The unhappy triad often occurs after a blow to the lateral (outside) of the knee when the foot is planted on the ground.

Common Fractures

Term	Pronunciation	Meaning
avulsion fracture	*uh*-VUHL-*shuhn*	broken bone that happens when a tendon or ligament detaches and pulls off a piece of bone
Colles fracture	KAWL-eez	breaking the distal part of the radius; most common injury caused by falling on an outstretched arm
complete fracture		complete break through a bone
compound fracture	KOM-pound	broken bone in which the skin is broken
compression fracture	*kuhm*-PRESH-*uhn*	broken bone that occurs due to forces directed along the longitudinal axis of the bone
oblique fracture	*uh*-BLEEK, oh-BLEEK	broken bone in which the fracture line is diagonal to the bone
Salter-Harris fracture	SAHL-*tuhr* HAIR-*uhs*	fracture involving the physis (FEYE-sis), or growth plate, in children
Torus fracture, buckle fracture	TAWR-*uhs*	partial fracture in which the end of one bone "buckles" into the growth plate in children

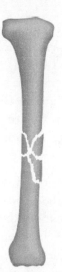

*A comminuted (KOM-uh-noot-ed)
fracture is a fracture in which the
bone has broken in several places.*
© Dorling Kindersley

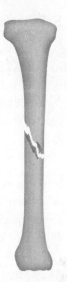

*A spiral fracture is a fracture in
which the bone is twisted.*
© Dorling Kindersley

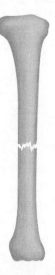

*A transverse (trans-VURS) fracture is a broken bone in which
the fracture plane is perpendicular to the bone.*
© Dorling Kindersley

Vascular Emergencies

Vascular emergencies can result from **hemorrhage** (HEM-rij), which is bleeding, and **occlusion** (*uh*-KLOO-*zhuhn*), which is obstruction of blood vessels. Highly vascular organs like the spleen, lungs, and digestive tract can cause life-threatening internal bleeding when they are injured or ruptured. Serious bleeding also can be caused by an aortic dissection or the rupture of an aortic aneurism. An **aortic dissection** (dih-SEK-*shuhn*) occurs when the walls of the aorta separate. An **aortic aneurism** (AN-*yuh*-riz-*uhm*) is a dilation in the aorta.

Vaso-occlusive (vas-oh-*uh*-KLOO-siv) **crisis** is a complication of sickle cell anemia and occurs when sickled red blood cells obstruct blood vessels, causing pain and infarcts in many organs. It is a common cause of **acute chest syndrome**, which impairs bleeding when the lung vessels become occluded, or blocked. **Pulmonary emboli** (EM-*buh*-leye), or blood clots in the vessels in the lungs, can also result when a **deep vein thrombosis** (throm-BOH-sis), or a blood clot in the deep veins of the lower extremities, dislodges and migrates to the lungs. An **embolism** (EM-*buh*-liz-*uhm*) is any substance that breaks loose from one part of the body and moves to another part, where it blocks blood vessels. Emboli can be made up of **amniotic** (am-nee-OT-ik) fluid, fat, air, and even talc used by intravenous drug users.

Cardiac and Pulmonary Emergencies

Cardiac and pulmonary emergencies often go together because of the intimate connection between the heart and lungs.

Cardiac Emergencies

One of the major cardiac emergencies is **myocardial infarction** (meye-*uh*-KAHR-dee-*uhl* in-FAHRK-*shuhn*), or a heart attack. Heart attacks most commonly occur when one of the coronary arteries becomes blocked, cutting off blood supply and resulting in **ischemia** (ih-SKEE-mee-*uh*), or lack of oxygen, to an area of the heart. This lack of oxygen can cause an infarction, or death, of that part of the **myocardium** (meye-*uh*-KAHR-dee-*uhm*), or heart muscle. Heart attacks have numerous symptoms, not all of which occur in all people all the time. These symptoms include **diaphoresis** (deye-*uh*-*fuh*-REE-sis), or sweating; **angina** (an-JEYE-*nuh*, AN-*juh*-*nuh*), or chest pain; pain or numbness down the left arm; vomiting; shortness of breath; anxiety; tiredness; and **palpitations** (pal-pi-TEY-*shuhnz*), or irregular heartbeats.

A **subendocardial** (suhb-en-doh-KAHR-dee-*uhl*) **infarct**, also called a non-ST-elevation myocardial infarction (NSTEMI), involves a small part of the inside of the wall of the heart and often affects the left ventricle. A **transmural** (tranz-MYOOR-*uhl*) infarct, or ST-elevation myocardial infarction (STEMI), is more serious because the entire thickness of the heart muscle dies, or becomes **necrotic** (*nuh*-KRAW-tik).

In severe heart attacks, cardiac rupture can occur, which means that the heart muscle bursts. A cardiac rupture can cause **pericardial tamponade** (tam-*puh*-NEYD), also called **cardiac tamponade,** in which blood fills the **pericardium** (per-i-KAHR-dee-*uhm*), or sac around the heart. Cardiac tamponade can also be due to hypothyroidism; trauma; or inflammation and infection of the pericardium, or **pericarditis** (per-i-kahr-DEYE-tis).

Other cardiac emergencies include **arrhythmias** (*uh*-RITH-mee-*uhs*, ey-RITH-mee-*uhz*), or irregular heartbeat. Ventricular arrhythmias are the most serious (see Chapters 12 and 19 for further discussion of arrhythmias). The arrhythmia that occurs most often during heart attacks is **ventricular fibrillation** (fib-*ruh*-LEY-*shuhn*), or v-fib, which is asynchronous contraction and quivering of the ventricular muscles. V-fib cannot be sustained for long and normally degenerates into **asystole** (ey-SIS-*tuh*-lee), or lack of a heartbeat, resulting in **cardiogenic** (*car*-dee-oh-GEN-ic) **shock** and sudden cardiac death. Ventricular flutter is a rapid heart rate of 180 to 250 beats per minute (bpm), that often becomes v-fib if left untreated. A cardiac **defibrillator** (dee-FIB-*ruh*-ley-ter) is a machine that uses electricity to shock the heart back into a normal rhythm.

WORDS OF WARNING

Drug abuse can also cause cardiac emergencies. Cocaine increases the heart rate while constricting the coronary blood vessels, causing cardiac ischemia, which can lead to a heart attack. Cocaine also can cause **atrial fibrillation** (a-fib), in which the atria contract out of synchrony. A-fib is a risk factor for stroke.

A **hypertensive** (heye-per-TEN-siv) **emergency,** formerly called **malignant hypertension** (heye-per-TEN-*shuhn*), refers to extremely high blood pressure accompanied by papilledema. **Papilledema** (pap-*uh*-*luh*-DEE-*muh*) is swelling of the **optic disc** (DISK), which is the head of the optic nerve. This swelling is due to increased intracranial pressure, which can cause blurred vision and vomiting. Hypertensive emergency can cause organ damage, especially of the kidneys, central nervous system, and heart. It can also increase the risk for stroke, seizure, and heart attack. **Hypertensive urgency** occurs when there is high blood pressure but no organ damage. **Hypertensive crisis** is a general term that refers to both hypertensive emergency and hypertensive urgency.

Pulmonary Emergencies

Pulmonary emergencies are indicated by respiratory distress, or difficulty breathing, and include pneumothorax and pulmonary emboli as described previously. **Asphyxia** (as-FIK-see-*uh*) is a respiratory emergency and is indicated by hypoxia, hypoxemia, and hypercapnia. **Hypoxia** (heye-POK-see-*uh*) is low oxygen levels in the tissues. **Hypoxemia** (heye-pok-SEE-mee-*uh*) is low oxygen levels in the blood, and **hypercapnia** (heye-per-KAP-nee-*yuh*) is a high level of carbon dioxide in the blood. **Cyanosis** (*seye*-uh-NOH-suhs) is blue discoloration of the lips and skin that happens due to inadequate oxygenation of the blood. The causes for asphyxia include drowning, smoke inhalation, and choking.

Angioedema (an-jee-oh-i-DEE-*muh*) can also cause asphyxia and is swelling of the face, tongue, and mucous membranes of the mouth and throat. The throat can swell so much that it blocks that airway, causing **stridor** (STREYE-der), or difficult breathing, which can be life-threatening. Hereditary illness or allergic reactions to food or medication can cause angioedema.

Respiratory emergencies in children are also common. **Epiglottitis** (ep-i-glot-TEYE-tis) is usually found in children and is a life-threatening swelling of the epiglottis, or the tissue at the base of the tongue that normally keeps food from entering the **trachea** (TREY-kee-*uh*), or windpipe. The epiglottis can swell so much that it interferes with breathing. Epiglottitis is most often caused by a bacterial respiratory infection, such as strep throat or *Haemophilus influenza*.

Croup (KROOP) is also called **laryngotracheobronchitis** (*luh*-RINJ-oh-TREY-kee-oh-brong-KEYE-*tuhs*) and is often caused by a viral infection in children that causes the vocal cords to swell. Croup causes a characteristic "barking" cough and can range from a mild illness to severe breathing difficulties that cause airway obstruction and require hospitalization.

An **asthma attack** is an acute **exacerbation** (ig-ZAS-er-bey-*shuhn*) of chronic asthma, characterized by shortness of breath, wheezing, and chest tightness. An asthma attack can progress to acute severe asthma, formerly called **status asthmaticus** (STAT-*uhs* az-MA-*tuh-cuhs*). In this condition, medication does not work and **intubation** (in-too-BEY-*shuhn*), or placement of a breathing tube, becomes necessary.

Internal Medicine Emergencies

There are many types of internal medicine emergencies, including infections, allergic reactions, poisoning, problems with internal organs, some hospital-acquired conditions, and exacerbations of chronic illnesses. Many of these emergencies cause metabolic abnormalities.

Metabolic Derangements

Internal medicine emergencies are often accompanied by metabolic **derangements** (dih-REYNJ-*muhntz*), or abnormalities that arise when the body cannot carry out vital processes. For example, **hyperthermia** (heye-per-THUR-mee-*uh*) happens when the body loses the ability to regulate its temperature and becomes overheated. **Heat-stroke** is a form of hyperthermia caused by extended exposure to high temperatures. **Sunstroke** is similar to heatstroke and results from overexposure to the sun.

Both heatstroke and sunstroke can be complicated by **dehydration** (dee-heye-DREY-*shuhn*), or inadequate amount of body water. Dehydration can cause blood abnormalities like **hypovolemia** (heye-*puh-vuh*-LEE-mee-*yuh*), which is low blood volume, and **hypernatremia** (heye-*puhr-nuh*-TREE-mee-*yuh*), which is too much sodium in the blood. Some types of dehydration also can cause **hyponatremia** (heye-*puh-nuh*-TREE-mee-*yuh*), or too little salt in the blood.

Hypothermia (heye-*puh*-THUR-mee-*yuh*) occurs when the body temperature falls too low to sustain normal body functioning. **Frostbite** (FRAWST-beyet) is tissue damage that results as a result of being frozen. **Chilblains** (CHIL-bleynz) are skin ulcers that develop after exposure to cold.

Hyperkalemia (hayh-per-key-LEE-mee-*yuh*) can be caused by a wide range of medical problems and is the presence of too much potassium in the blood. Markedly elevated blood potassium levels can cause deadly heart arrhythmias. **Hypoglycemia** (heye-poh-gleye-SEE-mee-*uh*) is a low blood sugar level. Severely low blood sugar can cause seizures, unconsciousness, brain damage, and death. Severe hypoglycemia is most often caused by an overdose of insulin or other diabetic medications.

Ketoacidosis

Diabetic ketoacidosis (kee-toh-a-si-DOH-sis) most often occurs when there is too little insulin in the blood of a person with type 1 diabetes. It is characterized by **hyperglycemia** (heye-per-gleye-SEE-mee-*uh*), or high blood sugar; **acidemia** (a-sid-ee-mee-*yuh*), or acid in the blood; and the presence of blood and urinary

ketone (KEE-tohn) bodies, which are formed when the body switches to breaking down fatty acids when there is not enough insulin. Dehydration and other blood chemistry abnormalities can also occur. Diabetic ketoacidosis can proceed to diabetic **coma** (KOH-*muh*) and death if left untreated. Ketoacidosis can also result from heavy alcohol abuse. This condition is called **alcoholic ketoacidosis**.

Shock

Shock is a condition in which there is insufficient blood flow to the vital organs, which can damage organs and cause death. There are different kinds of shock, including the following:

- **Cardiogenic** (kahr-dee-*uh*-JEN-ik) **shock** occurs when a damaged heart can no longer pump enough blood for the organs, as in a heart attack.
- **Hypovolemic** (heye-*puh-vuh*-LEE-mik) **shock** occurs when organs don't get enough blood, which can happen as a result of serious hemorrhages from gunshot wounds.
- **Neurogenic** (noor-*uh*-JEN-ik) **shock** can occur as a consequence of damage to parts of the nervous system that regulate blood pressure and heart rate.

Anaphylactic (an-*uh-fuh*-LAK-tik) **shock** is caused by allergic reactions. **Anaphylaxis** (an-*uh-fuh*-LAK-sis) is a serious allergic reaction that can occur in response to foods, medicines, and insect bites. Anaphylaxis causes the body to release **histamine.** The release of histamine results in **vasodilation** (vas-oh-deye-LEY-*shuhn*), which is the widening of blood vessels. This causes **hypotension** (heye-*puh*-TEN-*shuhn*), which is low blood pressure. Throat swelling also occurs and can cause breathing difficulties.

Septic (SEP-tik) **shock** can occur during serious infections, such as **septicemia** (sep-*tuh*-SEE-mee-*uh*), or bacterial infection of the blood. Bacteria and other organisms release toxins that damage tissues and can cause very low blood pressure that cannot adequately perfuse organs.

WORDS OF WARNING

Thyroid storm is a serious condition that results from **thyrotoxicosis** (theye-roh-tok-si-KOH-sis), or untreated hyperthyroidism. It can cause confusion, psychiatric symptoms, agitation, sweating, hypertension, tachycardia, fever, shock, and delirium. Left untreated, thyroid storm can cause congestive heart failure and pulmonary edema.

Infectious Diseases

Infectious diseases are also known as **transmissible** (trans-MIS-*uh-buhl*) or **communicable** (*kuh*-MYOO-ni-*kuh-buhl*) **diseases**. They are produced by **pathogens** (PATH-*uh-juhnz*), or organisms that cause disease. Pathogens can be contracted from the environment or passed from person to person.

GI infections are usually contracted by swallowing contaminated food or water. GI infections often produce diarrhea, and for this reason many of them are called **diarrheal** (deye-*uh*-REE-*uhl*) **diseases**. Diarrheal diseases can cause severe dehydration and are among the leading causes of death of children under age five.

Salmonella (sal-*muh*-NEL-*uh*) is a bacteria that can cause **Salmonella enteritis** (en-*tuh*-REYE-tis), or **salmonellosis** (sal-*muh*-nel-OH-sis). This condition is food poisoning accompanied by diarrhea that is bloody and **mucopurulent** (myoo-*kuh*-PYOOR-*yuh-luhnt*), which means that it contains pus and mucus. Salmonellosis can be more serious in babies and people who are **immunocompromised** (im-*yuh*-noh-KOM-*pruh*-meyezd), or who have impaired immune systems. It can cause severe dehydration and **sepsis** (SEP-sis), an overwhelming response to an infection in which the blood pressure drops and shock occurs.

Escherichia coli (esh-uh-RIK-ee-yuh COH-leye), or *E. coli* (EE-COH-leye), is a group of bacteria that range from benign (some types live in our gut and help us digest food) to disease-causing. The latter kind are called **pathogenic** (path-*uh*-JEN-ik) *E. coli* and include the strains that are often responsible for food recalls. These types cause gastroenteritis characterized by bloody diarrhea. *E. coli* 0157:H7 is a pathogenic strain that is known to cause **hemolytic uremic syndrome** (hee-*muh*-LIT-ik yoo-REE-mik SIN-drohm), or HUS, which can result in death. The main abnormalities of HUS include **hemolytic anemia** (*uh*-NEE-mee-*uh*), in which blood cells are destroyed; **uremia** (yoo-REE-mee-*uh*), or acute kidney failure; and **thrombocytopenia** (throm-boh-seye-*tuh*-PEE-nee-*uh*), or low levels of platelets in the blood.

Pneumonia (noo-MOHN-*yuh*) is often seen in the ER and can be caused by a number of respiratory organisms. Complications of HIV sometimes present as pneumonia. *Pneumocystis jiroveci* (noo-moh-SIS-*tuhs* yee-row-VET-zee), formerly known as *Pneumocystis carinii* (noo-moh-SIS-*tuhs* cuh-REYE-nee-ee), is one of the most common organisms that causes opportunistic infections in people with AIDS.

People with HIV can also develop active **tuberculosis** (*too*-bur-*kyuh*-LOH-sis), or TB. TB is caused by a type of bacteria that grows best in environments where there is a lot of oxygen, like the lungs. TB organisms are called **acid-fast bacilli** (*buh*-SIL-eye), or AFB. They can be seen under the microscope by treating them with a dye that lights up under fluorescent lights. TB infections usually appear in the lungs, but TB can also infect other areas like the bones, skin, and central nervous system. TB that spreads throughout the body is called **disseminated** (dih-SEM-*uh*-neyt-ed), or **miliary** (MIL-ee-er-ee), **TB**.

> **DID YOU KNOW?**
>
> TB is spread through the air by aerosolized droplets. It is considered a disease of poverty because it thrives among people who are malnourished or living in crowded conditions like refugee camps and homeless shelters. It also is common in prisons. Though the incidence of TB infections is declining slightly worldwide each year, in many areas of the world it is still **endemic** (en-DEM-ik), or occurs frequently and at a steady rate in the population.

Other infections seen in the ER include **necrotizing fasciitis** (NEK-*ruh*-teyez-ing fash-ee-EYE-tis). This rare skin condition is caused by flesh-destroying bacteria and often results in limb amputations.

Hospital-Acquired Conditions

Hospital-acquired conditions are ones that develop as a consequence of medical treatment or being exposed to organisms and other environmental risks present in the hospital. **Nosocomial** (nos-*uh*-KOH-mee-*uhl*), or hospital-acquired, infections can develop among hospitalized patients due to contaminated surfaces and medical instruments. Medical illnesses can also weaken patients' immune systems, making them less able to fight infection. Common nosocomial infections include pneumonia, urinary tract infections, and **bacteremia** (bak-*tuh*-REE-mee-*uh*), which is a bacterial infection of the blood. Other hospital-acquired conditions include falls; foreign objects left in the body during surgery; **pressure ulcers** (UHL-serz), commonly known as bedsores, which are skin erosions caused by prolonged inactivity; and **blood incompatibility** (in-*kuhm*-PAT-*uh*-bil-*uh*-tee), or receiving the wrong blood type during a transfusion.

Hepatic Encephalopathy

Hepatic encephalopathy (en-sef-*uh*-LOP-*uh*-thee) occurs due to liver failure. Toxins that are normally processed by the liver build up in the blood, causing confusion; psychiatric symptoms; sleepiness; **jaundice** (JAWN-dis), or yellow discoloration of the eyes and skin; peripheral edema; and **ascites** (*uh*-SEYE-teez), or fluid in the abdominal cavity. **Peritonitis** (per-i-tn-EYE-tis), or infection of the lining of the abdominal cavity, can also occur. **Asterixis** (as-*tuh*-RIK-*suhs*) is a characteristic flapping hand movement that occurs during hepatic encephalopathy. Left untreated, hepatic encephalopathy can lead to hepatic coma and death.

WORD ORIGINS

Hepatic encephalopathy is often accompanied by **fetor hepaticus** (FEE-awr hi-PAT-*uh-cuhs*), or the "breath of death," in which the breath has a fecal or corpselike odor. Fetor hepaticus is a sign of late-stage liver failure. It is caused by high blood pressure in the portal vein and **portosystemic** (PAWRT-oh-si-STEM-ik) venous shunts that develop during liver disease in order to allow blood to bypass the diseased liver.

Poisoning

Poisoning can be caused by food, snake venom, plants, medications, and household products. For example, **salicylate** (*suh*-LIS-*uh*-leyt) toxicity results from aspirin overdoses and can cause seizures, pulmonary edema, and heart attack. **Acetaminophen** (*uh*-see-*tuh*-MIN-*uh-fuhn*) **overdose** can cause altered consciousness and **hepatic** (hi-PAT-ik), or liver, injury. (Tylenol is a brand of acetaminophen.)

Ethyl alcohol (ETH-*uhl* AL-*kuh*-hawl), or **ethanol** (ETH-*uh*-nawl), is found in beer, wine, and hard liquor and is the most common form of alcohol poisoning. Ethanol impairs the central nervous system. Ethanol toxicity can cause respiratory failure and death.

Sedative hypnotics (SED-*uh*-tiv hip-NOT-iks) are medications that are sometimes used illicitly, like **benzodiazepines** (ben-zoh-deye-AZ-*uh*-peenz). They depress the central nervous system and can cause respiratory depression. **Opiates** (OH-pee-its), like **heroin** (HER-oh-in), can cause altered consciousness, pinpoint (constricted) pupils, and decreased heart and breathing rate. Overdoses of **stimulants** (STIM-*yuh-luhnts*), like **cocaine** (koh-KEYN) and **amphetamines** (am-FET-*uh*-meenz), can cause aggression, psychosis, rapid heart rates, irregular heart rhythms, and heart attack or stroke.

Overdose with a **tricyclic** (treye-SEYE-klik, treye-SIK-lik) **antidepressant** (TCA) can cause heart arrhythmias, urinary retention, seizures, hallucinations, and confusion. **Lithium** (LITH-ee-*uhm*) toxicity can cause seizures, coma, and kidney failure. For more pharmacological information, see Chapter 26.

Organophosphates (awr-*guh*-noh-FOS-feyts) are found in insecticides. Poisoning with organophosphates can result in muscle weakness, cramps, paralysis, seizures, coma, and respiratory difficulties.

Neurological and Neurosurgical Emergencies

Neurological and neurosurgical emergencies occur when there is sudden dysfunction in the brain, spinal cord, and other nerves.

Stroke

Stroke is also called a cerebrovascular accident (CVA). Emergency treatment of stroke is necessary in order to decrease damage to the brain. There are two types of strokes: ischemic and hemorrhagic. **Ischemic** (ih-SKEE-mik) **stroke** results when the blood supply to the brain is blocked, usually by a blood clot. **Hemorrhagic** (hem-er-AJ-ik) **stroke** is bleeding into the brain. The main aim of treatment is to increase blood supply to the brain for ischemic stroke or to stop the bleeding in hemorrhagic stroke. For more information on intracranial bleeds, see Chapter 19.

Seizure and Status Epilepticus

Seizures (SEE-zherz) occur because of sudden, abnormal discharges of electricity in the brain that cause sudden body movements or changes in behavior. The many causes for seizures include medical illness, head trauma, infection, cancer, fever, withdrawal from drugs, and sleep deprivation.

The many kinds of seizures produce different symptoms based on the part of the brain they affect. **Partial**, or **focal**, **seizures** affect only one body part or region. **Simple seizures** do not affect consciousness, but **complex seizures** do affect consciousness.

Generalized seizures affect the entire body and always affect consciousness. **Tonic-clonic** (TON-ik CLON-ik) **seizures** are generalized seizures that affect the entire brain and were formerly known as **grand mal** (GRAND MAWL) **seizures**. A generalized seizure can progress to **status epilepticus** (STAT-*uhs* ep-*uh*-LEP-tik-*uhs*), which is a continuous seizure that lasts for more than 5 minutes. It can cause brain damage and be life-threatening without treatment.

Traumatic Brain Injury

A **traumatic brain injury** (TBI) is caused by external trauma to the brain. A closed head injury is one which leaves intact the integrity of the skull and dura, or membrane covering the brain. These kinds of injuries include concussions, which cause transient brain dysfunction, often due to sports injuries; **intracranial hematoma** (hee-ma-TOH-*muh*), a clot which results from bleeding inside the skull; **cerebral contusion** (*kuhn*-TOO-*zhuhn*), in which the brain matter is bruised or injured; and **diffuse axonal** (AK-son-*uhl*) **injury**, in which the nerve axons are injured, usually from high-speed impacts, like car crashes. Diffuse axonal injury is one of the main causes of persistent coma and **vegetative** (VEJ-i-tey-tiv) **state**, from which most people never awake.

A penetrating head injury is one in which the skull and at least the dura mater is penetrated, such as by a stab wound. In **perforating** (PUR-*fuh*-reyt-ing) **head trauma**, the object passes completely through one side of the head and out the other side. Because the body's barriers have been breached, infection is a serious risk in penetrating head injuries. The object forms a **cavitation** (kav-i-TEY-*shuhn*), or pathway, through the brain that can be markedly wider than the object itself. Tissue around the pathway is also compressed and injured. For more information on intracranial hemorrhages, see Chapter 19.

Spinal Cord Compression and Injuries

Spinal cord compression can be caused by trauma, tumors, fractures, ruptured intervertebral discs, and abscesses. **Abscesses** (AB-ses-ez) are collections of pus caused by infections. Symptoms correlate with the level of the spinal cord that is compressed and can include paralysis, loss of sensation, areas of increased sensation, and urinary or fecal incontinence.

Cancers that often metastasize to the spinal cord include lung, breast, prostate, renal, and lymphoma. Surgical **decompression** (dee-*kuhm*-PRESH-uhn), or removal of the tumor, and radiation are used to relieve compression and preserve neural function. Chemotherapy is used for some types of cancers.

Spinal cord injury results from trauma to the spinal cord. In complete spinal cord injury, all motor and sensory function is lost below the level of the injury. In incomplete spinal cord injury, some function below the level of the injury is spared. A **spinal cord transection** (tran-SEK-*shuhn*) occurs when the spinal cord is cut completely through. A **spinal cord hemisection** (hem-i-SEK-*shuhn*) occurs when the spinal cord is cut halfway through. **Spinal shock** is loss of sensation accompanied by paralysis following a spinal cord injury, with gradual regain of function. **Central cord syndrome** is weakness or paralysis in the upper limbs, with the lower limbs being spared.

Meningitis and Encephalitis

Meningitis (men-in-JEYE-tis) is infection or inflammation of the meninges. Symptoms of meningitis include vomiting; stiff neck; **photophobia** (foh-*tuh*-FOH-bee-*uh*), or sensitivity to light; and **phonophobia** (foh-*nuh*-FOH-bee-*uh*), or sensitivity to sound. Meningitis in a baby can cause the **fontanel** (fon-tn-EL), or soft spot, to bulge. Meningitis typically is caused by many different types of bacteria. **Aseptic** (ey-SEP-tik) **meningitis** is meningitis in which no bacteria can be isolated and can be caused by viruses and fungi. **Noninfectious meningitis** can be caused by drug reactions, cancer, and autoimmune disorders.

Encephalitis (en-sef-*uh*-LEYE-tis) is an infection or inflammation of the brain. Symptoms can include headache, fever, fatigue, seizures, hallucinations, and increased intracranial pressure. Like meningitis, encephalitis can be caused by a variety of bacteria and viruses, as well as autoimmune conditions. Encephalitis is rare, and the leading cause of encephalitis is the herpes virus.

Psychiatric Emergencies

Mental health emergencies fall into three categories: psychosis, thoughts about injury to self or others, and psychiatric medication side effects.

As Chapter 17 explained, psychosis is a condition of impaired reality, often accompanied by delusions and hallucinations. Psychosis can also be accompanied by **catatonia** (kat-*uh*-TOH-nee-*uh*), which is a profound inner preoccupation in which the person becomes agitated and moves incessantly or stays still in one position. Psychosis has many causes, including medical, neurologic, and psychiatric illness. Poisoning, medication, and drug overdose or withdrawal can also cause psychosis, as can sleep deprivation and extreme stress. **Substance-induced psychosis** refers to a psychotic state that has been caused by a substance, such as amphetamines.

Suicidal ideation (eye-dee-EY-*shuhn*) refers to recurring thoughts or preoccupation with suicide, or killing oneself. Many people who experience suicidal ideation do not complete suicide, although a significant number do. Warning signs include a sense of hopelessness; fatigue; **psychomotor agitation** (seye-koh-MOH-ter aj-i-TEY-*shuhn*), which are movements caused by extreme anxiety; **insomnia** (in-SOM-nee-*uh*), or an inability to sleep; and **anhedonia** (an-hee-DOH-nee-*uh*), or the inability to experience pleasure from activities that were previously enjoyable. Suicidal ideation is associated with depression and stressful life events, as well as many other psychiatric disorders. Suicidal ideation is also related to side effects of certain antidepressant medications, especially **selective serotonin reuptake inhibitors (SSRIs)**.

Homicidal (hom-*uh*-SEYED-l) **ideation** refers to recurrent thoughts or preoccupation with **homicide** (HOM-*uh*-seyed), or killing another person. Homicidal ideation is common in psychosis, and is associated with many psychiatric disorders, including **schizophrenia** (skit-*suh*-FREE-nee-*uh*, skit-*suh*-FREN-ee-*uh*).

Neuroleptic, or **antipsychotic** (an-tee-seye-KOT-ik, an-teye-seye-KOT-ik), medications can cause **neuroleptic malignant** (noor-*uh*-LEP-tik *muh*-LIG-*nuhnt*) **syndrome**, or NMS. This syndrome can be life-threatening. Symptoms of NMS include fever, muscle rigidity, altered consciousness, and sometimes **delirium** (dih-LEER-ee-*uhm*), which is sudden altered mental functioning. NMS is also accompanied by autonomic instability, which refers to the abnormal activity of the autonomic nervous system and causes symptoms like high blood pressure and unstable vital signs. Levels of an enzyme called **creatinine phosphokinase** (kree-AT-n-een fos-foh-KEYE-neys), or CPK, become elevated in the blood due to muscle breakdown, called **rhabdomyolysis** (rab-doh-meye-AWL-*uh*-sis). **Leukocytosis** (loo-koh-seye-TOH-sis), or an elevated level of white blood cells in the blood, is also common.

> **STUDY TIP**
>
> One way to remember the symptoms of neuroleptic malignant syndrome is with the acronym FALTER: F for fever, A for autonomic instability, L for leukocytosis, T for tremor, E for elevated CPK enzyme levels and encephalopathy, and R for rigidity.

The Least You Need to Know

- Trauma refers to physical and psychological injury resulting from sudden events like accidents and violence.
- Cardiovascular emergencies include myocardial infarction and hypertensive emergencies.

- Pulmonary emergencies are indicated by respiratory distress, or difficulty breathing.

- Internal medicine emergencies are often accompanied by metabolic derangements and sometimes shock.

- Neurological and neurosurgical emergencies are often due to trauma, hemorrhages, blood clots, infections, cancer, and other medical illnesses.

- Psychiatric emergencies include psychosis, suicidal or homicidal ideation, and neuroleptic malignant syndrome.

Genetic Diseases

Chapter 21

In This Chapter

- Different ways that genes and chromosomes mutate
- Dominant and recessive autosomal disorders
- Disorders resulting from mutations in sex chromosomes
- Genetic diseases that usually affect adults only

Genetic diseases are caused by genetic mutations and chromosomal abnormalities. Different kinds of genetic mutations and chromosomal abnormalities produce different types of genetic diseases. The names of these diseases can stem from a variety of sources. Sometimes a name comes from the type of biological abnormality that causes it. Sometimes the name describes the physical symptoms of the disease. Learning genetic terms will help you understand more about what's going on in many different kinds of genetic diseases. Because genes affect every area of the body, learning genetic terminology also helps you learn about many types of diseases, even those that are not directly caused by genetic mutations and chromosomal abnormalities.

Genetic Mutations and Chromosomal Abnormalities

If you recall from the Chapter 4 overview of basic genetic terms, a chromosome is a structure inside our cells that carries genetic information. Humans carry two copies of each kind of chromosome in their cells. There are 22 pairs of autosomes and 1 pair of sex chromosomes. **Autosomes** (AW-*tuh*-sohmz) are chromosomes that do not code for sexual characteristics.

The pair of sex chromosomes contains at least one X chromosome; the other chromosome in the pair can be either an X or a Y. X chromosomes code for female characteristics, so someone with an XX genetic makeup is female. Y chromosomes code for male sexual characteristics, so someone with an XY genetic makeup is male. A gene contains segments of DNA and is a hereditary unit. Each chromosome contains lots of genes, which are found at particular locations on chromosomes.

Types of Genetic Mutations

Genetic disorders can be caused by various **gene mutations** (myoo-TEY-*shuhnz*), or changes in the DNA sequence on a chromosome. Some mutations occur *de novo* (DEY NOH-voh), or spontaneously. Others are **heritable** (HER-i-*tuh-buhl*), or passed from parent to offspring.

A **point mutation** is a DNA change that happens at a single location on the chromosome. A **deletion** results from the removal of a section of DNA from a chromosome. A **trinucleotide** (TREYE-NOO-klee-*uh*-teyed) **repeat** produces a gene that is extra-long. A **duplication** refers to doubling sections of the DNA.

A **translocation** (trans-loh-KEY-*shuhn*) refers to when genetic material is transferred from one chromosome to another. A **reciprocal** (ri-SIP-*ruh-kuhl*) **translocation** happens when two chromosomes swap genes. A **Robertsonian** (ROB-erts-OHN-ee-*yuhn*) **translocation** happens when an entire chromosome attaches to another.

An **inversion** (in-VUR-*zhuhnz*) is when part of a chromosome breaks off and reattaches to the same chromosome upside down. An **insertion** is when part of a chromosome breaks off and reinserts itself in a different location on the chromosome.

Missing and Extra Chromosomes

A **chromosomal** (KROH-*muh*-sohm-*uhl*) **abnormality** is when part of or an entire chromosome is missing or when an extra chromosome exists. Chromosomal abnormalities are also called **chromosomal aberrations** (ab-*uh*-REY-*shuhnz*).

Cri-du-chat (CREE-doo-SHAH) **syndrome** is an example of a genetic disease caused by a chromosomal aberration. In this case, a piece of chromosome 5 is missing. This syndrome causes infants to have a high-pitched cry (like a cat's cry) and also causes psychiatric symptoms, wide-set eyes, small head, and short stature.

Most chromosomal abnormalities occur in every cell. **Mosaicism** (moh-ZEY-*uh*-siz-*uhm*) can sometimes occur in which some cells express the abnormality, yet others do not. This can result in a milder form of the corresponding disease.

WORDS OF WARNING

A **chimera** (keye-MEER-*uh*) is an organism that has cells that are genetically different from each other. Chimeras are different from mosaics. A chimera contains genetic material from two or more zygotes that have fused during embryonic development. In contrast, a mosaic organism contains genetic information from only one zygote, and the genetic information is expressed in different manners in different cells. Chimerism is normally found only among animals and is extremely rare among humans. There have been reports of human blood chimerism, in which different types of blood are found in one person. This may happen during the development of twins, when cells of one twin continue to live in the body of the other twin.

The term **aneuploidy** (AN-yoo-PLOI-dee) describes an abnormal number of chromosomes. The term can refer to **monosomy** (MON-*uh*-soh-mee), or having only one chromosome in a chromosomal pair. For example, **Turner syndrome**, or monosomy X, is caused by a missing sex chromosome, resulting in only one X chromosome. This syndrome causes female sterility, heart and thyroid problems, diabetes, short stature, and cognitive and physical abnormalities.

Polysomy (POL-ee-soh-mee) refers to a condition in which a chromosomal pair has more than two chromosomes. The prefix indicates the abnormal number of chromosomes that are present. For example, having three chromosomes in a chromosomal pair is called **trisomy** (TREYE-*suh*-mee). An example is **Klinefelter** (KLEYEN-felt-er) **syndrome,** or XXY syndrome, which is a trisomy that causes long limbs, tall stature, male sterility, and learning disabilities. Having four sets of chromosomes in a chromosomal pair is called **tetrasomy** (TET-*truh*-soh-mee).

Trisomies that cause common syndromes often include the number of the affected chromosomal pair in the name. For example, trisomy 21 refers to having three copies of chromosome 21. Trisomy 21 is also known as **Down syndrome**. It is the most common chromosomal disorder, causing mental retardation, characteristic facial features, and many medical problems. **Edwards syndrome**, trisomy 18, is the second most common trisomy. It causes mental retardation and multiple medical problems. Most children with Edwards syndrome die during infancy.

Autosomal Conditions

Many genetic terms come from the principle of **Mendelian** (men-DEE-lee-*uhn*) **inheritance**. Gregor Mendel, the father of genetics, was an Austrian monk who developed his theories based on pea hybridization experiments in his cloister garden. He noticed that certain physical traits, like flower color, were dominant. In plants that were **heterozygous** (het-er-*uh*-ZEYE-*guhs*), or contained two different copies of a trait, flower colors did not blend. Instead, the dominant flower color hid the recessive color. Recessive traits "receded" when a plant with recessive colored flowers was crossed with one with dominant traits. Recessive traits reappeared when the plant was crossed with another plant with recessive traits, resulting in a **homozygous** (hoh-*muh*-ZEYE-*guhs*) plant, or one containing two copies of the same recessive trait. These experiments laid the groundwork for theories about dominant and recessive inheritance.

It's important to understand dominant and recessive inheritance when you are learning about autosomal conditions. **Autosomal** (AW-*tuh*-sohm-*uhl*) conditions result from mutations on autosomes, or chromosomes that don't contain genetic information for sexual characteristics. These conditions are classified as either dominant or recessive. The following figures show the process of how these conditions can be passed down from parents to offspring.

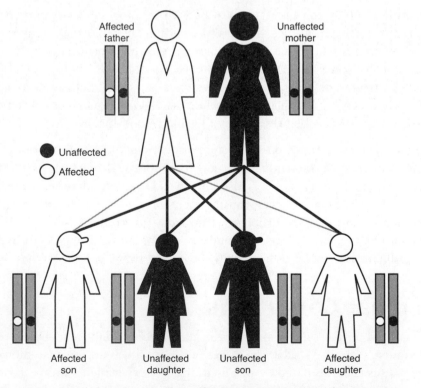

In autosomal dominant diseases, if an offspring receives one copy of a mutated gene from an affected parent, the offspring will develop the disease.

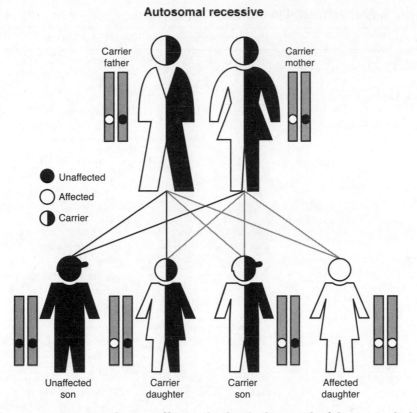

Autosomal recessive

Carrier father

Carrier mother

● Unaffected
○ Affected
◑ Carrier

Unaffected son

Carrier daughter

Carrier son

Affected daughter

In autosomal recessive diseases, offspring develop the disease only if they receive both copies of the mutated gene from their parents, each of whom must be a carrier of the affected gene.

Autosomal-Dominant Conditions

An autosomal-dominant condition is passed to offspring from either the mother or the father. Only one copy of the mutated gene is necessary to produce the disease. If an offspring receives a copy of the defective gene, she or he will develop the disease.

Common Autosomal-Dominant Conditions

Term	Pronunciation	Description
achondroplasia	ey-kon-*druh*-PLEY-*zhuh*	genetic dwarfism, can also be a sporadic mutation
factor V Leiden thrombophilia	LEYED-n thrawm-*buh*-FIL-ee-*yuh*	causes hypercoagulability (heye-per-koh-AG-*yuh*-*luh*-BIL-*uh*-tee), which greatly increases the risk for blood clots
familial hypercholesterolemia	*fuh*-MIL-*yuhl*, *fuh*-MIL-ee-*uhl* heye-per-kuh-les-ter-uh-LEE-mee-uh	causes very high blood levels of low-density lipoprotein cholesterol, leading to early-onset cardiovascular disease
hereditary spherocytosis	*huh*-RED-i-ter-ee sfee-roh-seye-TOH-sis	hemolytic anemia that results in the formation of sphere-shaped red blood cells that results in jaundice and **splenomegaly** (splee-noh-MEG-*uh*-lee), or an enlarged spleen
neurofibromatosis	noor-oh-feye-broh-*muh*-TOH-sis	disorder in which nerve tissues grow tumors, interfering with function
osteogenesis imperfecta	os-tee-*uh*-JEN-*uh*-sis im-*pur*-FEKT-*uh*	disorder of collagen synthesis characterized by weak, brittle bones that deform and break easily
polycystic kidney disease	POL-ee-SIS-tik	condition in which many cysts form in the kidneys, causing marked enlargement and loss of function; can also be autosomal recessive (more rare)
retinitis pigmentosa	ret-n-EYE-tis PIG-*muhnt*-OH-*suh*	most common cause of inherited retinal degeneration and blindness

Autosomal-Recessive Conditions

An autosomal-recessive condition is passed to offspring from either the mother or the father. Because the gene is not dominant, two copies of the mutated gene are necessary to produce the disease. In order for an offspring to be affected, both the mother and the father need to be genetic carriers of the disease, which means that they each carry a copy of the mutated gene.

DID YOU KNOW?

Autosomal-recessive disorders are more likely to appear in the offspring of **consanguineous** (kon-sang-GWIN-ee-*uhs*) unions, mating that occurs between two genetically related individuals. Recessive mutations are more likely to appear in certain populations due to the **founder effect**. This happens when a new population is "founded" by a small number of individuals. If one individual in the founding group carries the genetic mutation, the frequency of that mutation is likely to increase in later generations. For example, the higher frequency of the gene for Tay-Sachs disease among Ashkenazi Jews may in part have been caused by the founder effect.

Inborn Errors of Metabolism

Inborn errors of metabolism are also called **congenital metabolic diseases**, or **inherited metabolic diseases**. These terms refer to a group of diseases that are usually autosomal-recessive (though some are X-linked, see the section later in this chapter). The affected genes code for enzymes that are important in metabolism. Disease results when toxic waste products accumulate, or certain substances are unable to be metabolized. These diseases can affect numerous organ systems and have a wide variety of symptoms.

This group of diseases is broken into several categories. **Disorders of amino acid metabolism** interfere with the production or breakdown of amino acids. For example, **phenylketonuria** (fen-l-kee-toh-NOOR-ee-*uh*) is due to a nonfunctional liver enzyme that cannot metabolize phenylalanine. If untreated, this disease causes seizures and mental retardation.

Disorders of carbohydrate metabolism interfere with the production and breakdown of carbohydrates. **Glycogen** (GLEYE-*kuh-juhn*) **storage diseases** are a group of disorders of carbohydrate metabolism caused by a defective enzyme involved in glycogen breakdown or production. This group of diseases can cause muscle weakness, cramps, and sometimes liver and kidney problems.

Lysosomal (LEYE-*suh*-sohm-*uhl*) **storage diseases** are caused by malfunctioning **lysosomes,** which are **organelles** (awr-*guh*-NELZ) important in cellular digestion. One example is **Tay-Sachs** (TEY-SAKS) **disease**. This disease causes a characteristic "cherry red" spot on the retina, progressive deterioration in physical and mental functioning, and death in childhood. It also can occur in adolescents and adults.

Peroxisomal (*puh*-ROX-*uh*-zohm-*uhl*) **disorders** are caused by malfunctioning **peroxisomes**, which are organelles that are important in cellular lipid metabolism. An example of this type of disorder is **Zellweger** (ZEL-weg-ur) **syndrome**. In this syndrome, very-long-chain fatty acids accumulate in many organs, causing abnormal brain development and many other organ abnormalities.

WORD ORIGINS

Some names for inborn errors of metabolism are emblematic and come directly from the disease symptoms. For example, **maple syrup urine disease** is an autosomal-recessive disorder of amino acid metabolism that causes the urine to smell like maple syrup. **Swiss cheese cartilage dysplasia** (dis-PLEY-*zhuh*) is an autosomal-dominant disorder of amino acid metabolism that affects collagen synthesis. It causes abnormal bone growth, joint deformities, dwarfism, and problems with vision and hearing.

Autosomal-Recessive Disorders

Term	Pronunciation	Description
21-hydroxylase deficiency	heye-DROK-*suh*-leys	also called congenital adrenal hyperplasia because it results in the inability to make aldosterone; causes severe salt wasting, low cortisol level, excess androgens, and ambiguous genitalia in infants
albinism, achromia	AL-*buh*-niz-*uhm*, ey-KROH-mee-*uh*	defect in an enzyme that helps produce melanin, resulting in total lack of skin, hair, and eye pigment and vision problems
cystic fibrosis	SIS-tik feye-BROH-sis	disorder characterized by thick mucus that causes breathing difficulties and pancreatic enzyme insufficiency that causes digestive problems
galactosemia	*guh*-lak-*tuh*-SEE-mee-*uh*	disorder of carbohydrate metabolism in which an enzyme deficiency results in complete inability to metabolize galactose, causing an enlarged liver, cirrhosis, cataracts, brain damage, and ovarian failure in women

Term	Pronunciation	Description
Gaucher disease	GOU-chur	lysosomal storage disease in which fat builds up in various organs, causing an enlarged liver and spleen, anemia, and sometimes neurological symptoms
Niemann-Pick disease	NEE-*muhn*-PIK	lysosomal storage disease in which fat builds up in the liver, spleen, lungs, bone, marrow, and brain, causing an enlarged liver and spleen and neurological symptoms, including seizures

WORDS OF WARNING

Even though *lactose* sounds like *galactose*, don't confuse galactosemia with lactose intolerance. **Lactose intolerance** is a condition in which there is an acquired or inherited deficiency of the enzyme that metabolizes lactose. Many people with lactose intolerance can still partially metabolize lactose, and the condition does not result in long-term damage. Galactosemia is more serious and produces long-term damage if affected people do not follow a strict lactose- and galactose-free diet.

X-Linked Disorders

Sex-linked conditions result from mutations on sex chromosomes, which contain information for sexual characteristics. In X-linked disorders, the mutation causing the disease lies on the X chromosome and is most often passed from mother to child.

X-Linked Dominant Disorders

X-linked dominant disorders are passed down from parents who are affected by the disease. The father contributes either an X or a Y chromosome, and the mother contributes an X chromosome to offspring. In order to be affected, an offspring needs to receive an affected X chromosome from either a mother or father who has the disease. If the offspring receives an X chromosome with the mutated gene, he or she will develop the disease.

X-linked dominant disorders are extremely rare. An example is **X-linked hypophosphatemia** (heye-*puh*-FOS-fuh-TEE-mee-*yuh*), which is a genetic form of rickets.

Affected people develop **osteomalacia** (os-tee-oh-*muh*-LEY-*shuh*), or soft, easily deformable bones that respond poorly to vitamin D treatment.

X-Linked Recessive Disorders

X-linked recessive disorders are passed down to offspring from parents who are carriers of the gene. Mothers who are carriers for the mutation do not normally show symptoms of the disease. This is because they have two X chromosomes, and the second X chromosome compensates for the defective gene on the first X chromosome. Fathers who carry the mutation do show symptoms of the disease. This is because men have an X and a Y chromosome, and the Y chromosome cannot compensate for the defective gene on the single X chromosome.

X-linked recessive conditions most often affect male offspring. In order to develop the disease, female offspring would need to receive a copy of the mutated gene from both parents, meaning that the mother was an unaffected carrier and the father was an affected carrier. For example, **hemophilia A** (hee-*muh*-FIL-ee-*uh*, hee-*muh*-FEEL-*yuh*) affects mostly boys. People with this disease bleed easily because they cannot form normal blood clots due to insufficient levels of clotting factor VIII. Another example is **Duchenne muscular dystrophy** (doo-SHEN MUS-kyuh-ler DIS-troh-fee), which is caused by a mutation that codes for the protein **dystrophin** (dis-TROH-*fuhn*). The disorder causes progressive muscle weakness and wasting and eventual death. Other X-linked recessive conditions include male pattern baldness and red-green color blindness.

Y-Linked Disorders

There are few Y-linked human disorders because the small Y chromosome contains few genes. Some male infertility problems are caused by deletions on the Y chromosome.

Mitochondrial Diseases

Mitochondrial (meye-*tuh*-KON-dree-*uhl*) **diseases** result from malfunctioning or abnormal mitochondria, the energy-producing organelles of a cell. Mitochondria are present only in egg cells, so mitochondrial diseases can be passed only through the maternal line, from mother to child. **Mitochondrial myopathies** (meye-OP-*uh*-theez) are a group of mitochondrial diseases that affect muscle cells. A characteristic sign of these types of diseases is ragged red fibers, which are enlarged mitochondria present in muscle cells of affected people. The muscles of affected people degenerate, often accompanied by neurological problems such as seizures or dementia.

Diseases with Multifactorial Inheritance

Some genetic diseases are caused by only one gene mutation. Others are caused by many different genes that are expressed as a result of interactions with the environment and lifestyle choices, such as smoking. These types of genetic disorders are said to have **multifactorial** (muhl-tee-fak-TAWR-ee-*uhl*) **inheritance**, which is also called **complex** and **polygenic** (pol-ee-JEN-ik) **inheritance**. The pattern of inheritance for these types of disorders is often unclear. Some people with relatives affected by the disorder never develop it while others do. Examples of conditions with multifactorial inheritance include asthma, type 2 diabetes, heart disease, high blood pressure, inflammatory bowel disease, multiple sclerosis, obesity, schizophrenia, bipolar disorder, and some cancers.

Genetic Diseases of Adulthood

Many genetic mutations are present in the germline cells like the gametes (egg and sperm) that contain genetic material. Germline mutations can be passed along to offspring and usually affect every cell in the body. As a consequence, germline mutations often cause abnormalities in many different organ systems and appear early as diseases of childhood. Some genetic disorders, however, take longer to develop and primarily affect adults.

For example, **alpha-1 antitrypsin** (AL-*fuh wuhn* an-tee TRIP-*suhn*) **deficiency** is an autosomal-codominant disorder with two variations of the gene, each contributing to the disease. It causes asthmalike symptoms that don't respond to treatment and results in emphysema, impaired liver function, and liver failure. Versions of this disease are found in children also.

Huntington (HUHN-ting-*tuhn*) **disease** is an autosomal-dominant disorder that causes degeneration of brain cells, resulting in cognitive decline; poor muscle coordination; psychiatric symptoms; and **chorea** (*kuh*-REE-*uh*), or characteristic writhing, dancelike movements.

Familial Alzheimer (AHLZ-heye-merz) **disease** (FAD) is an autosomal-dominant disorder, also called early-onset Alzheimer disease. It begins before age 65 and has symptoms similar to those of **sporadic** (*spuh*-RAD-ik) **Alzheimer disease**, which is not heritable and starts at a later age. **Amyloid** (AM-*uh*-loid) plaques and **neurofibrillary** (noor-*uh*-FIB-*ruh*-leyr-ee) **tangles** form in the brain and destroy brain cells, causing memory loss; **aphasia** (*uh*-FEY-*zhuh*), or difficulty speaking and understanding words; mood swings; irritability; and other psychiatric symptoms.

Some types of cancer are linked to heritable mutations as well. These types of cancer appear earlier and may be more aggressive, with a worse **prognosis** (prog-NOH-sis), than cancers caused by sporadic genetic mutations. For example, some types of breast cancer are linked to the genes *BRCA1* and *BRCA2*. Women who carry one of these genes are more likely to develop breast cancer and/or ovarian cancer. Men who carry one of these genes are also more likely to develop breast and/or prostate cancer. **Retinoblastoma** (ret-noh-bla-STOH-*muh*) is a cancer of the retina that can cause blindness. Even though retinoblastoma is rare, it is the most common inherited childhood cancer and is highly treatable. Autosomal dominant retinoblastoma can occur earlier and be more aggressive than sporadic cases, which have a later age of onset and can also rarely occur in adulthood.

The Least You Need to Know

- Genetic disorders can be caused by various genetic mutations or changes to the sequence of DNA on a chromosome.
- Some genetic disorders are caused by chromosomal abnormalities, which occur when part or an entire chromosome is missing or there is an extra chromosome.
- Autosomal conditions can be recessive or dominant, and result from mutations on autosomes.
- Sex-linked conditions can be recessive or dominant, and result from mutations on sex chromosomes.
- Although many genetic diseases cause symptoms in childhood, some do not show up until adulthood.

Cancers

In This Chapter

- Cancer types, symptoms, diagnosis, and treatment
- Gastrointestinal cancer
- Lung, breast, and skin cancer
- Endocrine, reproductive, and urinary tract cancer
- Leukemia and lymphoma
- Cancer in children

Cancer occurs when cells become abnormal and their growth becomes chaotic. Genetic mutations initiate the development of cancer. Carcinogens produce mutations. Smoking is a carcinogen that is the number one risk factor for the development of cancer.

Cancer terms can be lengthy and look complicated. Most tumors are named after the type of cell whose growth goes awry. Knowing this general rule can help you decipher the names of many tumors. Likewise, learning the general terms that refer to cancer development and diagnosis will help you understand cancers in various organ systems.

General Cancer Terminology

The term **neoplasm** (NEE-*uh*-plaz-*uhm*) refers to abnormal or out-of-control cell growth, also called a **tumor** (TOO-mer). Neoplasms can be either benign or malignant. **Benign** (bih-NEYEN) neoplasms do not tend to produce dysfunction or disease. **Malignant** (*muh*-LIG-*nuhnt*) neoplasms tend to spread and cause disease.

Cancers can either be **solid**, which refers to organ tumors, or **liquid**, which refers to blood cancer. Cancers are named based on **histology** (hi-STOL-*uh*-jee), or the kind of tissue from which they originate. Cancers are also classified based on the type of cell that becomes **cancerous** (KAN-ser-*uhs*), or grows abnormally.

Carcinoma (kahr-*suh*-NOH-*muh*) refers to malignant tumors that arise from epithelial cells. This is the most common form of cancer in adults, but it's rare in children. **Squamous cell carcinoma** is a kind of carcinoma that arises from squamous cells found in the epithelium in various parts of the body.

Sarcoma (sahr-KOH-*muh*) refers to malignant tumors that arise from connective tissue (bone, fat, muscle, blood vessels) and **hematopoietic** (hi-mat-oh-poi-EE-tik), or blood-forming, tissue. **Leukemia** (loo-KEE-mee-*uh*) refers to liquid tumors that arise from hematopoietic cells in the bone marrow. **Lymphoma** (lim-FOH-*muh*) refers to solid tumors that usually arise from hematopoietic cells and are found in lymph nodes.

Germ cell tumors are tumors that arise from **pluripotent** (ploor-ee-POH-*tuhnt*), or nonspecialized, cells that can differentiate into specialized cells. **Blastoma** (bla-STOH-*muh*) arises from precursor cells, or embryonic tissues.

STUDY TIP

The ending –*oma* means tumor and is used in many cancer terms. Tumors are named for the types of cells or tissues from which they originate, plus the ending -*oma*. An example is **adenoma**, which is a tumor that originates from glandular tissue (recall that *adeno*- means gland).

Carcinogenesis

Carcinogenesis (kahr-*suh*-*nuh*-JEN-*uh*-sis) refers to the process by which cancer develops. Most cancer develops from DNA mutations. **Carcinogens** (kahr-SIN-*uh*-*juhnz*) and **mutagens** (MYOO-*tuh*-*juhnz*) are substances that can induce DNA mutations.

Recall from Chapter 2 that the word root *onco*- means tumor and is used in many terms describing cancer. For example, **oncology** is the study and treatment of cancer. An **oncovirus** (ong-*kuh*-VAHR-*uhs*) is a virus that can infect cells and cause cancer. An **oncogene** (ONG-*kuh*-jeen) is a gene that initiates cancer by promoting cell proliferation, inhibiting **apoptosis** (ap-*uh*-TOH-sis) or cell death, and promoting cellular immortality, which happens when cells acquire mutations that allow them to avoid cell death. Many oncogenes are inherited, though many others are produced through sporadic, or random, mutations in DNA. A **proto-oncogene** (PROH-toh-ONG-*kuh*-jeen) is a gene that becomes an oncogene when it mutates.

A **free radical** carries an electrical charge and is highly reactive. Free radicals damage DNA and contribute to the disease progression of cancer. An **antioxidant** (an-tee-OK-si-*duhnt*) can react with free radicals and decrease their damaging effects. **Tumor suppressor genes** keep cellular growth in check, direct DNA repair, and determine rate of cellular apoptosis and **senescence** (si-NES-*uhns*), or the natural die-off of cells.

Cancer Pathogenesis

Pathogenesis (path-*uh*-JEN-*uh*-sis) refers to the process by which disease develops. Cancer cells have the ability to go through uncontrolled **mitosis** (meye-TOH-sis), or cell division, and tend to invade other tissues and **metastasize** (*muh*-TAS-*tuh*-seyez), or spread, to other parts of the body. Cancer can develop when a mutation inactivates tumor suppressor genes and/or DNA repair genes, allowing cells to proliferate. Cellular proliferation leads to **neoplastic** (NEE-*uh*-plas-tik) **transformation** in which cells develop abnormal features. **Dysplasia** (dis-PLEY-*zhuh*) is the development of cell abnormalities that are sometimes precursors to cancer. **Hyperplasia** (heye-per-PLEY-*zhuh*) is an abnormal increase in cell number. It is sometimes a precursor to cancer, but not always.

A **polyp** (POL-ip) is an overgrowth of cells. It is usually benign but can become cancerous over time. A primary tumor is located at the original location of growth. A secondary tumor is also called a **metastatic** (met-*uh*-STAT-ik) **tumor** because it has spread beyond its initial location.

Exophytic (eks-oh-FIT-ik) refers to cancer that has grown out from the wall of a tubular organ, such as the colon, causing obstruction. **Circumferential** (ser-kuhm-*fuh*-REN-*shuhl*) **tumors** grow around tubular organs and can cause obstructions by narrowing the lumen.

Cancer cells grow quickly and require a blood supply to sustain their rapid metabolisms. Many cancers induce **angiogenesis** (an-jee-oh-JEN-*uh*-sis), or blood vessel formation, to bring more blood and oxygen to the area. **Neovascularization** (NEE-oh-VAS-*kyuh-luh*-ri-zey-*shuhn*), the development of new blood vessels, is why some tumors tend to bleed.

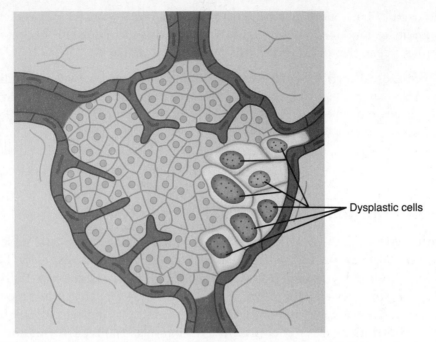

When cells undergo neoplastic transformation, they develop dysplastic features that can be the precursors to cancer.

Adam Howard © Dorling Kindersley

Cancer Symptomatology

Many early stage cancers, especially the most deadly kinds like pancreatic and lung cancer, are **asymptomatic** (ey-simp-*tuh*-MA-ik), meaning they don't have symptoms. They may also have nonspecific symptoms such as fatigue, malaise, weight loss, and nausea, which can hinder diagnosis. For example, fever of unknown origin is a nonspecific symptom that is found in many cancers.

As cancer grows, it tends to produce more symptoms. **Mass effect** refers to symptoms that are due to the physical presence of a tumor compressing or blocking a neighboring organ or tissue. **Infiltration** (in-fil-TREY-*shuhn*) occurs when a cancer grows into its parent organ, often disrupting the functioning of that organ. **Invasion** happens when the tumor grows into surrounding tissues and organs. **Metastasis** (*muh*-TASS-*tuh*-sis) is when the tumor spreads throughout the body, usually through the blood and lymphatics.

Some cancers produce **paraneoplastic** (par-*uh*-nee-*uh*-PLAS-tik) **syndromes,** a group of symptoms that are associated with a certain cancer. Symptoms are often related to hormone hypersecretion or **ectopic** (ek-TOP-ik-ic) hormone production away from the hormone's normal production site.

Cancer Diagnosis

Many cancers are diagnosed on **biopsy** (BEYE-op-see), or cutting off a small piece of tissue for analysis. In a **fine-needle aspiration** (FNA) biopsy, a hollow needle is used to collect cell samples from a **superficial lump,** or one near the surface of the skin. Tumor markers are also used. They are chemicals that cancerous cells release into the blood. Tumor markers can be used in diagnosis, monitoring, or determining response to treatment.

Biopsies are analyzed in the lab to determine **tumor classification,** or the types of cells the tumor has originated from. **Grading** identifies cancer by type and aggressiveness, from low to high grade. High-grade cancers have a poorer prognosis.

Cells are analyzed for differentiation. Undifferentiated cells are less mature, less specialized, and carry a worse prognosis than differentiated cells. **Anaplastic** (an-*uh*-PLAS-tik) cells are poorly differentiated cells. **Pleomorphic** (plee-*uh*-MAWR-fik) tumors have cells at various stages of development.

Staging classifies how far a cancer has spread beyond its original location. Analysis of lymph nodes adjacent to the tumor is used in staging. There are several systems of staging, which vary based on cancer type and how it presents. One commonly known system of staging is called the Roman Numeral system, also called the Overall Stage Grouping. This system has five stages. Stage 0 corresponds to **carcinoma in situ** (in SEYE-tyoo), which is a precursor of cancer that has remained within the boundaries of its original location. Stage I corresponds to **localized** cancers that have remained in their original site and are **noninvasive,** or have not invaded neighboring organs. Stage II corresponds to cancers that are still localized but have begun to invade adjacent tissue. Stage III corresponds to cancers that are also localized but have invaded adjacent tissue more extensively than Stage II cancers. The distinction between Stage II and Stage III cancers is complicated and varies based on the type of cancer involved. Stage IV refers to cancers that have metastasized, or spread to other parts of the body.

> **WORD ORIGINS**
>
> The term **cancer** comes from the Greek word *carcinos*, which means crab. Hippocrates was one of the first to describe the crablike appearance of malignant tumors. Humans have had cancer at least since Neolithic times and the dawn of agriculture. The first known record of cancer comes from 3,000-year-old Egyptian papyri, which describe breast cancer. The link between tobacco use and cancer was made as early as the eighteen century, though the ill health effects of tobacco were surmised as early as the seventeenth century.

Cancer Treatment

Cancer is treated with a variety of methods. Tumors are often surgically **excised** (EK-seyezd), or cut out of the surrounding tissue. Surgical **debulking** (dee-BUHLK-ing) is the removal of part of a tumor to improve symptoms when the tumor cannot be entirely removed or to make other treatments more effective.

Radiation therapy uses radiation to shrink tumors. **Brachytherapy** (BREY-kee-THER-*uh*-pee) is the internal placement of radiation near or directly in the tumor. **Chemotherapy** (kee-moh-THER-*uh*-pee) is the use of medications that are **cytotoxic** (seye-*tuh*-TOK-sik), which means that they kill cells or interfere with their growth. **Antineoplastic** (an-tee-nee-oh-PLAS-tik) is the general name for chemotherapy medications. **Hormone therapy** involves removing a gland that is producing too many hormones. Hormone therapy can also refer to medications that interfere with the ability of hormones to increase the growth of certain cancers. **Combined therapy** refers to the use of more than one cancer medication. **Adjuvant** (AJ-*uh*-vuhnt) chemotherapy is given after primary treatment to increase the likelihood of reaching **remission** (ri-MISH-*uhn*), which is the disappearance of all signs of cancer.

Regression (ri-GRESH-*uhn*) refers to when cancer shrinks. **Recurrence** (ri-KUR-*uhns*) and **relapse** (REE-laps) both refer to when cancer returns after having been successfully treated. **Refractory** (ri-FRAK-*tuh*-ree) **cancer** does not respond to treatment. **Palliative** (PAL-ee-ey-tiv, PAL-ee-*uh*-tiv) care refers to care that is given to patients with **terminal** cancer, or cancer that cannot be cured and will result in death. The aim of palliative care is to relieve symptoms and make the patient as comfortable as possible.

Cancer of the Digestive System

Cancer can occur anywhere in the digestive system. Many GI cancers are carcinomas, though other types of cancer also occur.

Colorectal Cancer

Colorectal cancer is cancer of the large intestine and rectum and is also called **bowel** (BOU-*uhl*, BOUL) **cancer**, or sometimes simply **colon** (KOH-*luhn*) **cancer**. Colorectal cancer is the second leading cause of cancer deaths in the United States. Development of colorectal cancer is linked to age and lifestyle choices. Smokers, sedentary people, heavy alcohol drinkers, and people who eat a lot of red meat are at increased risk. There are also genetic contributions.

Most colorectal cancers are **adenocarcinomas** (ad-n-oh-kahr-*suh*-NOH-*muhz*) that originate from the glandular cells in the epithelium lining the digestive tract. A small percentage are lymphomas.

Symptoms of colorectal cancer include changes in bowel habits; rectal bleeding; anemia; **cachexia** (*kuh*-KEK-see-*uh*), which is weight loss; **anorexia** (an-*uh*-REK-see-*uh*), which is loss of appetite; and bloating. Colorectal cancer can be diagnosed through screening **colonoscopy** (koh-*luh*-NOS-*kuh*-pee), which is recommended to begin at age 50.

Liver Cancer

Liver cancer is usually caused by infection with hepatitis B or C virus. It also results from **cirrhosis** (si-ROH-sis), or scarring of the liver most often caused by alcoholism. **Aflatoxin** (af-*luh*-TOK-sin) is a rare cause of liver cancer. Aflatoxin is found in a type of fungus that sometimes grows in small amounts in peanuts, wheat, and corn. Most tumors found in the liver result from metastasis from other organs.

The most common type of liver cancer is **hepatocellular** (hep-at-oh-SEL-*yuh*-ler) **carcinoma**, or HCC. A liver tumor is a **hepatoma** (hep-*uh*-TOH-*muh*), which can be benign or malignant. A **cholangiosarcoma** (koh-lang-ee-oh-sahr-KOH-*muh*) is a bile duct cancer that can start where the bile ducts begin inside the liver.

Symptoms of liver cancer can include jaundice; bloating caused by **ascites** (*uh*-SEYE-teez), or fluid in the abdomen; easy bruising due to blood clotting abnormalities; and right upper quadrant abdominal pain.

Pancreatic Cancer

Most pancreatic cancer is caused by **ductal** (DUHKT-*uhl*) **adenocarcinoma** that starts in the **exocrine** (EK-*suh*-krin) pancreas, or the part that excretes pancreatic enzymes through ducts. A small number of benign pancreatic cancers arise from the **islets of Langerhans** (LANG-ur-hanz), which make hormones. These types of tumors are called **neuroendocrine** (noor-oh-EN-*duh*-krin) **tumors**, because they arise from neural and endocrine cells.

Symptoms of pancreatic cancer can include upper abdominal pain that extends to the middle or lower back pain; **steatorrhea** (stee-at-*uh*-REE-*uh*), or greasy, pale-colored, and foul-smelling stool caused by the inability to digest fats; diabetes; and **migratory thrombophlebitis** (throm-boh-fli-BEYE-tis), also called **Trousseau** (troo-SOH) **syndrome**, which refers to tender nodules in veins that arise due to inflammation and hypercoagulability.

> **DID YOU KNOW?**
>
> Pancreatic cancer has one of highest fatality rates of all cancers. Only about 5 percent of all people diagnosed with pancreatic cancer survive beyond five years after diagnosis. People who smoke, are obese, eat diets high in red meat, and have a family history of pancreatic cancer are more at risk.

Stomach Cancer

Stomach cancer is also called **gastric** (GAS-trik) **cancer**. Most stomach cancers are classified as adenocarcinomas. A small percentage are lymphomas.

Stomach cancer is often asymptomatic in early stages or may have vague symptoms like indigestion, loss of appetite, and bloating after meals. By the time it is diagnosed, stomach cancer has usually spread and is quite advanced, causing symptoms like **hematemesis** (*huh*-MAT-*uh*-MEE-*suhs*), which is vomiting blood; **melena** (*muh*-LEE-*nuh*), which is tarry blood in the stool; and **dysphagia** (dis-FEY-*juh*), which is difficulty eating. Stomach cancer can also cause **acanthosis nigricans** (ey-kan-THOH-*suhs* ni-*gruh*-kanz), which is hyperplasia of the skin of the back of the neck and the **axilla** (ak-SIL-*uh*), or armpit. The rapid development of **seborrheic keratosis** (seb-*uh*-REE-ik ker-*uh*-TOH-sis), which are raised, brown skin spots that usually develop slowly with age, can indicate a paraneoplastic syndrome.

After lung cancer, stomach cancer causes the greatest amount of cancer deaths worldwide. Infection with the bacteria *Helicobacter pylori* (hee-lik-oh-BAK-tur peye-LOR-ee) causes most stomach cancers. Smoking substantially increases stomach cancer risk. Eating meats cured with **nitrates** (NEYE-treyts) and **nitrites** (NEYE-treyts) and smoked fish may also increase the risk for stomach cancer.

Esophageal Cancer

Most esophageal cancers are squamous cell carcinomas and develop from the cells that line the upper part of the esophagus. Almost all squamous cell carcinoma esophageal cancers are caused by smoking and alcohol consumption.

A fair number of other types of esophageal cancers are adenocarcinomas, which arise from the glandular cells near the junction between the esophagus and the stomach. Most esophageal adenocarcinomas develop as a result of long-standing gastroesophageal reflux disease (GERD) in the following manner:

1. Stomach acid reflux injures cells of the esophagus.

2. Over time, the injured cells undergo cellular **metaplasia** (met-*uh*-PLEY-*zhuh*), which means that they begin to grow abnormally and develop neoplastic changes.

3. These changes result in Barrett esophagus, which is a premalignant condition.

Symptoms of esophageal cancer include dysphagia and difficulty swallowing hard foods like bread and meat; **odynophagia** (oh-din-*uh*-FEY-*juh*), or painful swallowing; a hoarse cough; vomiting blood; and heartburnlike pain. **Superior vena cava** (VEE-*nuh* KEY-*vuh*) **syndrome** is a symptom of advanced esophageal cancer and refers to airway obstruction caused by the tumor.

Oral Cancer

Oral cancer refers to any cancer found in the mouth and can include adenocarcinomas, which are derived from salivary glands; lymphomas, which are derived from tonsil and lymphoid tissue; and melanomas, which are derived from melanocytes in oral mucosa. Mouth cancer mostly affects the tongue but can also affect the mucosa lining of the mouth. Most oral cancers are squamous cell carcinomas.

Mouth cancer symptoms include a skin lump or ulcer that is painless and doesn't heal. Other symptoms include **leukoplakia** (loo-*kuh*-PLEY-kee-*uh*), or white patches, and **erythroplakia** (ih-RITH-*ruh*-PLEY-kee-*uh*), or red patches, in the mouth.

Most oral cancers are linked to smoking and excessive alcohol use. Some are linked to infection with a type of human **papillomavirus** (pap-*uh*-LOH-*muh*-veye-*ruhs*), which also causes cervical cancer.

Lung Cancer

Lung cancer is the leading cause of cancer deaths worldwide in men and women. Smoking causes 90 percent of lung cancers. Most lung cancers are carcinomas, which are further classified into nonsmall cell carcinoma and small cell carcinoma, also called oat cell carcinoma.

Nonsmall cell lung carcinoma is further broken down by subtype, of which the most common is adenocarcinoma. Adenocarcinoma is the most common lung cancer found in lifelong smokers.

Small cell lung cancer contains **vesicles** (VES-i-*kuhlz*) with neuroendocrine hormones. For this reason, paraneoplastic syndromes with hormonal symptoms often accompany small cell lung cancer. These cancers can cause hypersecretion of **antidiuretic hormone** (ADH), causing the syndrome of inappropriate ADH (SIADH). Symptoms include **hyponatremia** (heye-*puh*-ney-TREE-mee-*yuh*), or low blood levels of sodium; and fluid overload, which causes edema, difficulty breathing, and high blood pressure.

Squamous cell lung carcinoma is the second most common type of lung cancer, followed by large cell lung carcinoma. Because the lungs have such an extensive blood and lymphatic supply, many tumors in other parts of the body metastasize to the lungs.

Symptoms of lung cancer can include **hemoptysis** (hi-MOP-*tuh*-sis), which is coughing up blood; and clubbing of the fingernails, which causes the nails to become rounded and whitish in color while the fingertips become enlarged due to inadequate levels of oxygen. Tumors in the top part of the lungs can damage sympathetic nerves, causing **Horner** (HAWRN-erz) **syndrome,** with symptoms that include **ptosis** (TOH-*suhs*), or drooping of the eyelid; **miosis** (meye-OH-sis), or pupil constriction; decreased sweating; and reddened **conjunctiva** (kon-juhngk-TEYE-*vuh*), or bloodshot eyes.

DID YOU KNOW?

Tobacco use is the number-one risk factor for developing cancer. According to the World Health Organization, about one person dies every 6 seconds due to tobacco. Tobacco causes 22 percent of cancer deaths, 71 percent of lung cancer deaths, and kills 6 million people worldwide each year. Of this number, 600,000 people never smoked but developed cancer through secondhand smoke exposure. Tobacco smoke contains 50 confirmed carcinogens, and 250 chemicals harmful to health. Tobacco can cause cancer of the lung, bladder, larynx, head, neck, mouth, stomach, kidney, esophagus, and pancreas. Tobacco is also a significant contributor to heart disease. Secondhand smoke causes lung cancer and asthma. Tobacco smoke causes low infant birth weight, birth complications, and sudden infant death.

Breast Cancer

Breast cancer is the fifth leading cause of cancer deaths worldwide. In the United States, roughly 1 in 8 women will be diagnosed with breast cancer at some point in their lifetime. Over the past decades, better diagnosis and treatment methods have improved the prognosis for those diagnosed with breast cancer.

Breast cancer usually arises from the milk ducts, through which milk passes to the nipples, and is called **ductal carcinoma**. Ductal carcinoma is further divided into two subtypes. Ductal carcinoma in situ is also called **intraductal** (IN-*truh* DUHKT-*uhl*) **carcinoma**. It is localized, noninvasive, and has **microcalcifications** (kal-*suh*-fi-KEY-*shuhnz*), or areas where the tissue has become hardened with small calcium deposits. Invasive ductal carcinoma invades and infiltrates the breast tissue.

Another common area for breast cancer is in the lobules, where milk is formed. These tumors are called **lobular** (LOB-*yuh*-ler) carcinomas. Lobular carcinoma in situ is characterized by abnormal cells in the breast lobules with the presence of microcalcifications. Even though it is a benign condition, lobular carcinoma in situ can increase the risk for breast cancer.

WORD ORIGINS

Phyllodes (feye-LOH-deez) tumors are rare and arise from the **stromal** (STROH-*muhl*) **cells** surrounding the breast ducts and lobules. They grow quickly and can be benign or malignant. The name *phyllodes* comes from the Greek word for leaf, which is what these tumors look like when they grow.

Atypical ductal hyperplasia (heye-per-PLEY-*zhuh*) refers to the overgrowth of breast cells. It is benign but increases breast cancer risk. A **fibroadenoma** (feye-broh-ad-n-OH-*muh*) is a hard, movable lump in the breast that is most often benign. **Mastitis** (ma-STEYE-tis) is infection in the breast that can cause a lump, nipple discharge, pain, and a fever.

Symptoms of breast cancer include the following:

- A palpable lump in the breast or armpits
- **Peau d'orange** (POH DAWR-ahnj), which means "skin of an orange" and refers to a change in breast skin color and texture, which becomes orange and thick
- Enlargement of one breast

- Changes in nipple position or size
- **Inversion** (in-VUR-*zhuhn*) of the nipple, in which the nipple tip points inward rather than outward
- Blood or other nipple discharge
- **Mastodynia** (mast-uh-DEYE-nee-*yuh*), or breast pain
- Armpit pain or swelling
- Skin dimpling caused by the tumor pulling on the skin

Left untreated, breast cancer can become a **fungating** (fung-EYT-ing) **lesion**, which looks like a fungus. The inside cells become **necrotic** (nuh-KRAW-tik), or die. The cancer can ulcerate through the skin and produce dark, strong-smelling fluid.

Risk factors for breast cancer include smoking; age; female sex; being **nulliparous** (*nuh-luh*-PAIR-*uhs*), which is never having borne a child; high hormone levels; obesity; and family history of breast cancer. Some genetic mutations are inherited through families and substantially increase the risk for breast cancer. (See Chapter 21 for a discussion of the *BRCA1* and *BRCA2* genes.)

Some breast cancer, called **hormone receptor–positive breast cancer**, depends on estrogen and progesterone for its growth. This type of breast cancer can often be treated with drugs that block the effect of estrogen. *HER2/neu* is an oncogene that can make breast cancer more aggressive. It is used as a biomarker to estimate the severity and prognosis of the cancer and help in treatment decisions. Certain drugs target HER2. See Chapter 26 for more information about antineoplastics.

Triple-negative breast cancer does not express cell-surface receptors for estrogen, progesterone, or *HER2/neu*. Some of these types of breast cancer are aggressive with poorer prognosis than hormone receptor–positive breast cancer. Others have a similar course. Triple-negative breast cancer has a much higher relapse rate during the first five years after diagnosis. Beyond five years, it has a lower relapse rate than hormone receptor–positive breast cancer.

Skin Cancer

Skin cancer can form from various types of cells in the different layers of the skin. **Basal** (BEY-*suhl*) **cell carcinoma** is the most common, least lethal skin cancer. It originates from the bottom layer of the epidermis and is pearly or translucent in color. **Squamous** (SKWEYs-*muhs*) **cell carcinoma** originates from the middle layer of epidermis and is likely to spread. It appears as an ulcer or reddish plaque on the skin. **Melanoma** (mel-*uh*-NOH-*muh*) originates from **melanocytes** (*muh*-LAN-*uh*-seyets), which make skin pigment, and is the most likely to spread, most lethal, but least common. Melanoma often appears as a change in the color, shape, or size of an existing mole.

Other types of skin lesions carry the risk of becoming cancerous. A **keratoacanthoma** (keyr-*uh*-TOH-AK-*uhn*-THOH-*muh*) arises from hair follicles. If left untreated, it often dies and peels off. Because some keratoacanthomas can become invasive and metastasize, most are treated. The appearance of **Kaposi** (KAP-oh-zee) **sarcoma** is an AIDS-defining event. It causes raised, brown skin lesions and also affects the mouth, GI tract, and lungs. Kaposi sarcoma is due to infection with human herpes virus 8. **Actinic keratosis** (ak-TIN-ik ker-*uh*-TOH-sis) is a premalignant condition that can progress to squamous cell carcinoma. It produces thick, scaly, crusty patches on the skin.

Endocrine Cancers

Endocrine cancers can arise in any part of the endocrine system. Because the endocrine system produces the body's network of hormonal messengers, endocrine cancers can produce many different symptoms throughout the body.

There are two main types of malignant thyroid cancers. **Papillary** (PAP-*uh*-ler-ee) **thyroid cancer** is the most common type and is more common in women. **Medullary** (MED-uhl-*er*-ee, MEJ-uh-*ler*-ee) **thyroid cancer** arises from **parafollicular** (PAIR-*uh*-*fuh*-LIK-*yuh*-ler) cells, which secrete calcitonin—important in calcium homeostasis. Medullary thyroid cancer tends to run in families.

Symptoms of thyroid cancer can include a palpable nodule and **goiter** (GOI-ter), or enlarged thyroid gland. People who have had previous radiation to the neck are at increased risk for developing thyroid cancer.

Adrenal cancer is rare. Adrenal carcinomas are extremely rare and originate from the adrenal cortex, the outer steroid-producing part of the adrenal gland. Adrenal carcinomas produce many hormonal symptoms, including **virilization** (VIR-*uh*-*luh*-ZEY-*shuhn*), or the production of male characteristics, and **feminization** (FEM-*uh*-*nuh*-ZEY-*shuhn*), or the production of female characteristics. Adrenal **adenomas** (ad-n-OH-*muhz*) are benign adrenal tumors that don't always cause symptoms. They sometimes secrete excess cortisol, causing Cushing syndrome (see Chapter 16). A **pheochromocytoma** (fee-oh-kroh-moh-seye-TOH-*muh*) is a tumor that develops in the adrenal medulla. It secretes adrenaline (epinephrine) and noradrenaline (norepinephrine), causing anxiety, sweating, racing heart, high blood pressure, and high blood sugar.

Carcinoid tumors are sometimes called **APUDomas** (a-*puhd*-OH-*muhs*), because they arise from endocrine APUD (amine precursor uptake and decarboxylation) cells. Carcinoid tumors can grow in the lung and digestive tracts, as well as other organs. Many are benign, but most have malignant potential. They produce hormones, especially serotonin, and can cause flushing, diarrhea, wheezing, abdominal cramping, and peripheral edema.

Cancer of the Female Reproductive System

Cancer can occur in any part of the female reproductive system. Many cancers of the female reproductive system are carcinomas, though cancer can also arise from other types of cells in this system, like germ cells.

Ovarian Cancer

Most ovarian cancer develops from epithelial cells of the ovaries and is called **ovarian epithelial carcinoma**. The most common subtypes are the following:

- **Serous** (SEEER-*uhs*) **tumors** can be benign or malignant.
- **Endometrioid** (en-doh-MEE-TREE-oid) **tumors** resemble the uterine lining.
- **Serous cystadenocarcinomas** (SIST-ad-n-oh-sahr-KOH-*muhs*) derive from glandular epithelium.

> **DID YOU KNOW?**
>
> **Dysgerminomas** (dis-jerm-*uh*-NOH-*muh*) are usually benign germ cell tumors that occur inside the ovary or testis. The most common in women is a **teratoma** (ter-*uh*-TOH-*muh*), which contains parts of all three germ cell layers (ectoderm, mesoderm, and endoderm). Teratomas can contain hair, teeth, eyes, hands, feet, and limbs. They are thought to be **congenital** (*kuhn*-JEN-i-tl), or present at birth. Teratomas have the potential to become malignant but rarely do so. They can be found in the ovaries, testes, and in areas along the body midline, including the skull, nose, tongue, and neck.

Symptoms of ovarian cancer can be vague and include bloating, pelvic pain, difficulty eating, frequent urination, back pain, constipation, abnormal vaginal bleeding, and ascites. The risk of ovarian cancer increases with a history of obesity and **polycystic** (POL-ee-SIST-ik) **ovarian syndrome**, in which the ovaries grow numerous cysts that produce estrogen. Obesity can increase the production of estrogen in fat cells and increase the risk for reproductive cancers like ovarian and endometrial cancer. Ovarian cancer is also linked to *BRCA1* and *BRCA2* mutations (see Chapter 21).

Endometrial Cancer

Endometrial (en-doh-MEE-tree-*uhl*) **cancer** is sometimes called **uterine** (YOO-ter-in, YOO-*tuh*-reyen) **cancer** and arises from the lining of the uterus. It is the fourth most common cancer in women, and the most common gynecological cancer in the United States. The most common type of endometrial cancer is called endometrial adenocarcinoma. There are three common subtypes: endometroid carcinoma (which is the least aggressive), uterine papillary serous carcinoma, and uterine clear cell carcinoma. The last two carry worse prognoses.

Symptoms of endometrial cancer include abnormal vaginal bleeding, or **metrorrhagia** (mee-*truh*-REY-jee-*uh*), especially after menopause or between periods. **Menometrorrhagia** (men-*uh*-mee-*truh*-REY-jee-*uh*) refers to excessive vaginal bleeding that can occur during menstruation, or abnormally between periods. Risk for endometrial cancer increases if there has been a history of endometrial hyperplasia and excessive estrogen exposure.

Cervical Cancer

Worldwide, **cervical** (SUR-vi-*kuhl*) **cancer** is the second most common and fifth deadliest of cancers among women. This is a tragedy, because the five-year survival rate is more than 90 percent for the earliest stages of invasive cervical cancer and more than 70 percent for all stages combined. Detection and early treatment are the keys to survival. Screening is easily done with **Papanicolaou smears**, or Pap smears, which check for abnormal cells. Infection with human papillomavirus (HPV) explains almost all cases of cervical cancer. An HPV vaccine exists that can protect against infection with HPV and cervical cancer.

Most cervical cancers are squamous cell carcinomas. The second most common are adenocarcinomas, which arise from glandular epithelial cells. A precancerous cervical lesion is called **cervical intraepithelial** (in-*truh*-ep-*uh*-THEE-lee-*uhl*) **neoplasia** (CIN). Low-grade squamous intraepithelial lesion (LGSIL) refers to mild dysplasia, which usually resolves without treatment but needs monitoring and follow-up exams because it sometimes becomes cancerous. High-grade squamous intraepithelial lesion (HGSIL) refers to carcinoma in situ that has not become invasive.

Cervical cancer is often asymptomatic. Symptoms can include abnormal vaginal bleeding or discharge, swollen legs, appetite loss, weight loss, and pelvic pain.

Cancer of the Male Reproductive System

Cancer can occur in any part of the male reproductive system. The most common types of male reproductive cancers are germ cell tumors and prostate cancer.

Testicular Cancer

Testicular (te-STIK-*yuh*-ler) **cancer** is cancer of the testes. It is the most common cancer in young adult men aged 15 to 35 and is highly treatable, with an overall five-year survival rate of about 95 percent.

Most testicular cancers are considered germ cell tumors, or **germinomas** (jerm-*uh*-NOH-*muh*). Testicular germ cell tumors are further divided into **nonseminomas** (NAWN-sem-*uh*-NOH-*muhz*) and **seminomas** (sem-*uh*-NOH-*muhz*). Nonseminomas are more common, more aggressive, and usually diagnosed in younger men. Subtypes of nonseminomas include **yolk sac** (YOHK SAK) **tumors** and **embryonal** (em-bree-OH-*nuhl*) **carcinomas**. Seminomas are more rare, slow growing, and diagnosed later in life. Seminomas can be pure seminomas, having only one type of cell, or can have **syncytiotrophoblast** (sin-SISH-oh-TROH-foh-blast) cells scattered throughout.

WORDS OF WARNING

The use of the prefix *non-* in *nonseminomas* can be confusing. Both types of cancers are considered germ cell tumors because they grow from the types of cells that make sperm. The distinction between seminoma and nonseminoma is based on the microscopic appearance of the cell and what kinds of germ cells they arise from. The distinction is important because the treatments are different for seminomas versus nonseminomas.

Symptoms of testicular cancer include heaviness and pain in the scrotum; an enlarged testicle or a testicular lump; and **gynecomastia** (geye-ni-koh-MAS-tee-*uh*), or swelling of breast tissue.

Prostate Cancer

Prostate (PROS-teyt) **cancer** is the second most common cause of cancer in men in the United States, and the second most common cause of cancer death among most racial groups in the United States.

Most cancers of the prostate are slow-growing adenocarcinomas. Prostate cancer sometimes doesn't cause symptoms. When it does, symptoms can be similar to those of **benign prostatic hypertrophy** (BPH), or **benign prostatic hyperplasia**, and include **dysuria** (dis-YOOR-ee-*uh*), or difficulty urinating; **nocturia** (nok-TOOR-ee-*uh*), or nighttime urination; hesitancy, or difficulty initiating a urine stream; **hematuria** (hee-*muh*-TOOR-ee-*uh*), or blood in the urine; painful intercourse; and erectile dysfunction.

Risk for prostate cancer is associated with obesity, age, family history, and African descent. **Prostate-specific antigen** (AN-ti-*juhn*), or PSA, is a tumor marker whose utility is controversial. PSA levels are often elevated in benign prostatic hypertrophy and can lead to false positives and unnecessary treatments, which can be injurious and cause long-term problems.

Cancer of the Urinary Tract

Most cancers of the urinary tract are types of carcinomas. Bladder cancer, for example, arises from the **urothelium** (yoor-*uh*-THEE-lee-*uhm*), or outer surface of the bladder lining, and is called **transitional** (tran-ZISH-*uhn-uhl*) **cell carcinoma**. Symptoms of bladder cancer include hematuria, dysuria, or increased urinary frequency.

Smoking causes more than half of bladder cancers in men and one third of bladder cancers in women. Risk is also linked to occupational exposure to carcinogens like **benzidine** (BEN-zi-deen) and **aniline** (AN-l-in, AN-l-eyen) dyes and **2-naphthalene** (NAP-*thuh*-LEEN), which is used in mothballs.

The majority of kidney cancers are caused by renal cell carcinoma of the renal tubules, of which most are **renal cell carcinoma** and **clear cell adenocarcinoma**. Kidney cancer can also appear in the renal pelvis and is called **urothelial** (yoor-oh-THEE-lee-*uhl*) **cell carcinoma**, most cases of which are **transitional cell carcinoma**.

Symptoms of kidney cancer can include a lump in the abdomen; hematuria; pain along the sides of the back, which is also called flank pain; and anemia due to suppression of **erythropoietin** (ih-rith-roh-POI-i-tn, ih-rith-roh-poi-EET-n), or **erythrocytosis** (ih-rith-rih-saht-OH-*suhs*), which is increased red blood cells due to increased erythropoietin.

Smoking increases the risk for kidney cancer, as does prior history of prostate or cervical cancer and a history of kidney disease and dialysis.

Blood and Immune System Cancers

Blood and immune system cancers belong to two groups: leukemia, which is liquid cancer; and lymphoma, which is solid cancer.

Leukemia

Leukemia is a liquid cancer that occurs when the bone marrow makes immature white blood cells, called **blasts**. Most leukemias occur in adults.

Leukemia is classified into acute versus chronic. **Acute leukemia** is the most common type found in children and is characterized by a rapid buildup of immature white blood cells. Immediate treatment is necessary because there is a high risk of metastasis to other organs. **Chronic leukemia** is characterized by a gradual accumulation of mature but still abnormal white blood cells. Chronic leukemia is usually found in older people and monitored rather than treated right away.

Acute and chronic leukemias are further classified on the basis of the kinds of cells that are affected. **Lymphoblastic** (lim-*fuh*-BLAST-ik)**/lymphocytic** (lim-*fuh*-SIT-ik) **leukemias** most often affect **lymphocytes** (lim-fuh-SEYET), which fight infections, especially precursor B cells. **Myelogenous** (meye-*uh*-LOJ-*uh*-*nuhs*) **leukemia** most often affects red blood cells, though some white blood cells and platelets can be affected.

Many subtypes exist. The most common in adults are the following:

- **Chronic lymphocytic leukemia (CLL)**
- **Acute myelogenous leukemia (AML)**
- **Chronic myelogenous leukemia (CML)**
- **Hairy cell leukemia (HCL):** the name comes from the hairy appearance of abnormal B cells under the microscope
- **Adult T-cell leukemia (ATL):** caused by the human T-lymphotropic virus (HTLV), which infects CD4+ T cells and induces abnormal cell proliferation

Symptoms of leukemia include easy bruising; **petechiae** (pi-TEE-kee-*uh*, pi-TEK-ee-*uh*), which are small, punctate bleeds under the skin; opportunistic infections; and swollen lymph nodes where blasts gather. Causes of leukemia include previous radiation and chemotherapy, infection with the human T-lymphotropic virus, exposure to the chemical **benzene** (BEN-zeen), and genetic disorders like Down syndrome.

Lymphoma

Lymphoma is a solid tumor that forms from lymphocytes (white blood cells) in lymph nodes, spleen, bone marrow, and other organs like the skin, brain, and digestive tract. The two main subtypes of lymphoma are **Hodgkin** (HODJ-kin) **lymphoma** and **non-Hodgkin** (NAWN-HODJ-kin) **lymphoma**. Hodgkin lymphoma is the least common type. It is typified by the presence of **Reed-Sternberg** (REED STURN-burg) **cells**, which are giant B cells that may have several nuclei and are not mature enough to produce antibodies. It is associated with a prior history of mononucleosis and infection with Epstein-Barr virus. Non-Hodgkin lymphoma is the most common type. It includes all lymphomas that do not contain Reed-Sternberg cells.

WORDS OF WARNING

The distinction between Hodgkin and non-Hodgkin lymphoma is a matter of controversy. Some experts would like to entirely dispense with the distinction. A 2008 World Health Organization classification also recommended getting rid of it. However, many people still use this terminology.

Lymphomas are common among people with AIDS, transplant patients taking immunosuppressive medications, and people with genetic conditions that impair the immune system. There are three main types of AIDS-related lymphomas: diffuse large B-cell lymphoma, B-cell immunoblastic lymphoma, and Burkitt lymphoma. Symptoms of lymphoma include **lymphadenopathy** (lim-fad-n-OP-*uh*-thee), or swelling of lymph nodes, and various nonspecific symptoms such as fever and night sweats.

Pediatric Cancer

Cancer is mainly a disease found in adults. Children who develop cancer usually have forms of it that are not found among adults. The most common form of cancer in children is leukemia. Among children with cancer, roughly 30 percent have leukemia.

The most common type of leukemia in children is acute lymphoblastic leukemia (ALL), also called acute lymphocytic leukemia.

Blastomas (bla-STOH-*muhz*) arise from embryonic cells and are more common in children. An example is **Wilms** (WILMS) **tumor**, which is a **nephroblastoma** (nef-roh-blast-OH-*muh*), or a cancer that develops from embryonic kidney cells. It is usually diagnosed around age three and is more common in people of African descent. Other common childhood blastomas include **retinoblastoma** (ret-*uh*-noh-blast-OH-*muh*), which is a tumor of the retina, and **medulloblastoma** (*muh-duh*-loh-blast-OH-*muh*), which are brain tumors.

Children also develop **sarcoma** (sahr-KOH-*muh*), or soft-tissue cancer. An example is **Ewing** (YOO-ing) **sarcoma**, a rare cancer that develops in the ribs, pelvis, and middle of the long leg bones.

Sex chord stromal tumors also develop in children but are rare. They develop from the supportive tissue in the ovary and testes. **Sertoli cell tumors** secrete estrogen and can cause early puberty in girls or feminization in boys. **Sertoli-Leydig** (sur-TOH-lee LEY-*duhg*) **cell tumors** make testosterone and can cause early puberty in boys or virilization in girls.

The Least You Need to Know

- The number-one risk factor for developing cancer is tobacco use, especially smoking.
- A neoplasm is an abnormal or out-of-control cell growth, also called a tumor, that can be benign or malignant.
- Carcinomas are malignant tumors that arise from epithelial cells, and are the most common form of cancer in adults.
- The most common types of cancer worldwide are cancer of the lung, stomach, liver, colon, and breast.
- Children develop different types of cancers than adults. The most common childhood cancer is leukemia.

Diagnostic Testing and Treatment

Part 5 is dedicated to diagnostic testing and treatment. Chapter 23 presents terms associated with all the various medical lab tests, from one of the simplest tests, a urine dipstick, to highly sophisticated tests like genetic and DNA analyses. Chapter 24 covers medical imaging like x-rays, CT scans, MRI, and PET scans. Other diagnostic tests are included, like an EEG (which detects brain waves and electrical activity in the brain) and an ECG (which detects electrical activity in the heart). Chapter 25 covers noninvasive and minimally invasive diagnostic techniques. Therapies are also covered, including interventional radiology, robotic surgery, and therapies like kidney dialysis. Chapter 26 provides a basic introduction to pharmacology. This chapter is just the tip of the iceberg in this vast field of medicine that cannot even begin to be presented in its entirety. Instead, this chapter is intended to provide a general introduction to pharmacological terms, how medicines are categorized by body systems, and examples of the names of individual medicines. For more complete listings, a pharmacology manual is required. This chapter also does not present medication side effects, although these are always important considerations in any medication regimen.

Clinical Laboratory Medicine

Chapter 23

In This Chapter

- Urine dipstick tests and urinalysis
- Metabolic panels, liver function tests, lipid panels, and thyroid tests
- Blood tests
- Body fluid analyses and cultures
- Cardiac enzyme tests, toxicology screens, serology, and DNA analysis

Clinical laboratory testing is essential for diagnosis and treatment of human disease. There are many different types of lab tests, and these can be done on samples from many different parts of the body. Certain results can help confirm a diagnosis. Others can help monitor the progression of disease or treatment. Interpreting the results of these tests can be complicated.

Many clinical laboratory terms stem from chemistry and biochemistry, so knowing some basic chemical terms can be beneficial. Other terms stem from other branches of science. Knowing the general terminology is the first step in navigating the morass of medical laboratory tests.

Urinalysis

Urinalysis (yoor-*uh*-NAL-*uh*-sis) is a screening test that looks at abnormalities of substances in urine. One of the cheapest and easiest urine tests can be done in minutes in a doctor's office and is called a urine dipstick test, shortened to Udip (YOO-dip). This test consists of placing a plastic strip into a urine sample. The strip has various boxes on it that change color after it sits in urine for a certain amount of time. The urine dipstick test measures the following:

- **Urine specific gravity**, which is the concentration of the urine
- Urine pH, which indicates acidity
- Protein in the urine
- Sugar in the urine
- **Nitrite** (NEYE-treyet), which can indicate the presence of bacteria
- **Ketones** (kee-TOHNZ), which result from fat breakdown
- Red and white bloods cells in the urine
- **Leukocyte esterase** (ES-*tuh*-reys), which can indicate white blood cells in the urine
- **Bilirubin** (BIL-ee-roo-bin), which can suggest liver disease or some kinds of anemia
- **Urobilinogen** (yoor-oh-beye-LIN-*uh-juhn*), which can suggest liver disease
- **Hemoglobin** (HEE-*muh*-gloh-bin), which suggests the presence of red blood cells

If the results of the urine dipstick test are abnormal, the urine is often sent to the lab for further analysis. During a urinalysis, the urine is examined with the naked eye to look for abnormal color and cloudiness. The urine is also examined under the microscope to look for cells, urine crystals, mucus, and bacteria. Urine is generally considered to be sterile, so the presence of any of these things can indicate infection or disease.

Sometimes a urine chemistry is performed, which looks for various chemicals in the urine. These include hormones and various types of acids and proteins that can help diagnose conditions like kidney and autoimmune diseases.

The presence of casts in urine is always abnormal. **Casts** are cylindrical groupings of cells that can consist of red blood cells, white blood cells, epithelial cells, bacteria, and various proteins. Each type of cast can indicate different disease processes in the kidney. If bacteria are found, urine is processed further.

Other urine tests include **fractional** (FRAK-*shuh*-nl) excretion of sodium, or FeNA, which is used in diagnosing kidney failure. **Human chorionic gonadotropin** (KAWR-ee-on-ik goh-nad-*uh*-TROH-pin), or HCG, can be measured in the urine and is used to determine pregnancy. Urine **osmolality** (oz-*muh*-LAL-*uh*-tcc) is another way to look at urine concentration and takes into the account the amount of dissolved substances in the urine.

Clinical Biochemistry

Panels are groups of tests that are usually run together as a group in the clinical laboratory. Several types of panels are used to help diagnose medical conditions.

Basic Metabolic Panel

A **basic metabolic panel**, or BMP, is a screening test that measures blood levels of **serum analytes** (SEER-*uhm* AN-*uh*-leyets), or substances in the noncellular liquid part of blood that can be measured to estimate and monitor health status. Tests for **electrolytes** (ih-LEK-*truh*-leyets) are important parts of the metabolic panel. Electrolytes are vital for muscle contraction, as well as body water and acid–base balance. Abnormal electrolytes can indicate dehydration and disease states, such as kidney disease or diabetes.

> **DID YOU KNOW?**
>
> Medical professionals use special language to indicate how quickly they need the results for laboratory tests. If they are needed as soon as possible, such as during an emergency, the word **stat** is added to the order. *Stat* comes from the Latin word *statim*, which means immediately.

Basic Metabolic Panel Tests

Test	Pronunciation	Importance/Assesses
blood urea nitrogen (BUN)	BLUHD yoo-REE-*uh* NEYE-*truh-juhn*	metabolic waste product, estimates kidney function
creatinine	kree-AT-n-een	waste product of muscle metabolism, estimates kidney function
glucose	GLOO-kohs	blood sugar measurement, indicates diabetes or prediabetes

continues

Basic Metabolic Panel Tests   (continued)

Test	Pronunciation	Importance/Assesses
calcium	KAL-see-*uhm*	electrolyte that plays a major role in muscle contraction, nerve conduction, and heart muscle contraction; can indicate bone or parathyroid disorders
carbon dioxide (CO2), bicarbonate	KAHR-*buhn* deye-OK-seyed, beye-KAHR-*buh*-neyt	electrolyte important for acid–base balance
chloride	KLAWR-eyed	electrolyte important for acid–base balance and body fluid homeostasis
potassium	*puh*-TAS-ee-*uhm*	electrolyte important for cellular metabolism and muscle contraction, especially cardiac
sodium	SOH-dee-*uhm*	electrolyte important for nerve and muscle function

Comprehensive Metabolic Panel

The **comprehensive metabolic panel**, or CMP, is similar to the BMP, only it includes more tests. The tests that are included in the CMP vary by facility, with the total number of tests ranging from 12 to 20. In general, the CMP includes the 8 tests in the BMP and adds some, but not always all, of the tests in the following table.

Common Comprehensive Metabolic Panel Tests

Term	Pronunciation	Importance
albumen	al-BYOO-*muhn*	assesses kidney and liver function
total protein	TOH-*tuhl* PROH-teen	assesses kidney and liver function
creatinine clearance	kree-AT-n-een KLEE-*uhns*	assesses kidney function
gamma glutamyl transferase (GGT)	GAM-*uh* gloot-uh-MIL TRANS-*fuh*-reys	assesses liver function; can indicate alcohol abuse and/or congestive heart failure
alkaline phosphatase (ALP)	ALK-*kuh*-leyen, ALK-*kuh*-lin FOS-*fuh*-teys	liver enzyme; assesses liver function and can indicate bone disease

Term	Pronunciation	Importance
alanine aminotransferase (ALT)	AL-*uh*-neen *uh*-MEE-noh TRANS-*fuh*-reys	liver enzyme; assesses liver function
aspartate aminotransferase (AST)	*uh*-SPAHR-teyt *uh*-MEE-noh TRANS-*fuh*-reys	liver enzyme; assesses liver function
cholesterol, triglycerides	*kuh*-LES-*tuh*-rawl, treye-GLIS-*uh*-reyedz	measures levels of fats in the blood
Lactate dehydrogenase (LDH)	LAK-teyt dee-heye-DRAW-*juh*-neys	found in many tissues; indicates tissue damage
phosphate (PO4)	FOS-feyt	electrolyte important for acid–base balance; can indicate parathyroid, bone, malnutrition, kidney, and liver disorders
total bilirubin (tbili)	TOH-*tuhl* BIL-ee-*roo-bin*	waste product of red blood cell breakdown; assesses liver function and can indicate some types of anemia
uric acid	YOOR-ik AS-id	waste product of protein breakdown; assesses kidney function and presence of gout

WORDS OF WARNING

The types and numbers of tests included in BMPs and CMPs vary by facility. The BMP was originally named SMA, which is short for sequential multiple analysis. A BMP is sometimes called a CHEM-7 or SMA-7 even though some hospitals include eight tests in this panel. A CMP can include 12, 14, or 20 tests. Some hospitals call a CMP a CHEM-12, CHEM-14, or CHEM-20, even though the numbers in these terms don't always indicate the total number of tests in each panel. The take-home message is: don't rely on the name to figure out the number and types of tests included in BMPs and CMPs.

Liver Function Tests

Liver function tests, or LFTs, are used to assess and monitor the health of the liver. A set of LFTs is called a **hepatic function panel.** LFTs are often included in BMPs and CMPs. Because the liver is the major producer of clotting factors, some coagulation tests like PT and INR can be used to assess liver function (see coagulation tests section). Other tests that can assess liver function include the ones listed in the following table.

Common Liver Function Tests

Test	Pronunciation	Importance
alpha-1 antitrypsin	AL-*fuh* WUHN an-tee-TRIP-*suhn*	helps diagnose alpha-1 antitrypsin deficiency, a rare genetic cause for emphysema and liver disease
urine bilirubin	YOOR-*uhn* BIL-ee-roo-bin	part of a urinalysis; can indicate liver damage or blockage of bile ducts
urine urobilinogen	YOOR-*uhn* yoor-oh-beye-LIN-*uh-juhn*	part of urinalysis; can indicate liver disease
conjugated or direct bilirubin (dbili)	KON-*juh*-gey-ted	can indicate liver diseases, especially alcoholic liver disease, drug reactions, and bile duct disorders
unconjugated indirect or bilirubin (ibili)	*uhn* KON-*juh*-gey-ted	can indicate some types of liver diseases, transfusion reactions, and hemolytic anemia
hepatitis A, B, and C	hep-*uh*-TEYE-tis	tests for infectious causes of hepatitis, cirrhosis, and/or liver cancer
ammonia	*uh*-MOHN-*yuh*	toxic waste product of protein catabolism; builds up in liver failure and can help determine the cause of coma
copper		can help diagnose Wilson disease, a rare genetic disease in which copper accumulates in the liver and other organs
ceruloplasmin	suh-roo-*luh*-PLAZ-min	protein that carries copper in the blood; can help diagnose Wilson disease

Lipid Panel

A lipid panel is a group of tests that measure several types of blood fats. Lipid tests are helpful in determining risk and treatment for cardiovascular disease. The lipid panel usually measures:

- **Total cholesterol** (*kuh*-LES-*tuh*-rawl): total amount of fat in blood
- **Low-density cholesterol, LDL:** "bad" cholesterol that can build up in the blood vessels, causing atherosclerosis and cardiovascular disease

- **High-density cholesterol, HDL:** "good" cholesterol
- **Triglycerides** (treye-GLIS-*uh*-reyedz): blood fats that are linked to heart disease, diabetes, and stroke

Thyroid Function Tests

Thyroid function tests look for hypothyroidism and hyperthyroidism and are used as screening tests for newborns. Different types of thyroid and pituitary disorders produce characteristic elevations or decreases in thyroid hormone levels.

Thyroid-stimulating hormone (TSH) or **thyrotropin** (theye-*ruh*-TROH-pin) is an initial screening test for the hormone that stimulates the thyroid to release thyroid hormones. **Total thyroxine** (theye-ROK-sin) or **T4** test measures the total amount of thyroxine in the blood that is unbound plus the amount bound to **thyroxine-binding globulin** (GLOB-*yuh*-lin). **Free thyroxine** or **Free T4** measures the amount of unbound thyroxine in the blood. Thyroxine is a **prohormone** (PRO-HOR-mohn), the inactive form of thyroid hormone, and is converted into triiodothyronine, the active form, in tissues. **Triiodothyronine** (treye-eye-oh-doh-THEYE-*ruh*-neen) or **T3** measures the active form of the thyroid hormone.

Hematology

Hematology tests analyze red blood cells, white blood cells, and the blood's clotting ability.

WORD ORIGINS

The term that describes the process of drawing blood samples for laboratory analysis is **phlebotomy** (*fluh*-BOT-*uh*-mee). It comes from the Greek word *phlebo*, which means vein, and the ending *-tomy*, which means "to cut." So *phlebotomy* literally means to cut into a vein. A similar word is **venipuncture** (VEEN-*uh*-puhngk-cher), which means to access a vein for the purpose of providing medical treatment or sampling blood for analysis.

Complete Blood Count

The complete blood count, or CBC, gives an estimate of anemia, bleeding, and the level of immune cells in the body. The CBC usually includes the following:

- **Red blood cell count** (RBCs): measures the number of red blood cells in the blood, useful in diagnosing anemia and red blood cell disorders
- **White blood cell counts** (WBCs): measures the number of white blood cells in the blood, useful in diagnosing infection and immune disorders
- **Platelet count:** blood cells capable of clotting
- **Hemoglobin** (HEE-*muh*-gloh-bin): the oxygen-carrying part of red blood cells; can indicate anemia, malnutrition, bleeding, and other blood disorders
- **Hematocrit** (hi-MAT-*uh*-krit): the proportion of blood that is made up of red blood cells; a rapidly falling hematocrit often indicates bleeding
- **Mean cell volume** (MCV): indicates the average volume of red blood cells
- **Mean cell hemoglobin concentration** (MCHC): an estimate of the amount of hemoglobin in each red blood cell

If the white blood cell count is abnormal, or there is other cause to suspect infection or immune system dysfunction, a white blood cell differential can be done. This test analyzes the following:

- **Abnormal and immature cells**: such as blasts, or large, immature cells; and **poikilocytes** (poi-*kuh-luh*-SEYETS), or abnormally shaped cells
- **Eosinophils** (ee-*uh*-SIN-*uh*-fils): important in allergy and parasitic infections
- **Neutrophils** (NOO-*truh*-fils): fight bacteria, important in acute inflammation and some cancers
- **Bands:** immature neutrophils
- **Lymphocytes** (LIM-*fuh*-seyets): B and T cells; make antibodies; important in fighting viral infection and tumors
- **Monocytes** (MON-*uh*-seyets): help fight infection, active in inflammation
- **Basophils** (BEY-*suh*-fils): active in inflammation and parasitic infections

Coagulation

Several blood tests measures **blood coagulation** (koh-AG-*yuh*-ley-*shuhn*), or how quickly or slowly the blood clots. Recall from Chapter 10 that blood requires coagulation factors in order to form clots. These factors are activated via two coagulation pathways: the **extrinsic** (ik-STRIN-sik) **pathway** and the **intrinsic** (in-TRIN-sik) **pathway**. These two pathways unite in a final common pathway, which leads to a blood clot.

Blood Coagulation Tests

Test	Pronunciation	Importance
prothrombin time (PT)	proh-THROM-bin	measures how long it takes for blood to clot; assesses liver production of clotting factors; measures the extrinsic pathway
international normalized ratio (INR)		compares the patient's clotting time via the extrinsic pathway to a standard international value
partial thromboplastin time (PTT)	PAHR-*shuhl* throm-*buh*-PLAS-tin	measures blood clotting time; measures the intrinsic and common coagulation pathways
activated partial thromboplastin time (aPTT)	AK-*tuh*-veyt-ed PAHR-*shuhl* throm-*buh*-PLAS-tin	measures the intrinsic coagulation pathway

Body Fluid Analysis

Laboratory tests are also done on other body fluids to look for pathogens and other abnormal processes. **Cultures** are microorganisms grown in the lab for purposes of identifying them and for **sensitivity testing**, to determine effective medications. For example, some bacteria are resistant to certain antibiotics and grow even in the presence of that antibiotic.

Microorganisms can be grown on special **growth media**, which contain nutrients that help them to grow, and also contain antibiotics and other medications to test growth inhibition. Bacterial, fungal, and yeast cultures can be grown in liquid media in test tubes or plated on solid **agar** (AG-er) on **Petri** (pee-tree) dishes, which are round, flat disks.

Virology cultures are used to identify viruses. The patient sample is introduced to test cells that certain viruses are known to infect. After a certain amount of time, the sample is analyzed for cell death or viral growth.

Stool cultures are also called **fecal** (FEE-*kuhl*) **cultures**. Stool cultures usually look for parasites and **ova** (OH-*vuh*), which are eggs left by parasites, and white blood cells, red blood cells, and bacterial toxins. Sometimes a stool analysis is also done. The physical appearance of the stool is examined for consistency, color, odor, and presence of mucus. Stool analysis also looks for **occult** (*uh*-KUHLT) **blood,** which is blood not visible to the eye, and fat, undigested meat, bile, white blood cells, sugars, and pH (acid level).

A **urine culture** is usually done after abnormalities are found on a urine dipstick test or urinalysis. Urine cultures look for bacteria, yeast, or fungi that may be causing a urinary tract or bladder infection. If bacteria grow in the culture, antibiotic sensitivity testing and **Gram stains** are performed. Gram stains help identify two general types of bacteria. Gram-positive bacteria have a thick outer cell membrane that takes up the stain, making them appear blue. Gram-negative bacteria lack this thick outer cell membrane, so they do not take up the stain and appear pink.

Blood cultures are done when there is suspicion of a blood infection, such as **bacteremia** (bak-*tuh*-REE-mee-*uh*) or **septicemia** (sep-*tuh*-SEE-mee-*uh*). Blood cultures help identify the causal organism. Gram stains and sensitivity testing are also done on blood cultures that grow organisms.

Cerebrospinal fluid (CSF) **cultures** are done when meningitis or encephalitis is suspected. A **lumbar** (LUHM-bahr) **puncture** is used to obtain CSF for analysis. A needle is inserted through the space between the vertebrae and through the meninges surrounding the spinal cord. CSF is withdrawn from the space between the meninges and spinal cord.

CSF cultures look for bacteria, viruses, yeast, and fungi that could infect the central nervous system. CSF analysis can also be done for other reasons, such as suspected hydrocephalus and autoimmune disorders. CSF analysis looks at the appearance and color of the CSF, presence of bacteria, white blood cells, red blood cells, cancerous cells, chloride, glucose, **glutamine** (GLOO-*tuh*-meen), protein, lactate dehydrogenase, **cryptococcal** (krip-*tuh*-KOK-*uhl*) **antigen** (a common cause of meningitis), and **oligoclonal** (awl-ig-oh-KLOH-*nuhl*) bands, which indicate the presence of antibodies. Opening pressure is also measured when the meningeal covering of the spinal cord is first punctured to extract the CSF sample.

Sputum (SPYOO-*tuhm*) **cultures** are grown from sputum, which is a secretion produced by the lungs and bronchi. Sputum cultures look for causes of respiratory infections. Sputum cultures look for bacteria, particularly **acid-fast bacilli** (*buh*-SIL-eye), or AFB. The presence of AFB usually indicates the presence of tuberculosis.

Synovial (si-NOH-vee-*uhl*) **fluid** lubricates the joints. It is analyzed if the joints are swollen, red, painful, or inflamed. Synovial cultures look for bacteria and fungi. AFB smears and cultures are sometimes done because tuberculosis can grow in joints. Synovial fluid analysis looks at the color; **viscosity** (vi-SKOS-i-tee), which is how easily the liquid flows; total counts of white blood cells and red blood cells; white blood cell differential; crystals; glucose; protein; lactate dehydrogenase; and uric acid.

Cytology (seye-TOL-*uh*-jee) is the study of cells. **Pathology** (*puh*-THOL-*uh*-jee) is the study of disease. So **cytopathology** (seye-toh-*puh*-THOL-*uh*-jee) refers to the diagnosis of diseases by examining cells. Cell samples can be obtained from various body fluids, as well as through **tissue biopsy** (BEYE-op-see), which surgically removes a small piece of tissue for analysis in the lab. Cells can also be sampled through **exfoliation** (eks-foh-lee-EY-*shuhn*), or scraping cells off a body surface, such as during a Papanicolaou smear, or Pap smear. Cytopathology is especially important during cancer diagnosis.

Other Laboratory Tests

Several other laboratory tests can be done to assess various physiological parameters not measured in the previous tests.

Cardiac Enzymes

When the heart muscle is injured, it leaks certain enzymes into the blood. These enzymes can be measured and indicate whether damage has occurred to the heart muscle, such as during a heart attack. Cardiac enzyme tests are also called **cardiac markers.**

Damaged heart muscle releases **troponin** (*truh*-POH-*nuhn*), which can be used as an early test for a heart attack because the enzyme level can be measured early in the blood. The heart ventricles secrete **brain natriuretic** (ney-*truh-yoo*-REE-tik) **peptide**, which is used for diagnosing and monitoring heart failure.

Creatine kinase (KREE-*uh*-teen KEYE-neys) or **creatine phosphokinase** (FOS-*fuh*-KEYE-neys) is found in blood when both skeletal and cardiac muscle are damaged. It can help determine whether a heart attack has occurred within the past day. **Creatine kinase isoenzyme** (eyes-oh-EN-zeyem) is a variant of creatine kinase. The ratio of creatine kinase isoenzyme to total creatine kinase gives further information about heart muscle damage.

Lactate dehydrogenase (LAK-teyt dee-HEYE-draw-*juh*-neys) is elevated in many types of tissue damage. It is imprecise for indicating whether a heart attack has occurred.

Toxicology

Toxicology screens look for legal and illegal substances in the blood or urine. They can help determine the type of treatment needed in the case of an overdose or acute intoxication. Toxicology screens often look for the following substances:

> **amphetamines** (am-FET-*uh*-meenz)
>
> **barbiturates** (bahr-BICH-er-its)
>
> **benzodiazepines** (ben-zoh-deye-AZ-*uh*-peenz)
>
> **codeine** (KOH-deen)
>
> **ethanol** (ETH-*uh*-nawl), or alcohol
>
> **heroin** (HER-oh-in)
>
> **hydromorphone** (heye-droh-MOR-fohn)
>
> **methadone** (METH-*uh*-dohn)
>
> **morphine** (MAWR-feen)
>
> **phencyclidine** (fen-SIK-li-deen), or PCP
>
> **propoxyphene** (proh-POK-*suh*-feen)
>
> **tetrahydrocannabinol** (te-*truh*-heye-*druh*-*kuh*-NAB-*uh*-nawl), the substance found in marijuana

Serology

Serology (si-ROL-*uh*-jee) refers to the study of blood serum in general and is often used to refer to the analysis of antibodies in blood serum. Serology is used to aid diagnosis of autoimmune disorders.

Various **autoantibodies** (aw-toh-AN-ti-bod-eez) are associated with autoimmune diseases. For example, **rheumatoid** (ROO-*muh*-toid) **factor**, or RF, is commonly found in patients with rheumatoid arthritis. Likewise, **antinuclear** (an-tee-NOO-klee-er) **antibodies** are often found in people with systemic lupus erythematosus, but these antibodies can be found in people with other types of autoimmune diseases.

Tumor markers are usually antigens from tumor cells that can be used to screen, diagnose, and monitor different types of cancer. For example, CA-125 (cancer antigen 125) can indicate ovarian cancer, but can also indicate other female reproductive cancers, as well as lung and breast cancer.

Immunohematology (im-yoo-noh-hee-*muh*-TOL-*uh*-jee) deals with antibody-antigen reactions in the blood. An important function of immunohematology is blood typing. Blood is typed by whether it is A, B, AB, or O and negative or positive status. Blood typing is necessary for matching a person's tissue to a donor's tissue in preparation for blood transfusions or organ transplantation. There are many other types of blood groups, some of which are used in tissue typing for organ transplantation.

Cytogenetics and DNA Analysis

Cytogenetics (seye-toh-*juh*-NET-iks) is the study of chromosomes, which uses **karyotyping** (KAIR-ee-*uh*-teyep-ing) to look at the number and appearance of chromosomes within cells. Karyotyping uses band patterns on specific chromosomes to identify chromosomal disorders, such as Down syndrome, or trisomy 21. DNA analysis can be done to identify mutations that are known to occur with certain diseases. DNA **polymerase** (POL-*uh*-*muh*-reys) **chain reaction**, or PCR, is a test used in DNA analysis.

Genetic tests can be done on DNA, protein, and **metabolites** (*muh*-TAB-*uh*-leyets). Samples for genetic testing can be obtained from blood; cheek cells obtained from swabbing the inside of the cheek; **amniocentesis** (am-nee-oh-sen-TEE-sis), which samples the amniotic fluid inside the placenta during pregnancy; and **chorionic villus** (KAWR-ee-on-ik VIL-*uhs*) sampling, which samples part of the placenta during pregnancy.

Chromosomal karyotypes are used to look at the number and appearance of chromosomes. In this figure, the karyotype shows that there is an extra chromosome in one of the chromosomal pairs.

© Dorling Kindersley

The Least You Need to Know

- Urinalysis is a screening test that can reveal urinary tract infections and other disease states in the body.
- Clinical biochemistry and liver function tests measure many substances in the blood that can assess disease states, especially concerning the liver and kidneys.
- Body fluids can be analyzed for chemical abnormalities and cultured for microorganisms.
- Serology is used to diagnose autoimmune disorders and cancer; immunohematology is used to match blood and tissues for transfusions and transplants.
- Cytogenetics and DNA analysis help diagnose genetic conditions.

Diagnostic Tests and Imaging

In This Chapter

- X-rays, fluoroscopy, and mammograms
- Sonograms and echocardiograms
- CT scans and MRIs
- Scintigraphy, SPECT scans, and PET scans
- Electroencephalograms and electrocardiograms

Medical imaging techniques are generally considered **noninvasive** (nawn-in-VEY-siv), because they do not cut through the skin. Some medical imaging modalities use low-dose radiation capable of penetrating the skin barrier without making an incision. Radiation is absorbed to varying degrees in different tissues, which explains how some types of medical images are recorded. Radiography, computed tomography (CT) scans, and nuclear medicine all use radiation to create an image of internal organs and structures.

Other types of medical imaging use nonradioactive means to record images of internal structures. Ultrasound uses sound waves, and electroencephalograms (EEGs) and electrocardiograms (ECGs) measure electrical impulses. Advances in medical imaging grew out of discoveries in physics, so medical terms related to medical imaging share many terms with physics.

Radiography

Radiography (rey-dee-OG-*ruh*-fee) is the use of radioactive **x-rays**, which are a form of electromagnetic radiation, to take one-dimensional images of the inside of the body. A **radiograph** (REY-dee-oh-graf) is the image produced by this process. Different types of techniques are used in radiography.

WORD ORIGINS

German physicist Wilhelm Röntgen is credited with the discovery of x-rays, for which he won the Nobel Prize in 1901. X-ray radiograms were originally called Röntgenograms. In 1895, Röntgen published the first scientific paper about an unknown type of radiation, which he preliminarily called x-rays. For many years this type of radiation was called Röntgen rays, though the term *x-ray* became more popular over the years. The medical applications of x-rays were first realized when Röntgen used them to photograph the bones in his wife's hand.

Plain-Film Radiology

Plain-film radiographs are commonly known as x-rays. Calcium in bones absorbs more radiation; soft tissues absorb less. For this reason, bones show up more clearly on x-rays than other types of tissues do. Bones look white on an x-ray while soft tissues look gray. Because the air in the lungs does not absorb much radiation, the lungs usually look black, unless a disease process is occurring. X-rays are often the preferred method for imaging problems with bones, such as fractures. Because x-rays are relatively inexpensive, can be done quickly, and use only a small amount of radiation, they also are used as initial screening tests for problems with lungs and the digestive tract.

Density refers to the amount of darkening of the x-ray image and is an indication of the quality of the image. **Contrast** refers to how much gray is on the x-ray. Contrast describes how clearly different structures can be seen and is also an indication of the quality of the image. **Radiodensity** (REY-dee-oh-DEN-si-tee) refers to the inability of x-rays to pass through a structure. Radiodensities show up white on x-rays. **Radiolucency** (REY-dee-oh-LOO-*suhn*-see) refers to the ability of x-rays to pass through a structure, which shows up black on an x-ray. A **shadow** refers to an area of the x-ray that appears gray or white. A shadow can be a normal finding, as in the cardiac shadow, or **silhouette**, that shows up in the middle of an x-ray of a healthy chest. Other shadows can be abnormal, as in abnormalities on a chest x-ray that can indicate pneumonia.

The term **view** refers to how an x-ray is taken. Views show different parts of the body. The following terms apply to x-ray views:

- In the **anteroposterior** (an-TEYR-oh-po-STEER-ee-er) view, the x-ray source enters the anterior (front) of the body and exits the posterior (back).

- In the **posteroanterior** (poh-STEYR-oh-an-TEER-ee-er) view, the x-ray enters the posterior (back) and exits the anterior (front).

- In the **lateral** (LAT-er-*uhl*) view, the x-ray enters perpendicular to the mid-sagittal plane (the vertical midline plane), in other words, the side view.

- In the **oblique** (oh-BLEEK) view, the x-ray enters perpendicular to any of the body's planes.

- **Flexion** (FLEK-*shuhn*) is the view taken with a flexed joint.

- **Extension** (ik-STEN-*shuhn*) is the view taken with an extended joint.

- **Prone** (PROHN) is the view taken when the patient lies frontside down.

- **Supine** (soo-PEYEN) is the view taken when patient lies backside down.

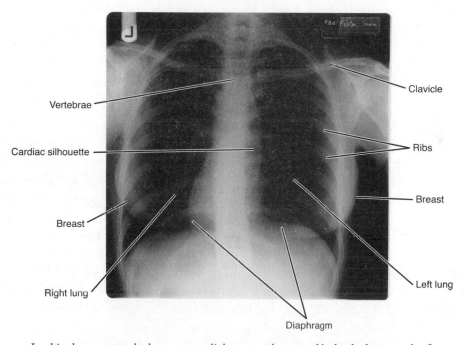

In this chest x-ray, the lungs are radiolucent and appear black; the bones and soft tissues are radiodense and their appearance ranges from gray to white.

Andy Crawford © Dorling Kindersley

Contrast X-Rays

Contrast x-rays use **radiocontrast** (REY-dee-oh-CON-trast) agents to create an image of hollow or fluid-filled structures of the body, such as the blood vessels and the digestive and urinary tracts. Radiocontrast agents are usually injected or ingested (swallowed). They light up when x-rayed. Radiocontrast agents are used in many types of medical imaging studies, including computed tomography (CT), magnetic resonance imaging (MRI), and nuclear imaging (see the section "Computed Tomography Scanning and Magnetic Resonance Imaging" in this chapter). Common contrast agents used in radiography include **iodine** (EYE-*uh*-deyen) and **barium sulfate** (BAIR-ee-*uhm* SULF-eyt).

Fluoroscopy

Fluoroscopy (flaw-ROS-*kuh*-pee) uses x-rays and contrast agents, also called contrast medium, to take images of moving body parts in real time. A **fluoroscope** (FLAWR-*uh*-skohp) is a machine that includes a radiation source and a screen to record the image. Fluoroscopes are often connected to video cameras, which can show real-time images of the movement of internal organs. Fluoroscopy is also used for medical tests such as **angiography** (an-jee-OG-*ruh*-fee), which shows blood flow inside vessels, and **pyelography** (peye-*uh*-LOG-*ruh*-fee), which looks at fluid movement in the urinary tract. Fluoroscopy is especially useful for imaging the motions of the digestive tract, such as swallowing or peristalsis of the intestine.

An **upper GI and small bowel series** shows how well contrast fluid moves through the digestive tract. This type of study can show **strictures** (STRIK-cherz), or areas of narrowing, and **obstructions** (*uhb*-STRUHK-shunz), or areas of blockage. For an upper GI series, the patient swallows a contrast medium, such as **barium sulfate** (SUHL-feyt), to introduce it into the digestive system. Imaging the colon for a lower GI series requires introducing the contrast into the colon using an **enema** (EN-*uh*-muh), which is a process by which liquid material is introduced into the digestive tract via the anus. **Positive contrast studies** generally use barium sulfate; **negative contrast studies** use air to visualize different problems in the digestive tract. **Double-contrast studies** first administer barium contrast, followed by air. This kind of study gives a better image of the intestinal lining than a **single-contrast study**.

Mammography

Mammography (ma-MOG-*ruh*-fee) uses x-rays to diagnose and screen for cancer and conditions of the breast. Normally, lower-energy x-rays are used in mammography than are used to image bones. **Mammograms** (MAM-*uh*-gramz) can provide early detection of cancer because they are able to show microcalcifications and other abnormalities associated with breast masses.

Dual-Energy X-Ray Absorptiometry

DEXA stands for **dual-energy x-ray absorptiometry** (ab-ZAWRP-tee-AWM-*uh*-tree). DEXA uses two types of x-ray beams, each containing different levels of energy, to create images of bone mineral density. The primary use of DEXA scans is to evaluate and monitor **osteoporosis** (os-tee-oh-*puh*-ROH-sis), or the weakening of bones due to age or disease.

Ultrasound and Echocardiography

Ultrasound (UHL-*truh*-sound) uses high-frequency sound waves to visualize soft-tissue structures, like the ovaries. The image produced by ultrasound is called a **sonogram** (SON-*uh*-gram, SOH-*nuh*-gram). A disadvantage of ultrasound is that it produces an image that is less distinct than images obtained with CT or MRI and relies heavily on the skill of the practitioner. However, ultrasound is inexpensive, is quick, is noninvasive, does not use radiation, can be done at the bedside, and can be used to show real-time images (such as a beating heart), all of which makes it a popular medical/screening test.

Common uses of ultrasound include the following:

- **Prenatal** (pree-NEYT-l) **imaging** helps detect fetal **anomalies** (*uh*-NOM-*uh*-leez), or abnormalities, and track the progress of the pregnancy.
- In the emergency room, ultrasound is used to diagnose internal bleeding and abdominal emergencies.
- **Abdominal ultrasound** is used to diagnose conditions of the kidneys, liver, gallbladder, spleen, bile ducts, and inferior vena cava.
- **Pelvic ultrasound** is used to image the pelvic organs, especially the male prostate, epididymis, bladder, and testicles.
- **Transvaginal** (TRANZ-VAJ-*uh*-nl) **ultrasound** is used to image the ovaries, endometrium, and bladder in women.
- **Doppler** (DOP-ler) **ultrasound** measures the velocity of blood flow. It is used to diagnose blood clots, vascular stenosis, and other blood vessel abnormalities.

Echocardiography (ek-oh-kahr-dee-AWG-*ruf*-ee) is a special kind of ultrasound that is used to create images of the heart. It is also called **cardiac echo** (EK-oh). Cardiac echo gives information about chamber size, which is the dimensions of the inside of the ventricles and atria; cardiac muscle damage; abnormalities in heart valve functioning; and measurements of heart function. Cardiac echo can also be used to assess **vegetations** (vej-i-TEY-*shuhnz*), such as bacterial growths, on heart valves or blood clots in the atria.

There are different types of cardiac echoes. **Transthoracic** (tranz-thaw-RAS-ik) **echocardiogram (TTE)** is performed through the chest wall to give a quick assessment of the heart. **Transesophageal** (tranz-ih-sof-*uh*-JEE-*uhl*) **echocardiogram (TEE)** is performed by introducing a probe into the esophagus. Images of the heart are taken through the esophagus wall. This procedure provides more accurate images than a TTE. **Stress echocardiography** or **cardiac stress test** assesses cardiac function in response to stress placed on the heart by exercise or taking a medication, in which case it's called a **nuclear** (NOO-clee-*uhr*) **stress test** (see the "Scintigraphy" section in this chapter).

Computed Tomography Scanning and Magnetic Resonance Imaging

Differentiating CT scans from MRI scans can sometimes be confusing. Both create more accurate, two-dimensional cross-sectional **tomograms** (TOH-*muh*-gramz), or slices of internal organs, than plain-film x-rays. CT and MRI scans can even be reconstructed to produce three-dimensional images. But CT and MRI have different advantages and risks associated with them.

Computed tomography (*tuh*-MAW-*gruh*-fee) **scanning**, or CT scanning, was once called computed axial tomography scanning, or CAT scanning. CT uses x-rays to create images of body cross sections. CT scans provide much greater resolution than plain-film x-rays do and are especially useful in emergency situations, such as the diagnosis of strokes. CT scans are capable of showing fluid quite well, and for this reason are useful in the diagnosis of hemorrhagic stroke. CT is especially good for imaging bone, calcifications, and structures like blood vessels and solid tumors in the bowel. For this reason, CT is often used for imaging thoracic and abdominal organs and fractured spinal vertebrae.

CT scans are quicker and less expensive than MRI scans but use ionizing radiation, which can damage DNA and cause a small increased risk for cancer. Also, CT scans usually involve administration of an intravenous contrast agent. CT contrast agents can be **nephrotoxic** (nef-roh-TOX-ik), or injurious to the kidney, and carry the risk of **contrast-induced nephropathy** (*nuh*-FROP-*uh*-thee), or kidney disease, especially among people who already have kidney impairment.

DID YOU KNOW?

Incidentaloma (IN-si-dent-*uh*-LOH-*muh*) is the term sometimes applied to a tumor that is incidentally found while doing medical imaging for another reason. Incidentalomas generally do not cause any symptoms and do not give any cause for suspicion about their presence. They are most often found in the adrenal glands. The use of whole-body CT scanning may increase the detection of symptomless and usually harmless incidentalomas. The discovery of such structures can lead to costly and anxiety-provoking medical tests in order to prove that the tumors are not disease causing.

Magnetic resonance (mag-NET-ik REZ-*uh-nuhns*) **imaging**, or MRI, is based on the concept of nuclear magnetic resonance. MRI uses magnetic fields to align the nuclei within the body's cells, which in turn create magnetic fields that are recorded by a scanner. MRIs are especially good for looking at soft tissues, especially the brain, spinal cord, muscles, tendons, ligaments, and many types of tumors.

One advantage of MRI is that it does not use radiation. In addition, the intravenous contrast agents commonly used in MRIs, such as **gadolinium** (gad-l-IN-ee-*uhm*), are not as nephrotoxic as CT contrast agents. However, MRI contrast agents can still cause problems for people with severe renal impairment, such as kidney failure.

Because of the use of a strong magnetic field, MRI is also **contraindicated** (kon-*truh*-IN-di-keyt-ed), or should not be used, in people who have metal in their bodies. Examples include people with cochlear implants, insulin pumps, cardiac pacemakers, metal plates or bolts, or other types of metal like shrapnel or a bullet. MRIs also require patients to sit still in a cramped space, where many people may feel claustrophobic.

Different types of MRIs include the following:

- **T_1-weighted MRI:** water looks dark, fat looks bright; good for differentiating fat from water and gray and white matter in the brain
- **T_2-weighted MRI:** fat looks darker, water looks brighter; good for showing edema

- **Diffusion** (dih-FYOO-*zhuhn*) **MRI:** measures the diffusion, or spread, of water throughout tissues; good for diagnosing ischemic stroke and multiple sclerosis
- **Functional MRI:** looks at changes in neural activity in the brain that cause an increased demand for oxygen; records signals from oxygenated and deoxygenated hemoglobin in red blood cells

Nuclear Imaging

Nuclear imaging uses **radioactive tracers** to produce images of various internal organs. **Gamma** (GAM-*uh*) **cameras** detect the radiation emitted by the tracers from inside the body and form an image of it. **Radionuclides** (rey-dee-oh-NOO-kleyeds) in the tracers are taken up more readily by some organs than others and can even bind to certain cell surface receptors. This allows nuclear imaging to identify certain types of disease processes earlier than other types of medical imaging.

In general, nuclear imaging shows physiological functions, such as brain glucose metabolism, rather than anatomical structures. Nuclear medicine scans tend to be organ-specific rather than region-specific like CTs and MRIs. A **hot spot** is an area of increased radionuclide uptake, which often corresponds to metabolically more active tissues. A **cold spot** is an area where certain disease processes prevent uptake of the tracer. Types of nuclear imaging include scintigraphy, single-photon emission computed tomography, and positron-emission tomography.

Scintigraphy

Scintigraphy (sin-TIG-*ruh*-fee) detects radionuclide probes to create two-dimensional images. Common uses of scintigraphy include **cholescintigraphy** (KOH-lee-sin-TIG-*ruh*-fee) or **hepatobiliary iminodiacetic** (*huh*-PAT-oh-BIL-ee-eyr-ee im-in-oh-DEYE-*uh*-SEE-tik) **acid scan**, or HIDA scan. This scan images the bile duct system and is useful in diagnosing biliary and gallbladder disease.

Other uses include the **ventilation-perfusion** (ven-tl-EY-*shuhn* per-FYOO-*zhuhn*) **scan,** which assesses breathing and circulation of blood in the lungs. The **whole-body bone scan** helps in diagnosing metabolic abnormalities of the bone, such as those that occur when cancer starts in the bone or metastases to it.

The **cardiac perfusion scan** uses radioactive **thallium** (THAL-ee-*uhm*) to evaluate coronary artery disease and provide a prognosis about cardiac function during a nuclear stress test. **Sestamibi** (sest-*uh*-MIB-ee) **parathyroid scan** uses a radioactive compound called sestamibi to diagnose parathyroid abnormalities, such as adenomas. **Radioactive iodine** (EYE-*uh*-deyen) **thyroid uptake test** uses radioactive iodine to diagnose diseases of the thyroid.

Single-Photon Emission Computed Tomography

SPECT stands for **single-photon emission** (FOH-ton ih-MISH-*uhn*) **computed tomography** (*tuh*-MAW-*gruh*-fee). SPECT uses gamma rays emitted from contrast administered to the patient to create three-dimensional images, usually of cross sections of the body. SPECT images are limited because they generally provide lower resolution images than positron-emission tomography (PET) scans do. SPECT scans are used to assess myocardial perfusion, which is another type of stress test to assess cardiac ischemia. SPECT scans also are used to assess functional brain imaging, which assesses cerebral blood flow and brain metabolism, and has been used to diagnose Alzheimer disease and epilepsy.

Positron-Emission Tomography

PET stands for **positron-emission tomography** (POZ-i-tron ih-MISH-*uhn tuh*-MAW-*gruh*-fee). PET uses positrons, or subatomic particles, and injected radioactive dye to image metabolically active tissues, such as cancer. PET is especially useful in showing cerebral blood flow and glucose metabolism in the brain. PET scans are limited because they can be used to show only short, time-limited tasks. They are most often used to assess cancer metastasis. PET scans are also useful in showing amyloid plaques typical in Alzheimer disease and showing seizure foci in epilepsy. PET scans can also show brain receptors for substances such as serotonin and dopamine in people with schizophrenia and drug addiction.

Other Diagnostic Tests

Medical professionals also make diagnoses and monitor medical conditions using electroencephalography and electrocardiography. These tests both rely on measuring electrical activity in the body.

Electroencephalography

EEG stands for **electroencephalogram** (ih-lek-troh-en-SEF-*uh*-luh-gram). EEGs use **electrodes** (ih-LEK-trohds), which are devices capable of conducting electricity, applied to the scalp to measure brain wave and electrical activity. EEGs are used often in the diagnosis of epilepsy, sleep disorders, coma, and the evaluation of brain death.

DID YOU KNOW?

Brain death happens when all brain activity, including involuntary activity needed for vital functions, ceases. Brain death is often used legally as confirmation of death, especially when concerning issues such as artificial life support and organ donation. The rigorous medical and legal stipulations regarding the definition of brain death include lack of specific findings on a series of physical exams done by separate physicians over a specified period of time. The person also should have a normal temperature and be free of drugs or medication that can suppress brain wave activity. Lack of brain wave activity, or flat lines, on an EEG is considered confirmation of brain death but is not required to certify death in the United States.

Electrocardiography

ECG stands for **electrocardiogram** (ih-lek-troh-KAHR-dee-*uh*-gram). ECGs use electrodes applied to the skin on the outside of the chest to measure the electrical activity of the heart. ECGs are inexpensive, quick tests that can measure the heart rate. They can also be used to estimate abnormalities such as enlarged heart chambers and damage to the heart muscle. They can even indicate certain lung problems, such as pulmonary embolism.

The term **lead** (LEED) is commonly used to refer to the electrical cable that connects the chest electrode to the ECG recording machine. **Precordial** (pree-KORD-ee-*uhl*) leads are placed at certain points on the chest right that correspond to certain areas of the heart. **Limb** leads are placed on the right and left wrists and the right and left ankles. An ECG **tracing** is a graph showing the electrical activity during a cardiac cycle. Specific waves are associated with different electrical events during the cardiac cycle. Certain abnormal waves are considered **pathognomonic** (*path*-uh-*nuh*-MON-ik), or characteristic, for specific heart abnormalities. (See Chapter 12 for an explanation of ECG waves.)

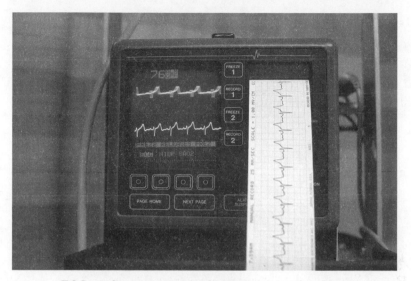

ECG machines measure the electrical activity of the heart.
Jim Ziv © Dorling Kindersley

The Least You Need to Know

- Radiography uses x-rays to take one-dimensional images of the inside of the body.
- Ultrasound uses high-frequency sound waves to image soft-tissue structures.
- Computed tomography scans use x-rays to create cross-sectional images of internal organs.
- Magnetic resonance imaging uses strong magnetic fields that align the nuclei within the body's cells to create an image of internal structures in the body.
- Nuclear imaging like scintigraphy, single-photon emission computed tomography, and positron-emission tomography uses radioactive tracers to produce images of the physiological functioning of various organs.
- Electroencephalography uses electrodes to record electrical activity in the brain; electrocardiography uses electrodes to record electrical activity in the heart.

Diagnostic Procedures and Therapeutic Surgery

Chapter 25

In This Chapter

- Diagnostic and therapeutic noninvasive procedures
- Endoscopy, laparoscopy, and other minimally invasive procedures
- Surgical radiology
- Surgery using computers and robots
- Hemodialysis, plasmapheresis, and other extracorporeal procedures

Modern medicine draws on many procedures beyond traditional surgery to diagnose and heal disease. Noninvasive techniques and minimally invasive techniques have many advantages, including quicker healing times and fewer days spent in the hospital. For these reasons, these types of techniques have become popular. As the number of these techniques expands, so does the number of medical terms used to describe them.

Interventional radiology is a separate branch of medicine that uses many types of minimally invasive techniques, each of which has a specific name. Technological advances have introduced computers and robots into the treatment of human disease. These types of procedures also have specific medical terms associated with them. Extracorporeal techniques are also used, in which parts of the body, like the blood, are removed for treatment, and then returned to the body.

Noninvasive Procedures

Noninvasive (non-in-VEY-siv) **procedures** refer to diagnostic and therapeutic procedures that do not break the skin or do not enter the body beyond bodily **orifices** (AWR-*uh*-fis-ez), or openings, such as the nose or ear.

Noninvasive Diagnostic Techniques

Examples of noninvasive diagnostic procedures include the following:

- During **auscultation** (aw-*skuhl*-TEY-*shuhn*), an examiner uses a **stethoscope** (STETH-*uh*-skohp), an instrument that transmits sound to the ears, to listen to heart, lung, bowel, and other body sounds.

- Blood pressure measurement involves using a **sphygmomanometer** (sfig-moh-*muh*-NOM-i-ter), or blood pressure cuff and measurement device.

- Body volume measurement involves using a **plethysmograph** (*pluh*-THIZ-*muh*-graf), or device that can measure changes in body volumes.

- Medical imaging techniques use various means to record images of internal organs and structures. Examples include x-rays, CT, ultrasound, cardiac echo, MRI, PET, and SPECT (see Chapter 24).

- **Pulse oximetry** (ok-SIM-i-tree) measures the amount of oxygen in the blood by placing a device on the fingertip or ear lobe.

- **Capnigraphy** (cap-NI-*gruh*-fee) measures carbon dioxide concentration in exhaled air.

- **Holter** (HAWL-ter) **monitoring** involves wearing a portable device on the chest that continuously monitors electrical activity, mainly of the heart, over a period of time.

Other types of noninvasive diagnostic techniques measure chemical, electrical, and other signals generated by bodily processes. Chapter 24 described two such measurements: ECGs and EEGs. Another example is **electromyography** (ih-lek-troh-mayh-AW-*gruh*-fee), or EMG, which measures electrical signals produced by skeletal muscle contraction. **Transcranial** (tranz-KREY-nee-*uhl*) **magnetic stimulation,** or TMS, is a related noninvasive diagnostic technique. It uses a magnet to induce small electrical currents in the brain. This procedure is used to study regions of the brain. Possible therapeutic applications lie in treating psychiatric disorders and neurological disorders such as Parkinson disease.

Noninvasive Therapeutic Techniques

Noninvasive techniques can also be used for therapeutic means. For example, **radiation** (rey-dee-EY-*shuhn*) **therapy** uses radiation waves to treat disease, especially cancer. **Photodynamic** (foh-toh-deye-NAM-ik) **therapy** uses selectively applied compounds that become toxic to certain cells when exposed to light. This technique is used to treat acne.

Lithotripsy (LITH-uh-*trip*-see) uses sound waves to break up abnormal collections of material, especially renal **calculi** (KAL-kyuh-leye). **Therapeutic ultrasound** (UHL-*truh*-sound) uses high-frequency sound waves for many applications, including treating ligament tears, joint inflammation, and cancer.

Continuous positive airway pressure, or CPAP (SEE-pap) is the use of a constant airflow to keep the airway open. This technique is often used to treat people with sleep apnea. **Bilevel positive airway pressure**, or BiPAP (BAHY-pap) uses two different preset pressures (inspiratory and expiratory). This technique is used for people with chronic obstructive pulmonary disease or respiratory failure.

Defibrillation (dee-FIB-*ruh*-ley-*shuhn*) uses electrical energy to block cardiac fibrillation and restore normal sinus rhythm. **Transcutaneous** (trans-kyoo-TEY-nee-*uhs*) **electrical nerve stimulation** or TENS (TENZ) uses an electrical current applied to the outside of the skin to stimulate nerves and to treat pain. **Electroconvulsive** (ih-LEK-troh-*kuhn*-VUHL-siv) **therapy**, or **electroshock** (ih-LEK-*truh*-shok), is the use of electrical currents to cause seizures in psychiatric patients under general anesthesia. This technique is used most often for treatment-resistant depression.

Hyperbaric (heye-per-BAR-ik) **oxygen therapy** uses a special room called a **pressure chamber** in which the air pressure is increased to deliver more oxygen to the lungs and other tissues. This treatment is used to treat air or gas embolisms found in decompression sickness; **osteomyelitis** (os-tee-oh-meye-*uh*-LEYE-tis), or bone infections; and nonhealing wounds such as **gangrene** (gang-GREEN) and diabetic ulcers. **Negative pressure wound therapy** uses a sealed wound compartment and special dressing connected to a vacuum pump to speed healing of second-degree and third-degree burns.

DID YOU KNOW?

While some medical treatments stand the test of time, others fall out of favor, either because they provide no benefit to the patient or because they are found to be downright dangerous. One such treatment is **insulin** (IN-*suh*-lin) **shock therapy**, which was used in the 1950s and 1960s, mainly to treat schizophrenia. Considered to be a noninvasive procedure, insulin shock therapy entailed the injection of high doses of insulin to produce seizures and coma. It fell out of favor when scientific papers showed very little treatment success, combined with such risks as brain damage and death. Insulin shock therapy has been largely replaced by neuroleptic medication (see Chapter 26).

Minimally Invasive Procedures

Minimally invasive procedures produce minimal damage to body tissues by making the smallest cuts possible or entering body cavities through natural orifices. Healing time is quicker and days spent in the hospital are fewer following minimally invasive surgery, as compared to **open surgery**, which involves breaking the skin and other tissues to enter a body cavity. Some minimally invasive procedures can even be done in a clinic on an outpatient basis.

Minimally invasive procedures use special minimal incision techniques, which are small incisions that are used to excise masses or insert small surgical instruments. **Fiberoptic** (feye-ber-OP-tik) cables, miniature video cameras, and video monitors are also used during minimally invasive procedures.

Endoscopy (en-DOS-*kuh*-pee) is an example of a minimally invasive procedure. An **endoscope** (EN-*duh*-skohp) is a device with a tube, light source, and a lens that is inserted into the body for diagnostic purposes. This procedure can also be used for treatments and certain surgeries, such as cauterizing bleeding vessels or sinus surgery. **Arthroscopic** (ahr-*thruh*-SKAW-pik) **surgery** or **arthroscopy** (ahr-THRAW-*skuh*-pee) is an endoscopic technique in which an endoscope is inserted into a joint for diagnostic and therapeutic purposes, such as anterior cruciate ligament reconstruction.

Laparoscopy (lap-*uh*-ROS-*kuh*-pee) or **keyhole** (KEE-hohl) **surgery** uses a small incision and camera assistance to insert instruments into the abdomen or pelvis. This procedure is used for diagnosis and surgical purposes, such as a cholecystectomy.

Percutaneous (pur-kyoo-TEY-nee-*uhs*) **surgery** uses a small needle to puncture the skin in order to reach internal organs and tissues. This procedure is used often in vascular procedures. In these procedures, a needle **catheter** (KATH-i-ter), or thin tube, is used to puncture blood vessels, a wire is threaded through the catheter, and other catheters are threaded over this wire.

Cryosurgery (kreye-oh-SUR-*juh*-ree) uses very cold substances, such as **liquid nitrogen** (NEYE-*truh-juhn*), to freeze abnormal tissues. This procedure is used for skin conditions such as warts and moles, for cervical disorders, and for some cancers.

Microsurgery (MEYE-kroh-sur-*juh*-ree) refers to the use of a microscope to assist surgical operations. This type of procedure is used when **anastomoses** (*uh*-nas-*tuh*-MOH-seez), or connections, need to be created between tiny blood vessels and nerves. For this reason, microsurgery is used often in plastic and reconstructive surgery and in transplantation and **replantation** (ree-PLANT-ey-*shuhn*), or reattachment, of body parts.

DID YOU KNOW?

Mohs (MOHZ) **micrographic surgery** is a minimally invasive technique used to treat certain types of skin cancer. It was originally called **chemosurgery** (kee-moh-SUR-*juh*-ree) because it used a paste that was applied to the skin cancer and the area surrounding it the night before surgery, which resulted in anesthesia. Today local anesthetic is used instead, and the procedure is performed in one day. In Mohs surgery, the surgeon removes small parts of the cancer, which is examined during the procedure by a pathologist to identify cancerous cells and guide tissue removal. Mohs surgery is especially useful for skin cancers on the face because it produces minimal disfigurement.

Stereotactic (ster-ee-*uh*-TAK-tik) **surgery** uses a special device to locate small targets within the body. Medical imaging, such as CT scans and plain x-rays, guides these types of procedures. Its use is limited to brain surgery.

Laser (LEY-zer) **therapy** uses high-intensity light to precisely cut or burn tissue. This procedure is used to remove tissue growths or **cauterize** (KAW-*tuh*-reyez), which means to burn, blood vessels to stop bleeding.

Interventional Radiology

Interventional radiology, also called **surgical radiology**, treats disease using minimally invasive techniques, often by using needles and catheters to avoid large incisions. Interventional radiologists use medical imaging to guide instruments through the body in order to perform therapeutic and diagnostic procedures. They use needles and **catheters** (KATH-i-terz), or thin, flexible tubes through which other instruments are threaded. Interventional radiologists use many different types of catheters whose names describe their functions. Examples include diagnostic **angiographic** (an-jee-*uh*-GRAF-ik) **catheters**, **microcatheters**, **drainage catheters**, **balloon catheters**, and **central venous** (VEE-*nuhs*) **catheters**. Interventional radiology is used to diagnose and treat a wide range of conditions in various fields of medicine, including oncology, neurology, gastroenterology, nephrology, and gynecology.

Examples of the types of abnormalities treated by interventional radiology include stenosis, aneurisms, and dissections. Interventional radiology also can be used to maintain and repair a **dialysis fistula** or **arteriovenous** (ahr-TEER-ee-oh-VEE-*nuhs*) **graft** (shortened to AV graft). An AV graft is a surgically created connection between an artery and a vein that is placed in an extremity, usually the arm, to provide venous access during kidney dialysis. AV grafts sometimes need declotting, which can be done using angioplasty and thrombolysis (see following table).

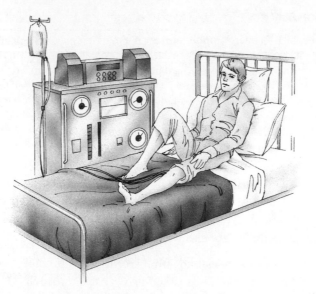

Hemodialysis involves removal of blood so that the toxins can be filtered by an external machine that takes the place of diseased kidneys.
© Dorling Kindersley

Interventional radiologists employ a variety of techniques that deal with blood vessels. **Angiography** (an-jee-OG-ruh-fee) is a procedure that takes images of blood vessels. **Angioplasty** (AN-jee-uh-plas-tee) is the repair of blocked blood vessels and often uses a "balloon" that inflates inside the vessel. During **cardiac catheterization** (KATH-i-tuh-ruh-ZEY-shuhn), a catheter is threaded into a peripheral blood vessel until it reaches the heart. This procedure is done to assess cardiac functioning and look at the coronary arteries. Coronary stenosis can be treated with stent placement, which is insertion of a tube that props open the blocked blood vessel.

Rather than reopening a blocked vessel, sometimes the treatment calls for the opposite. This technique is called **embolization** (em-buh-luh-ZEY-shuhn), and it blocks blood vessels in order to stop bleeding or cut off blood supply to tissue growths and tumors. **Radioembolization** (REY-dee-oh-em-buh-luh-ZEY-shuhn) delivers radiation to a tumor. In **transarterial chemoembolization** (Tranz-ahr-TEER-ee-uhl KEEM-oh-em-buh-luh-ZEY-shuhn), anticancer drugs are injected to block blood supply to tumors. In **uterine fibroid embolization** (YOO-ter-in FEYE-broid em-buh-luh-ZEY-shuhn), or UFE, substances are injected into uterine arteries to cut off blood supply to fibroids.

Interventional Radiology Procedures

Procedure	Pronunciation	Importance
cholangiography	*kuh*-lan-jee-OG-*ruh*-fee	images biliary abnormalities
cholecystostomy	koh-*luh*-si-STOS-*tuh*-mee	a hole is created in the gallbladder and a tube is placed to remove infected bile in someone with cholecystitis who is too sick to undergo surgery
radiologically inserted gastrostomy	ga-STROS-*tuh*-mee	placement of a feeding tube through the skin and directly into the stomach
endovascular aneurism repair	EN-doh-VAS-*kyuh*-ler AN-*yuh*-riz-*uhm*	angioplasty, stenting, and other surgical techniques are used to repair aneurisms and prevent their growth, often used for abdominal and thoracic aneurism repair
catheter-directed thrombolysis	throm-BOL-*uh*-sis	dissolves clots with pharmaceuticals and mechanical methods; used for pulmonary emboli and intra-arterial thrombolysis in ischemic stroke
thrombectomy	throm-BEK-*tuh*-mee	lyses intra-arterial clots; used to treat limb ischemia due to a blood clot
atherectomy	ath-*uh*-REK-*tuh*-mee	removal of atherosclerosis from large blood vessels; most often used in vessels of the lower limbs to relieve symptoms of peripheral arterial disease
dialysis catheter placement	deye-AL-*uh*-sis	establishes dialysis access for people with renal failure
inferior vena cava filter placement		places a device in the inferior vena cava to prevent propagation of a deep vein thrombosis, or blood clot
nephrostomy tube placement	*nuf*-RAW-*stuh*-mee	tubes are placed in nondraining kidneys to relieve urinary obstruction
percutaneous drain placement	pur-kyoo-TEY-nee-*uhs*	drains fluid from body compartments; for example, pleural drains allow pus and blood to flow out of the chest cavity

continues

Interventional Radiology Procedures   (continued)

Procedure	Pronunciation	Importance
kyphoplasty	KEYE-*fuh*-PLAS-tee	percutaneous injection of substances to repair vertebral compression fractures or collapsed vertebrae
vertebroplasty	ver-TEE-*bruh*-PLAS-tee	percutaneous injection of substances to fix vertebral fractures
transjugular intrahepatic portosystemic shunt (TIPS)	tranz-JUHG-*yuh*-ler IN-*truh*-hi-PAT-ik PAWRT-oh-si-STEM-ik SHUHNT	creates bypass channels to improve blood flow in a scarred liver
endovenous laser treatment/ sclerotherapy	EN-doh-VEE-*nuhs* LEY-zur, skleer-*uh*-THER-*uh*-pee	treats varicose veins from the inside of blood vessels
cryoablation	krey-oh-a-BLEY-*shuhn*	uses extreme cold to destroy discrete, localized sections of abnormal tissues
microwave ablation	MEYE-kroh-weyv a-BLEY-*shuhn*	destroys abnormal tissue using extreme heat emitted by high-frequency electrical currents generated by microwaves; used for tumors
radiofrequency ablation (RFA)	REY-dee-oh-FREE-*kwuhn*-see a-BLEY-*shuhn*	destroys abnormal tissue using extreme heat emitted by high-frequency electrical currents; used for tumors, varicose veins, and conduction abnormalities in the heart
high-intensity focused ultrasound (HIFU)	HEYE in-TEN-si-tee FOH-*kuhsd* UHL-*truh*-sound	uses high-intensity, focused sound waves to heat and destroy abnormal tissue, such as uterine fibroids, prostate cancer, and other tumors

Computer-Assisted and Robotic Surgery

Computer-assisted surgery is also called **computer-aided surgery**, **computer-assisted intervention**, **image-guided surgery**, and **surgical navigation**. Computer-assisted surgery provides better visualization of the surgical environment than traditional surgical methods. It also improves presurgical planning and reduces surgical errors and operating time.

Computer-assisted surgery uses medical imaging to create a three-dimensional image of a patient's internal structures and organs prior to surgery. The surgeon can manipulate the computer image to see internal structures from different angles. These images are used in presurgical planning to virtually simulate the surgery before it actually occurs. Along with special computer software, the three-dimensional images can be used to preprogram surgical robots prior to the operation.

The actual computer-assisted intervention is called surgical navigation, during which the surgeon uses a special instrument connected to a computer navigation system. Computer-assisted surgery has been used in neurosurgery, brain microsurgery, oral and maxillofacial surgery, orthopedic surgery, abdominal laparoscopy, gynecological surgery, and urology.

Robotic surgery is a surgical technique in which a surgeon operates using the assistance of a robot. There are three main types of robotic surgery. In **supervisory controlled** surgery, a robot performs preprogrammed surgery. In **telesurgical** (*tel*-uh-SUR-ji-kuhl)**, remote surgery**, the surgeon operates using a **telemanipulator** (*tel-uh-muh*-NIP-*yuh*-ley-ter) that controls the movements of the robot remotely. The surgeon performs the movements while the robot does the actual operation. In **shared control surgery**, the surgeon performs the procedure with assistance from the robot.

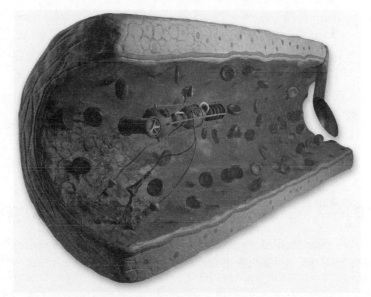

A tiny robot called a nanorobot can be used to remove an arterial plaque.
Geoff Brightling © Dorling Kindersley

Extracorporeal Therapies

Extracorporeal (ek-*struh*-kawr-PAWR-ee-*uhl*) **therapies** involve removal of part of the body, such as blood, for treatment outside the body, usually followed by returning it to the body. For example, **hemodialysis** (hee-moh-deye-AL-*uh*-sis) is removal of blood from the body so that wastes such as urea and nitrogen can be filtered out before the blood is returned to the body. This therapy is used in renal failure.

Plasmapheresis (PLAZ-*muh-fuh*-REE-*suhs*) is removal of blood plasma for treatment outside of the body, after which it is returned to the circulation. This therapy is used to remove autoantibodies in autoimmune disorders such as myasthenia gravis.

> **WORD ORIGINS**
>
> The word part *-pheresis* (*fuh*-REE-*suhs*) comes from the Greek word *apheiresis*, which means "taking away," so words that contain *-apheresis* refer to techniques that separate and remove parts from a whole. Several medical terms use this word part. For example, **plasmapheresis** (PLAZ-*muh-fuh*-REE-*suhs*) refers to the removal of blood plasma. **Plateletpheresis** (PLEYT-lit-*fuh*-REE-*suhs*) refers to the removal of platelets. **Leukapheresis** (LOO-*kuh-fuh*-REE-*suhs*) refers to the removal of white blood cells, and **erythrocytapheresis** (ih-RITH-*ruh*-seyet-*uh*-*fuh*-REE-*suhs*) refers to the removal of red blood cells.

Extracorporeal membrane oxygenation or ECMO (EK-moh) removes blood for oxygenation in a machine outside the body and takes the place of the heart and lungs when they are unable to function. This therapy is used in intensive care settings.

The Least You Need to Know

- Noninvasive procedures refer to diagnostic and therapeutic procedures that do not break the skin or enter the body beyond bodily orifices.
- Minimally invasive procedures produce minimal damage to body tissues by making the smallest cuts possible or entering body cavities through natural orifices.
- Interventional radiology treats disease using minimally invasive techniques, often by using needles and catheters to avoid large incisions.

- Computer-assisted and robotic surgery enable the creation of three-dimensional images of the internal organs, presurgical virtual simulation of the operation, and remote-controlled operations.

- Extracorporeal therapies involve removal of part of the body, such as blood, for treatment outside the body, usually followed by returning it to the body.

Pharmacology: Medications

Chapter 26

In This Chapter

- Medicines that fight infections
- Medicines that treat heart and breathing conditions
- Drugs for diabetes, hormonal conditions, and digestive problems
- Urinary and reproductive medications
- Seizure and mental health medications, painkillers, and muscle relaxants
- Drugs that fight cancer and treat overactive immune systems

Modern medicine draws on a vast pharmacopeia of drugs with which to treat human disease. These medications are divided into general categories usually based on the body system they treat. They are further divided into classes based on how they act to fight disease. Medications within classes are further divided into subclasses. Each subclass typically has several different individual types of medication, each of which usually has two different names: a generic name and a trade name.

Suffice it to say that there are thousands of terms associated with medical pharmacology. Learning the general categorization of medications will help you make sense of them. Keep in mind that this chapter is just an introduction. It presents examples of the names of some of the drugs associated with different types of medications, but by no means mentions all of them. Also, side effects are not discussed.

General Pharmacology Terms

Pharmacology (fahr-*muh*-KOL-*uh*-jee) is the study of medications and their use in treating disease. **Pharmacokinetics** (FAHRM-*uh*-koh-kin-ET-iks) refers to how the body processes the medication. **Pharmacodynamics** (FAHRM-*uh*-koh-deye-NAM-iks) refers to how the medication affects the body, such as whether the medication is successful in treating the disease and what toxic side effects the medication might have.

The term **therapeutic** (ther-*uh*-PYOO-tik) **index**, or **therapeutic window**, is used to describe the ratio of therapeutic effect to toxic side effects. A medication with a narrow therapeutic index is therapeutic only at nearly toxic doses, such as many anticancer drugs. A medication with a wide therapeutic index has a therapeutic effect far below its toxic dose.

WORD ORIGINS

Most medications become toxic in high-enough doses. The toxic dose often varies by individual. The Greeks recognized that the cure can almost be as bad as the disease. The word *toxic* originates from the Greek word *toxicon* and refers to any substance that can injure the body. The ancient Greek word for pharmacology is *pharmakon*, which can be translated as both drug and poison. Medieval physicians also recognized the toxic potential of medications. Swiss physician Paracelsus is considered the father of toxicology and is credited with the saying, *Sola dosis facit venenum* ("The dose makes the poison").

Absorption refers to how the body absorbs the medication. Routes of absorption include the skin, mucosa, eyes, and intestines. **Distribution** describes how well the medication spreads throughout the body. **Metabolism** (*muh*-TAB-*uh*-liz-*uhm*) describes how the body breaks down medication into active or toxic **metabolites** (*muh*-TAB-*uh*-leyets). Most medications are metabolized in the liver and, to a certain extent, in the kidney. **Excretion** (ik-SKREE-*shuhn*) refers to the route by which a medication and its by-products pass out of the body. Most medications are eliminated through the kidneys; others are excreted through the bile, breath, and skin.

Medications come in preparations that can be administered through different routes:

- **Transdermal** (tranz-DURM-*uhl*) refers to medications that are applied and absorbed through the skin. A common way to administer these types of medications is with skin patches and creams.
- **Ophthalmic** (off-THAWL-mik) medications are applied to the eyes, often with eye drops or ointments.
- **Otic** (otic (OH-tik, OT-ik) medications are administered into the ears, usually with ear drops.
- **Mucosal** (myoo-KOH-*suhl*) medication is administered via the mucous membranes, often with nasal and throat sprays.

- **Sublingual** (sub-LING-*gwuhl*) medications are placed under the tongue.

- **Oral** medications are taken by mouth, usually in tablet or liquid form.

- An **injection** is given via a shot.

- **Intravenous** (in-*truh*-VEEN-*uhs*-lee), or IV, medications are administered directly into the veins.

Antibiotics

Antibiotics (an-ti-beye-OT-iks) are medicines that either kill bacteria and are described as **bactericidal** (bak-TEER-ee-*uh*-SEYE-*duhl*) or inhibit their growth and are described as **bacteriostatic** (bak-TEER-ee-*uh*-STAT-ik). Antibiotics are effective only against bacteria, some fungi, and some parasites. They are not effective against viruses like the one that causes the common cold.

WORDS OF WARNING

There are fewer medications available for fighting viruses than for fighting bacteria. Viral medications include **acyclovir** (ey-SIK-*luh*-veer), which is used to treat the herpes virus. Another example is ribavirin, which is used to treat respiratory syncytial virus, a serious viral respiratory infection in children. **Highly active antiretroviral** (AN-tee-ret-roh-VAHY-*ruhl*) **therapy**, or HAART, is the AIDS cocktail composed of at least three medications that is used to decrease the level of HIV virus in the blood.

Antibiotic Classes

Antibiotics are grouped into classes on the basis of their mechanism of action, which refers to how they are able to kill or inhibit bacteria. Antibiotics have different **coverages**, which refers to the types of bacteria a given antibiotic can kill. Narrow-spectrum antibiotics target specific type of bacteria. Broad-spectrum antibiotics target a broader range of bacteria.

There are many types of antibiotic classes. One of the widest used classes are the **beta-lactams** (BEY-*tuh* LAKT-*uhms*), which take their name from the fact that they have a beta-lactam ring nucleus. Beta-lactams are bactericidal and inhibit bacterial enzymes important for cell wall synthesis.

Subclasses of beta-lactams have different bacterial coverage and include the following:

- **Penicillins** (pen-*uh*-SIL-inz): penicillin, **ampicillin** (amp-*uh*-SIL-in), **amoxicillin** (*uh*-MOKS-*uh*-SIL-in)
- **Carbacephems** (karb-*uh*-SEEF-*uhms*): **loracarbef** (lawr-*uh*-KARB-ef)
- **Clavams** (KLAV-*uhms*): **clavulanic** (klav-yoo-LAN-ik) **acid**
- **Carbapenems** (karb-*uh*-PEN-*uhms*): **imipenem** (im-ee-PEN-*uhm*)
- **Monobactams** (mawn-oh-BAKT-*uhms*): **aztreonam** (az-TREE-*uh*-nam)

Another beta-lactam subclass, **cephalosporins** (sef-uh-luh-SPOR-inz) and **cephamycins** (sef-uh-MEYE-sinz), is further broken down into five more subclasses. These subclasses are first-generation **cefazolin** (sef-uh-ZOHL-in); second-generation **cefaclor** (sef-uh-KLAWR); third-generation **cefixime** (sef-IKS-eem) and **ceftriaxone** (sef-treye-AKS-ohn); fourth-generation **cefepime** (SEF-uh-peem); and fifth-generation **ceftobiprole** (sef-*tuh*-BEYE-prohl).

Common Antibiotic Classes

Antibiotic Class	Pronunciation	What They Do	Examples
aminoglycosides	*uh*-MEE-noh-GLEYE-koh-seyeds	bactericidal; inhibit bacterial protein synthesis	neomycin (nee oh-MEYE- sin), streptomycin (strep-toh-MEYE-sin), gentamicin (gent-*uh*-MEYE-sin)
chloramphenicol	KLAWR-am-FEN-*uh*-kawl	bacteriostatic, inhibits bacterial protein synthesis	chloramphenicol (KLAWR-am-FEN-*uh*-kawl)
fluoroquinolones/ quinolones	flawr-oh-KWIN-*uh*-lohnz, KWIN-*uh*-lohnz	bactericidal; target enzymes important in bacterial DNA replication	ciprofloxacin (sip-roh-FLOKS-*uh*-sin), levofloxacin (leev-oh-FLOKS-*uh*-sin)
glycopeptides	gleye-koh-PEP-teyedz	bactericidal, inhibits cell wall synthesis; used in serious drug-resistant infections	vancomycin (van-koh-MEYE-sin)
lincosamides	Lin-KOW-*suh-meyedz*	bacteriostatic; inhibit bacterial protein synthesis	clindamycin (klin-*duh*-MEYE-sin)
lipopeptides	LIP-oh-PEPT-teyedz	bactericidal, bind to bacterial cell membranes; disrupt DNA, RNA, and protein synthesis	daptomycin (dapt-oh-MEYE-sin)

Antibiotic Class	Pronunciation	What They Do	Examples
macrolides	MAK-*ruh*-leyedz	bacteriostatic; inhibits bacterial protein synthesis	erythromycin (*uh*-RITH-roh-MEYE-sin), azithromycin (*uh*-ZITH-roh-MEYE-sin)
metronidazole	met-*ruh*-NEYEZ-*uh*-dawl,	interrupts DNA; treats parasitic infections like amebiasis, giardiasis	trade name: Flagyl (FLAJ-*uhl*)
nitrofurans	neye-troh-FYOOR-*uhnz*	bactericidal, mechanism unknown; treats uropathogens	nitrofurantoin (neye-troh-fyoor-an-TOH-in)
oxazolidinones	oks-az-*uh*-LID-een-ohnz	bacteriostatic, inhibit bacterial protein synthesis	linezolid (lin-EYZ-*uh*-lid)
polyketides	POL-ee-KEE-teyed	bacteriostatic, inhibit bacterial protein synthesis	tetracylcines (tet-*ruh*-SEYE-kleenz)
polypeptides	POL-ee-PEP-teyeds	bactericidal; disrupt bacterial cell walls	bacitracin (bas-*uh*-TREY-sin), polymyxin B (POL-ee-MIX-in BEE)
rifamycins	rif-*uh*-MEYE-sinz	bactericidal, suppress RNA synthesis	rifampin (rif-AMP-in), used to treat tuberculosis
sulfonamides	sulf-AWN-*uh*-meyedz	bacteriostatic; interfere with enzymes needed for folate synthesis; ultimately interfere with DNA synthesis	trimethoprim-sulfamethoxazole (treye-METH-*uh*-prim sulf-*uh*-meth-OX-*uh*-zawl), TMP/SMX; trade name: Bactrim (BAK-*truhm*)

STUDY TIP

One way to remember drugs that belong to the same class is to look at the beginnings or endings of their generic names. Often ones in the same class share common word beginnings and endings. This guideline does not hold true across the board for all antibiotics, but it often works. For example, drugs in the aminoglycoside class usually end with *-cin* or *-mycin* (gentamicin, neomycin). Cephalosporins usually begin with *cef-* (cefazolin, ceftriaxone, cefaclor). Carbapenems usually end in *-penem* (ertapenem). Penicillins usually end in *-cillin* (amoxicillin, ampicillin).

Antibiotic Resistance

Bacterial resistance refers to the ability of bacteria to become resistant to certain antibiotics. This can happen during antibiotic treatment when bacteria with certain genetic mutations are selected for the antibiotic itself. Some bacteria may randomly have mutations that enable them to survive in the presence of the antibiotic. They pass these mutations to subsequent generations of bacteria, producing superstrains of bacteria that are resistant to that antibiotic. This characteristic is called **intrinsic bacterial resistance** and is a heritable form of resistance. Bacteria can also become resistant through **acquired resistance**, in which they acquire spontaneous mutations during the course of antibiotic treatment. Antibiotic resistance can be passed between bacteria on plasmids, which are small, circular pieces of DNA that are separate from the bacterial chromosome.

Antibiotic resistance is spread by the overuse and misuse of antibiotics, which undermines the effectiveness of antibiotics. Infections that were once easily treatable have become resistant to several medications, making them deadly once again. An example is multidrug-resistant tuberculosis.

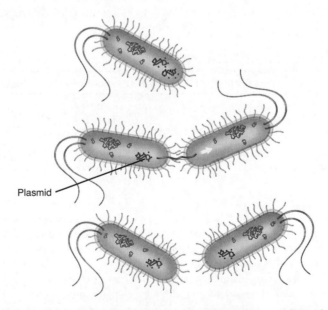

Plasmid

Some bacteria become antibiotic resistant when they acquire a plasmid that has antibiotic resistance genes on it.

© Dorling Kindersley

Cardiovascular and Respiratory Agents

Medical professionals can choose from a large inventory of medications to treat heart and respiratory conditions. This section provides the general categories of these types of agents.

> **STUDY TIP**
>
> In addition to the broader class to which most medications belong, drugs have at least two different names. The **generic name** is assigned to the chemical compound, which can be produced and manufactured by different companies. Generic names are used broadly, sometimes even across countries. **Trade name** refers to the brand name of a drug, which is assigned by different companies often for marketing purposes. The same chemical compound can have different trade names if it is produced by different companies. Trade names often vary across countries.

Antihypertensives

Antihypertensives (an-tee-heye-per-TEN-sivz) are used to decrease blood pressure.

Common Types of Antihypertensives

Type	Pronunciation	What They Do	Example
alpha-blockers	ALF-*uh* BLOK-urz	relax the muscles in the walls of small blood vessels; also improve urine flow in men with benign prostatic hypertrophy (BPH)	tamsulosin (tam-soo-LOH-sin), trade name: Flomax (FLOH-max) doxazosin (doks-AZ-*uh*-sin), trade name: Cardura (kar-DYOOR-*uh*)
angiotensin-converting enzyme inhibitors, ACE inhibitors	anj-ee-*uh*-TEN-sin	expand blood vessels so the heart doesn't need to pump so hard	enalapril (en-AL-*uh*-pril), trade name: Vaso-tec (VEYS-*uh*-tek)
angiotensin II receptor blockers	anj-ee-*uh*-TEN-sin	block the affect of angiotensin II on the heart and inhibit increases in blood pressure	losartan (loh-SAHR-tan), trade name: Cozaar (KOH-zawr)

continues

Common Types of Antihypertensives   (continued)

Type	Pronunciation	What They Do	Example
antiarrhythmics	AN-tee-ey-RITH-miks	help control abnormal heart rhythms by slowing or blocking abnormal electrical conduction in the heart	amiodarone (am-ee-OH-*duh*-ROHN), verapamil (*vuh*-RAP-*uh*-mil)
beta-blockers	BEY-*tuh* BLOK-urz	decrease rate and force of cardiac contraction and lower cardiac output	atenolol (*uh*-TEN-*uh*-lawl), trade name: Tenormin (ten-OR-*muhn*)
calcium-channel blockers		inhibit movement of calcium into cells in the heart and blood vessels, decrease the force of cardiac contraction, relax blood vessels	amlodipine (am-LOH-*duh*-peen), trade name: Norvasc (NOR-vask)
digitalis preparations, digoxin, digitoxin	dij-*uh*-TAL-is, dij-OKS-in, dij-*uh*-TOKS-in	increase the force of cardiac contraction in people with heart failure and arrhythmias	digoxin
vasodilators, nitrates	vey-zoh-DEYE-ley-turs, NEYE-treyts	relax blood vessels, increase oxygen supply to the heart, ease cardiac workload and relieve the chest pain of angina	hydralazine (heye-DRAL-*uh*-zeen), minoxidil (*muh*-NOX-*uh*-dil)

Blood Thinners

Blood thinners decrease the clotting ability of the blood. People with irregular heartbeats are at risk for blood clots and stroke because the blood collects in the chambers of the heart, where it can clot. There are two basic types of blood thinners: anticoagulants and antiplatelet agents. **Anticoagulants** (AN-tee-ko-AG-*yuh*-luhnts) increase the amount of time that it takes for blood to clot. Examples include **heparin** (HEP-uh-rin) and **warfarin** (WAHR-*fuh*-rin), sold under the trade name: **Coumadin** (KOO-*muh*-din). **Antiplatelet** (AN-tee-PLEYT-*luht*) **agents** interfere with the formation of a platelet plug. Aspirin is one example, as is **clopidogrel** (kloh-PID-*uh*-gruhl), with the trade name: **Plavix** (PLAV-iks).

Diuretics

Diuretics (deye-yoo-RET-iks) increase the amount of fluid excreted through the urine. This decreases fluid retention, blood volume, fluid in the lungs, and peripheral edema. The end result is that the heart doesn't have to pump so hard.

Common Types of Diuretics

Type	Pronunciation	What They Doe	Example
carbonic anhydrase inhibitors	kar-BAWN-ik an-HEYE-dreys	decrease activity of an enzyme to decrease sodium and water reabsorption, increase potassium and bicarbonate excretion in the urine	acetazolamide (*uh*-SEET-*uh*-ZOHL-*uh*-meyed)
loop diuretics		work on the ascending loop of the nephron to decrease sodium and water reabsorption	furosemide (fyoor-OH-*suh*-meyed), trade name: Lasix (LEY-ziks)
osmotic diuretics	oz-MAW-tik	increase urine output by increasing the osmolarity (oz-*muh*-LAR-i-tee) of the kidney filtrate, which pulls water out of the kidney	mannitol (MAN-*uh*-tawl)
potassium-sparing diuretics	*puh*-TAZ-ee-*uhm*	unlike other types of diuretics, decrease the amount of potassium lost in the urine	spironolactone (*spuh*-RAWN-*uh*-LAK-tohn)
thiazide diuretics	THAY-uh-zeyed	work on the distal convoluted tubule to decrease water retention	hydrochlorothiazide (HEYE-droh-klawr-THEYE-uh-zeyed)

Cholesterol Medications

Cholesterol (*kuh*-LES-*tuh*-rawl) **medications** decrease the amount of cholesterol in the blood. The aim is to decrease the formation of atherosclerosis in order to decrease the risk of cardiovascular disease.

Cholesterol medications include **HMG-CoA reductase** (*ruh*-DUK-teys) **inhibitors** and **statins** (STAT-*uhnz*). These medications inhibit the enzyme that plays a key role in cholesterol formation in the liver. An example is **simvastatin** (SIM-*vuh*-STAT-*uhn*).

Bile acid-binding resins and **bile acid sequestrants** (*suh*-KWES-*truhnts*) bind with bile acids to inhibit their reabsorption from the gut. **Colestipol** (koh-lee-STEYE-pawl) is an example. **Cholesterol absorption inhibitors** interfere with absorption of cholesterol from the small intestine into the blood. **Ezetimibe** (*uh*-ZET-*uh*-meyeb) is an example.

Nicotinic (nik-*uh*-TIN-ik) **acid** and **niacin** (NEYE-*uh*-sin) interfere with fatty acid breakdown, lower very-low-density lipoprotein (VLDL) levels in the blood, and increase high-density lipoprotein (HDL) levels. **Fibrates** (FEYE-breyts) decrease production of triglycerides and increase HDL levels through various mechanisms. An example is **gemfibrozil** (jem-FEYE-*bruh*-zil). **Omega-3 (**oh-MEG-*uh* THREE**) fatty acids** also lower triglycerides, but their mechanism is unclear.

Asthma Medications

Medications for asthma target the main problems of this disorder: inflammation and **bronchoconstriction** (BRAWN-koh-*kuhn*-STRIK-*shuhn*). Controlling asthma is a two-tiered strategy. A controller medication targets inflammation and controls chronic symptoms. A rescue or quick-relief medication is used for asthma exacerbations, or attacks. Sometimes asthma medication is placed in a **nebulizer** (NEB-yoo-leyez-ur), which makes the medication into a mist so that it can be inhaled into the lungs.

Asthma-control medications include the following:

- **Inhaled corticosteroids** (kawr-tik-oh-STEYR-oidz) target inflammation. Example: **fluticasone** (floo-TIK-*uh*-zohn), trade name: **Flovent** (FLOH-vent).
- **Long-acting beta agonists** (AG-*uhn*-ists) relax the muscles that line the airways to keep them open. Example: **salmeterol** (sal-MET-*uh*-rawl).
- **Theophylline** (thee-AWF-*uh*-leen) dilates the bronchi and bronchioles.
- **Leukotriene** (loo-koh-TREYE-een) **modifiers** target inflammatory chemicals that cause excess mucus production and swelling of the airways. Example: **montelukast** (mon-TEY-*luh*-kast), trade name: **Singulair** (SIN-gyoo-lair).

Allergy medications such as antihistamines (AN-tee-HIS-*tuh*-meenz), allergy shots, and immune modulators like **omalizumab** (oh-*muh*-LIZ-*uh*-mab) and **cromolyn** (KROH-*muh*-lin) nasal spray also help to control asthma symptoms.

Quick-relief asthma medications include the following:

- **Short-acting beta-agonists** provide fast-acting relief of bronchoconstriction and relax airways. Example: **albuterol** (al-BYOO-*tuh*-rawl).

- **Short-acting bronchodilators** (brawn-koh-DEYE-leyt-urz) quickly dilate bronchi. Example: **ipratropium** (ip-*ruh*-TROH-pree-*uhm*), trade name: **Atrovent** (AT-*ruh*-vent).

- **Oral corticosteroids** (kawr-tik-oh-STEYR-oidz) provide quick relief of inflammation during asthma attacks. Example: **prednisone** (PRED-*nuh*-zohn).

Cough Medicines

Antitussives (AN-tee-TUS-*uhvz*) are cough medicines. They are generally used for nonproductive, or dry, coughs. **Expectorants** (eks-PEK-*tuh-ruhnts*) are often used to treat wet coughs because they increase the amount of water in mucus, making it thinner and easier to cough up. A **mucolytic** (myoo-*kuh*-LIT-ik) thins bronchial secretions by breaking chemical bonds in mucus. Examples of these cough medications include the following:

- **Dextromethorphan** (DEKS-troh-*muh*-THAWR-fan) is a non-narcotic found in many over-the-counter cough suppressants.

- **Codeine** (KOH-deen) is a narcotic cough suppressant available only by prescription that decreases coughing by acting directly on the brain center that initiates coughing.

- **Acetylcysteine** (*uh*-SEE-*tuhl*-SIS-teen) is a mucolytic that is usually available only by prescription.

- **Guaifenesin** (gweye-FEN-*uh*-sin) is an expectorant commonly available over the counter.

DID YOU KNOW?

Complementary and alternative medicine includes many types of herbal and traditional remedies, such as those found in Chinese medicine and the Ayurvedic medicine of India. Many of these treatments are biologically active, and some are under investigation to determine their mechanism of action for new drug discovery. Many herbal medicines can interact with Western medicines. Some can even be dangerous by increasing or decreasing the effect of other medicines. Patients using such treatments are advised to inform all healthcare providers about this use. Examples of complementary herbal remedies include **echinacea** (ek-*uh*-NEY-*shuh*) for the common cold, ginger for digestive complaints like nausea and vomiting, and **St. John's wort** (WAWRT) for depression.

Diabetes, Gastrointestinal, and Hormonal Drugs

Many types of medications can be used to treat conditions that affect the digestive and endocrine systems. There are many types of diabetic medications, and they are used in different ways depending on the type of diabetes being treated.

Diabetic Medications

The aim of treatment is different for type 1 diabetes as compared to type 2 diabetes. Treatment for type 1 diabetes focuses on insulin replacement, mainly by using insulin injections. Some people have the option of using an insulin pump, which is a device with an insulin reservoir that is worn on the body and is connected to a catheter inserted into the abdomen. The pump can be programmed and administers extra insulin to help control blood sugar.

Medications for the treatment of type 1 diabetes include the following:

- **Rapid-acting insulin:** regular insulin, trade names: **Humulin** (HYOO-*myuh*-lin) 70/30 and **Novolin** (NOH-*vuh*-lin) 70/30; **lispro** (LIS-proh), trade name: **Humalog** (HYOO-*muh*-log); **aspart** (AS-pahrt), trade name: **NovoLog** (NOH-*vuh*-log)

- **Intermediate-acting insulin:** NPH, trade names: **isophane** (EYS-*uh*-feyn), Humulin N, Novolin N

- **Long-acting insulin: glargine** (GLAR-jeen), trade name: **Lantus** (LAN-*tuhs)*; **detemir** (DET-*uh*-meer), trade name: **Levemir** (LEEV-*uh*-meer)

Treatment for type 2 diabetes focuses on lowering the blood sugar through various means: stimulating the pancreas to increase insulin production, decreasing the amount of glucose released into the blood, and improving the sensitivity of the body's cells to the effects of insulin. For example, **meglitinides** (*muh*-GLIT-*uh*-neyeds) and **sulfonylureas** (sulf-AWN-*uhl*-yoor-ee-*uhs*) are both given orally and stimulate the pancreas to release insulin. **Repaglinide** (*ruh*-PAG-*luh*-neyed), trade name: **Prandin** (PRAND-in), is an example of a meglitinide. **Glipizide** (GLIP-*uh*-zeyed), trade name: **Glucotrol** (gloo-*kuh*-trawl), is an example of a sulfonylurea.

Dipeptydyl peptidase-4 (deye-PEP-*tuh*-dil PEP-ti-deys) **inhibitors** and **gliptins** (GLIP-tinz) are also given orally. They stimulate insulin release and inhibit glucose release from the liver. An example is **sitagliptin** (sit-*uh*-GLIP-tin), trade name: **Januvia** (jan-OOV-ee-*uh*).

Both **biguanides** (beye-GWAHN-eyedz) and **thiazolidinediones** (theye-uh-zoh-LID-een-deye-ohnz) are given orally. They inhibit glucose release from the liver and improve cell sensitivity to insulin. An example of a biguanide is **metformin** (met-FAWR-min). An example of a thiazolidinedione is **rosiglitazone** (roh-*suh*-GLIT-*uh*-zohn), trade name: **Avandia** (ey-VAN-dee-*yuh*).

Alpha-glucosidase (ALF-*uh* gloo-koh-SEYED-eys) **inhibitors** are given orally and decrease the rate of breakdown of starches and some sugars. An example is **acarbose** (ey-KARB-ohs), trade name: **Precose** (PREE-kohs).

Both **amylin mimetics** (am-*uh*-lin meye-MEET-iks) and **incretin mimetics** (in-KREET-in meye-MEET-iks) are injectable and stimulate insulin release. An example of an amylin mimetic is **pramlintide** (PARM-lin-teyed), trade name: **Symlin** (SIM-lin). An example of an incretin mimetic is exenatide (eks-EN-*uh*-teyed), trade name: **Byetta** (beye-ET-*uh*).

Thyroid and Adrenal Medications

Treatment for **hyperthyroidism** (hayh-pur-THAYH-roid-izm) aims to decrease the excessive output of thyroid hormones. Medications that do this are called **antithyroid** (AN-tee-THAYH-roid) medications. They act as **hormone antagonists** (an-TAG-*uhn*-ists) to reduce the thyroid's output of hormones. Examples include **methimazole** (*muh*-IM-*uh*-zohl) and **propylthiouracil** (proh-*puhl*-theye-*uh*-YOOR-*uh*-sil).

Hypothyroidism is treated by replacement therapy using a synthetic thyroid hormone called **levothyroxine** (lee-voh-theye-ROX-in), trade name: **Synthroid** (SIN-throid).

Adrenal insufficiency is usually treated with hormone replacement as well. Too little cortisol can be replaced with **exogenous glucocorticoids** (gloo-koh-KORT-*uh*-koidz), such as **hydrocortisone** (heye-droh-KORT-*uh*-zohn), **dexamethasone** (deks-*uh*-METH-*uh*-zohn), and **prednisone** (PRED-*nuh*-zohn). Too little aldosterone can be replaced with **fludrocortisone** (floo-droh-KORT-*uh*-zohn).

Heartburn Medications

Gastroesophageal reflux disease (GERD) is also known as heartburn or stomach reflux. It is treated with a variety of medications, including the following:

- **Antacids** (ant-AS-idz) neutralize stomach acid. Example: **aluminum hydroxide** (*uh*-LOO-*muh-nuhm* heye-DROK-seyed), trade name: **Maalox** (MEY-loks).

- **Histamine-2** (his-*tuh*-meen TOO) or **H-2 blockers** decrease acid production in the stomach. Example: **famotidine** (*fuh*-MOH-*tuh*-deen), trade name: **Pepcid** (PEP-sid).

- **Proton** (PROH-ton) **pump inhibitors** or **PPIs** inhibit acid production in the stomach. They are more effective than H-2 blockers. Example: **esomeprazole** (ES-*uh*-MEP-*ruh*-zawl), trade name: **Nexium** (NEKS-ee-*uhm*).

Digestive promotility (proh-MOH-TIL-*uh*-tee) **agents** increase the contractions of muscles in the digestive tract to relieve constipation, delayed stomach emptying, and symptoms of GERD. An example is **metoclopramide** (met-*uh*-KLOH-*pruh*-meyed), trade name: **Reglan** (REG-lan).

Antiemetics

Antiemetics (AN-tee-ee-MIT-iks) decrease nausea and vomiting. They are used for a variety of reasons, including motion sickness and side effects from general anesthesia and chemotherapy. There are many types of antiemetics, some of which are used for other conditions, such as psychiatry.

Common Antiemetics

Type	Pronunciation	What They Do	Example
5-HT₃ serotonin receptor blockers	ser-uh-TOH-nin	block serotonin receptors in the digestive tract and central nervous system	ondansetron (on-DAN-*suh*-trawn), trade name: Zofran (ZOH-fran)
antihistamines	AN-tee-HIS-*tuh*-meenz	block histamine receptors	promethazine (proh-METH-*uh*-zeen), trade name: Phenergan (FEN-ur-gan); diphenhydramine (deye-fen-HEYE-*druh*-meen), trade name: Benadryl (BEN-*uh*-dril)
cannabinoids	*kuh*-NAB-*uh*-noidz	derived from marijuana; used to treat nausea, vomiting, and loss of appetite in patients unresponsive to other types of medications	dronabinol (*druh*-NAB-*uh*-nawl), trade name: Marinol (MAIR-*uh*-nawl)

Type	Pronunciation	What They Do	Example
dopamine antagonists	DOH-puh-meen	block dopamine receptors to treat severe nausea and vomiting associated with cancer and radiation treatment	prochlorperazine (proh-klawr-PAIR-*uh*-zeen), trade name: Compazine (KOMP-*uh*-zeen)
steroids	STER-oidz	used to prevent vomiting during general anesthesia	dexamethasone (DEX-*uh*-METH-*uh*-zohn), trade name: Decadron (DEK-*uh*-drawn)

> **DID YOU KNOW?**
>
> **Antidiarrheal** (AN-tee-deye-*uh*-REE-*uhl*) **medications** are used for symptoms of diarrhea but do not usually cure the underlying disorder. An example is **loperamide** (loh-PAIR-*uh*-meyed), trade name: **Imodium** (im-OH-dee-*uhm*). This opioid affects only the intestine and does not affect the central nervous system because it cannot cross the blood–brain barrier.

Genitourinary and Reproductive Medications

Many types of medications are used to treat genitourinary symptoms. Overactive bladder and urinary incontinence are sometimes treated with **anticholinergic** (AN-tee-KOH-*luh*-NER-jik) **medications** like **oxybutynin** (oks-ee-byoo-TIN-in), trade name: **Ditropan** (DI-*truh*-pan), or **antimuscarinic** (AN-tee-musk-*uh*-RIN-ik) **medications** like **tolterodine** (tohl-TER-*uh*-deen), trade name: **Detrol** (DET-rawl). Both of these types of medications decrease bladder muscle spasms.

Urinary retention caused by benign prostatic hypertrophy (BPH) can be treated with alpha-blockers such as doxazosin (trade name: Cardura) and tamsulosin (trade name: Flomax), both of which relax the muscles in the neck of the bladder. BPH can also be treated with **finasteride** (fin-AS-*tuh*-reyed), trade name: **Proscar** (PROH-skahr), which decreases the size of the prostate.

Reproductive medications are used to treat the female and male reproductive systems. **Hormonal contraception** (kon-*truh*-SEP-*shuhn*), or birth control, interacts with the female endocrine system to produce a state of pseudo-pregnancy so that actual pregnancy cannot occur. Manufactured steroid hormones, called **synthetic steroid analogs** (AN-*uh*-lawgz), include **progestins** (proh-JEST-inz), which mimic natural progesterone. Use of progestins induces **anovulatory** (an-OV-yuh-luh-tohr-ee) cycles so that pregnancy cannot occur. There are many forms of birth control, including an oral pill, medroxyprogesterone (Depo-Provera) injection, a skin patch, skin implants, and a hormonal ring inserted into the vagina. Emergency contraception is available in the form of a **progestogen-only** (proh-JEST-*uh-juhn*) pill, or synthetic progesterone, taken after intercourse.

There are two general types of hormonal contraception. **Combined hormonal contraception** contains estrogen and progestogens, suppresses ovulation, and thickens cervical mucus. The Pill is an example of this type of hormonal contraception. **Progestogen-only contraception** contains only progestins, and suppresses ovulation only. The mini-pill is an example.

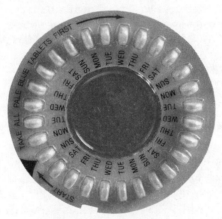

Oral contraceptives are given in pill form and often taken one each day throughout a woman's monthly cycle.
Susanna Price © Dorling Kindersley

WORDS OF WARNING

Hormone replacement therapy, or HRT, uses synthetic estrogen and progestin. This therapy was formerly used routinely to relieve symptoms of menopause such as hot flashes and to prevent osteoporosis (os-tee-oh-*puh*-ROH-sis), or thinning of the bones. However, large clinical trials showed that the risks of hormone therapy outweighed its benefits. Risks of HRT include heart attack, stroke, blood clots, and breast cancer. HRT is still sometimes used in certain circumstances, but it is no longer routine.

Male erectile dysfunction is treated with several medications: **sildenafil** (sil-DEN-*uh*-fil), trade name: **Viagra** (veye-AG-*ruh*); **vardenafil** (vahr-DEN-*uh*-fil), trade name: **Levitra** (*luh*-VEE-tree); and **tadalafil** (*tuh*-DAL-*uh*-fil), trade name: **Cialis** (seye-AL-*uhs*). These types of medications inhibit a type of enzyme, leading to increased blood flow into the penis and causing an erection.

Several medications are used to treat infertility. These medications are used in combination with assisted reproduction techniques, such as artificial insemination. **Clomiphene** (klo-*muh*-feen) **citrate** (SI-treyet), trade name: **Clomid** (KLO-mid), is an anti-estrogen medication that induces ovulation in women who are not ovulating normally. Other types of medications stimulate ovulation by using hormone agonists and various types of sexual hormones, such as follicle-stimulating hormone (FSH) and gonadotropin-releasing hormone (GnRH).

Brain and Nervous System Medications

There is often overlap between medications that are used to treat neurological disorders, psychiatric illnesses, and even some types of pain.

Antiepileptics

Antiepileptic (AN-tee-ep-*uh*-LEP-tik) **drugs** are also called **anticonvulsants** (AN-tee-con-VULS-*uhnts*) and **neuroleptics** (noor-*uh*-LEP-tiks). Many antiepileptics are effective not just in controlling seizures but also in treating muscle spasms, psychiatric conditions like bipolar disorder, and chronic **neuropathic** (noor-*uh*-PATH-ik) pain, which is pain that is caused by nerve damage.

Types of Antiepileptics

Type	Pronunciation	What They Do	Example
barbiturates	bahr-BICH-er-its	CNS depressants	phenobarbital (fee-noh-BARHB-*uh*-tawl); used in the early half of the 20th century, now rarely used
benzodiazepines	benz-oh-deye-AZ-*uh*-peenz	CNS depressants; also relax muscles	lorazepam (lawr-AZ-*uh*-pam)

continues

Types of Antiepileptics   (continued)

Type	Pronunciation	What They Do	Example
carboxamides	kahr-BOKS-*uh*-meyedz	decrease the excitability of nerve cells	carbamazepine (KAHR-*buh*-MAZ-*uh*-peen), oxcarbazepine (oks-kahr-BAZ-*uh*-peen)
fatty acids		broad-spectrum anticonvulsants that affect the function of the neurotransmitter gamma-aminobutyric (GAM-muh uh-MEEN-oh-byoo-teer-ik) acid and voltage-gated sodium channels	divalproex (deye-val-PROH-eks) sodium, trade name: Depakote (DEP-*uh*-koht)
fructose derivatives	FROOK-tohs	unknown mechanism of action	topiramate (toh-PEER-*uh*-meyt)
gamma-aminobutyric acid analogs	*GAM-uh uh*-MEE-noh-byoo-TEER-ik	used to control seizures and for neuropathic pain	gabapentin (GAB-*uh*-PEN-tin), trade name:Neurontin (noor-ON-tin)
hydantoins	heye-dan-TOH-inz	decrease electrical activity in the brain by stabilizing sodium channels	phenytoin (fen-ee-TOH-in)
pyrrolidines	peer-OH-*luh*-deenz	unknown mechanism of action	levetiracetam (lev-*uh*-teer-*uh*-SEET-*uhm*), trade name:Keppra (KEP-*ruh*)
succinimides	suk-SIN-*uh*-meyedz	contested mechanism of action	ethosuximide (eth-oh-SUKS-*uh*-meyed)
triazines	TREYE-*uh*-zeenz	block sodium channels	lamotrigine (*luh*-MOH-*truh*-jeen), trade name: Lamictal (*luh*-MIK-*tuhl*)

Psychotropics

Psychotropic (seye-*kuh*-TROH-pik) **medications** are used to treat psychiatric disorders. There is much overlap between psychotropic medications and several of the neuroleptics listed above. Many psychotropics work on neurotransmitters in the brain. Some block certain neurotransmitter receptors or affect cell channels through which neurotransmitters and other molecules pass. Psychotropics are separated into the following categories according to the types of conditions they treat.

Antidepressants (AN-tee-*duh*-PRES-*uhnts*) treat clinical depression. This category includes selective serotonin reuptake inhibitors (SSRIs), norepinephrine reuptake inhibitors (NRIs), selective serotonin-norepinepephrine reuptake inhibitors (SSN-RIs), tricyclic antidepressants (TCAs), and monoamine oxidase inhibitors (MOAs).

Stimulants (STIM-*yuh-luhnts*) treat attention deficit disorder. This category includes amphetamines and norepinephrine-dopamine reuptake inhibitors such as **methylphenidate** (meth-*uhl*-FEN-*uh*-deyt), trade name: **Ritalin** (RIT-*uh*-lin).

Antipsychotics (AN-tee-seye-KAWT-iks) treat psychosis and are divided into first-, second-, third-, and fourth-generation antipsychotics. Examples include **quetiapine** (*kwuh*-TEYE-*uh*-peen); **clozapine** (KLOZ-*uh*-peen); and **aripiprazole** (AIR-*uh*-PIP-*ruh*-zawl), trade name: **Abilify** (*uh*-BIL-*uh*-feye).

Mood stabilizers treat mood symptoms of bipolar disorder and include various types, such as minerals like **lithium** (LI-thee-*uhm*), anticonvulsants, and some antipsychotics.

Anxiolytics (anks-ee-*uh*-LIT-iks) treat anxiety and include benzodiazepines, SSRIs, barbiturates, and hydroxyzine.

Depressants (*duh*-PRES-*uhnts*) calm down the CNS and include hypnotics, sedatives, anesthetics, barbiturates, benzodiazepines, and opioids.

Dementia medications are used to slow the progress of dementia symptoms in Alzheimer disease. An example is donepezil (dawn-EP-*uh*-zil), trade name: **Aricept** (AIR-*uh*-sept).

Pain Medications

Pain medications are also called **analgesics** (AN-*uhl*-JEEZ-iks). **Nonsteroidal anti-inflammatory** (nawn-ster-OID-*uhl* an-tee-in-FLAM-*uh*-tawr-ee) **drugs** (NSAIDs) are one category of pain medication. This group includes aspirin; ibuprofen, trade name: **Motrin** (MOH-trin); and naproxen, trade name: **Aleve** (*uh*-LEEV).

Another category of pain medication is **anticonvulsants** (AN-tee-kuhn-VULS-*uhnts*). These types of medications are used for neuropathic pain (see "Antiepileptics" section). An example is gabapentin, trade name: **Neurontin**.

Opioids (OH-pee-oidz) are narcotics that depress the CNS and have addictive potential. Examples include **fentanyl** (FEN-*tuh*-nil), **morphine** (MAWR-feen), **codeine** (KOH-deen), and **oxycodone** (oks-ee-KOH-DOHN).

Muscle Relaxants

A **muscle relaxant** (*ruh*-LAX-*uhnt*) works on skeletal muscles to reduce pain and spasms that can cause **hyperreflexia** (heye-pur-*ruh*-FLEX-ee-*uh*), or heightened reflexes caused by paralysis and other neuromuscular disorders. There are two categories of muscle relaxants: neuromuscular blockers and spasmolytics. **Neuromuscular** (noor-oh-MUSK-*yuh*-ler) **blockers** work peripherally at the neuromuscular junction and do not affect the CNS. They are used in surgery to induce paralysis. An example is **succinylcholine** (SUKS-*uh*-*nuhl*-KOH-leen).

Spasmolytics (SPAZ-*muh*-LIT-iks) usually work in the CNS to decrease muscular spasms and spasticity caused by paralysis. Some examples are **cyclobenzaprine** (seye-kloh-BENZ-*uh*-preen) and **baclofen** (BAK-*luh*-fen).

Chemotherapy and Immunosuppressants

Chemotherapy (kee-moh-THAIR-*uh*-pee) refers to **cytotoxic** (seye-*tuh*-TOKS-ik) **medications** capable of killing cancer cells. Another name for these types of medications is **antineoplastics** (AN-tee-nee-*uh*-PLAS-tiks). Chemotherapy is often used in conjunction with radiation therapy and surgery. Chemotherapy indiscriminately targets rapidly dividing cells. This group includes cancer cells and normal cells that rapidly divide, such as those in bone marrow, the digestive tract, and hair follicles. Some types of chemotherapy, such as monoclonal antibodies, have been developed to target specific proteins on cancer cells.

Types of chemotherapy include **alkylating** (AL-*kuhl*-EYT-ing) **agents**. These attach an alkyl group to DNA, causing DNA damage. Cells that are more sensitive to DNA damage, like cancer cells, are preferentially killed. Some examples are **cyclophosphamide** (seye-kloh-FOS-*fuh*-meyed) and **cisplatin** (sis-PLAT-in).

Other types include the following:

- **Antimetabolites** (AN-tee-*muh*-TAB-*uh*-leyets) take the place of some of the building blocks of DNA, stopping cell division and growth. Example: **mercaptopurine** (mer-kapt-*uh*-PYOOR-eenz).

- **Vinka alkaloids** (VIN-*kuh* ALK-*uh*-loidz) are derived from plants. They interfere with mitosis and block cell division. Examples: **vincristine** (vin-KRIS-teen) and **vinblastine** (vin-BLAS-teem).

- **Taxanes** (TAKS-eynz) are derived from plants. They interfere with mitosis and block cell division. Examples: **paclitaxel** (*pak*-lih-TAK-suhl), trade name: **Taxol** (TAKS-awl).

- **Topoisomerase** (top-oh-eye-SAWM-er-eys) **inhibitors** interfere with DNA replication and transcription. Example: **etoposide** (*uh*-TOH-puh-seyed).

- **Cytotoxic antibiotics** kill cells by various mechanisms of action. Example: **mitomycin** (MEYE-*tuh*-MEYE-sin).

Immunosuppressants (im-myoo-noh-*suh*-PRES-*uhnts*) depress the immune system and are used to treat medical conditions caused by overactive immune responses, such as autoimmune disorders, rejection of organ transplants, and other conditions like asthma. For example, **glucocorticoids** (gloo-koh-KORT-*uh*-koidz) suppress cell-mediated immunity, including cytokine function, T-cell expansion, and B-cell antibody synthesis. **Prednisone** (PRED-*nuh*-zohn) and **cortisone** (KOR-*tuh*-zohn) are examples.

Cytostatics (seye-toh-STAT-iks) interfere with cell division and include chemotherapy drugs that are used in smaller doses for autoimmune diseases and to decrease organ transplant rejection. Examples include **methotrexate** (meth-*uh*-TREX-eyt) and **azathioprine** (AZ-*uh*-THEYE-*uh*-preen).

Monoclonal (maw-*nuh*-KLOH-*nuhl*) antibodies target specific antigens. They are used to treat cancer, autoimmune diseases, and asthma. **Tumor necrosis** (*nuh*-KROH-*suhs*) **factor alpha, also referred to as a binding protein**, is a monoclonal antibody that binds tumor necrosis factor alpha and prevents the synthesis of certain interleukins. An example is **infliximab** (in-FLIKS-*uh*-mab), trade name: **Remicade** (REM-*uh*-keyd).

- Other types of immunosuppressants include the following:
- **Polyclonal** (POL-ee-KLOH-*nuhl*) **antibodies** inhibit cell-mediated immune reactions. For example, **Rho(d)** (ROH-DEE) **immunoglobulin** helps to prevent hemolytic disease of the newborn.
- **Cyclosporin** (seye-*kluh*-SPAWR-*uhn*) decreases T cell activity. It is used to prevent transplant rejection.

- **Tacrolimus** (tak-*ruh*-LEYE-*muhs*) interferes with T-cell receptor activation. It is used to prevent organ transplant rejection and as a topical treatment for eczema.

- **Interferons** (in-ter-FEER-awnz) suppress cytokine production. They are used to treat multiple sclerosis.

- **Mycophenolate** (meye-*kuh*-FEN-*uh*-leyt) targets an enzyme important in DNA synthesis. B and T cells are especially sensitive to this type of interference in DNA synthesis.

The Least You Need to Know

- Antibiotics are medicines that kill bacteria or inhibit their growth.

- Cardiovascular agents include blood thinners and cholesterol medications. Respiratory medications include bronchodilators and antitussives.

- Gastrointestinal drugs include diabetic medications and antiemetics.

- Genitourinary medications are used to treat overactive bladder and urinary incontinence. Reproductive medications include oral contraceptives and fertility medications.

- Brain and nervous system medications include antiepileptics, psychotropics, and analgesics.

- Antineoplastics are chemotherapy drugs. Immunosuppressants are used to treat medical conditions caused by overactive immune responses.

Index

Symbols